COVID-19 AND THE RIGHT TO HEALTH IN AFRICA

This collection draws upon a range of thematic and regional case studies and uses the right to health as a normative framework to explore the devastating impact of the COVID-19 pandemic in Africa.

Drawing lessons from across the continent, the book discusses the challenges faced by African states seeking to ensure the availability, accessibility, and quality of health care in the context of the COVID-19 pandemic. In particular, the volume explores the impact of the pandemic on the right to health of vulnerable and marginalized groups, such as women, children, elderly persons with disabilities, refugees and asylum seekers, and people from disadvantaged communities. Due to the poor funding of the healthcare systems, access to health-related services was limited to these groups in many African countries, thereby leading to avoidable COVID-19-related deaths through shortages of vital supplies, including diagnostic tests, ventilators, and oxygen cylinders. Chapters in the volume also explore the contentious issues of vaccine mandates, equity, resource allocation, and the rights of healthcare providers during the pandemic.

This collection will be of interest to students of public health, human rights, and the social sciences, as well as to academics and policymakers with an interest in the nexus between the COVID-19 pandemic and public health policy in Africa.

Ebenezer Durojaye is a professor of law at the Centre for Human Rights, University of Pretoria, South Africa. His areas of research include human rights, socio-economic rights, sexual and reproductive health and rights, gender, and constitutionalism. He is the editor of *Litigating the Right to Health in Africa: Challenges and Prospects* (Routledge 2015) and co-editor of *International Law and the Framework Convention on Tobacco Control: Lessons from Africa and Beyond* (Routledge 2022), *Constitutional Resilience and the COVID-19 Pandemic: Perspectives from Sub-Saharan Africa* (2022), and *Sexual Harassment, Law and Human Rights in Africa* (2023).

Roopanand Mahadew is an associate professor of law at the Department of Law, University of Mauritius, Mauritius. His research and teaching explore international human rights law, public international law, and legal research methodology. He is the author of numerous journal articles and book chapters.

The COVID-19 Pandemic Series

Series Editor: J. Michael Ryan

This series examines the impact of the COVID-19 pandemic on individuals, communities, countries, and the larger global society from a social scientific perspective. It represents a timely and critical advance in knowledge related to what many believe to be the greatest threat to global ways of being in more than a century. It is imperative that academics take their rightful place alongside medical professionals as the world attempts to figure out how to deal with the current global pandemic, and how society might move forward in the future. This series represents a response to that imperative.

Titles in this Series:

Transformations in Social Science Research Methods during the COVID-19 Pandemic
Edited by J. Michael Ryan, Valerie Visanich and Gaspar Brändle

Social Structure Adaptation to COVID-19
Impact on Humanity
Edited by Suresh Nanwani and William Loxley

COVID-19 and the Right to Health in Africa
Edited by Ebenezer Durojaye and Roopanand Mahadew

For more information about this series, please visit: www.routledge.com

COVID-19 AND THE RIGHT TO HEALTH IN AFRICA

Edited by Ebenezer Durojaye and Roopanand Mahadew

Routledge
Taylor & Francis Group
LONDON AND NEW YORK

Designed cover image: @ Getty Images

First published 2024
by Routledge
4 Park Square, Milton Park, Abingdon, Oxon OX14 4RN

and by Routledge
605 Third Avenue, New York, NY 10158

Routledge is an imprint of the Taylor & Francis Group, an informa business

British Library Cataloguing-in-Publication Data
A catalogue record for this book is available from the British Library

ISBN: 978-1-032-67141-3 (hbk)
ISBN: 978-1-032-67142-0 (pbk)
ISBN: 978-1-032-67143-7 (ebk)

DOI: 10.4324/9781032671437

Typeset in Sabon
by Apex CoVantage, LLC

CONTENTS

CONTRIBUTORS

Adetoun T. Adebanjo (LLD, UFS) is a legal researcher and consultant in Queensland, Australia. Her research areas include human rights, with a focus on women's rights, and sexual and reproductive health and rights; public health law and policy; company and insolvency law; and international law and constitutional law, and she has published extensively in these areas. She is a co-editor of the book *Sexual Harassment, Law and Human Rights in Africa* (Palgrave Macmillan 2023).

Benson Chakaya Atonga is currently a PhD candidate, researcher, and tutor at the University of Pretoria Centre for Human Rights and holds a Master of Philosophy degree in Sexual and Reproductive Health and Rights from University of Pretoria (South Africa) and a bachelor's degree in Social Sciences from Maseno University (Kenya). He has held several positions including managing and coordinating National Advocacy coalition on Sexual and Reproductive Health Rights (Kenya). He previously worked at the Swedish International Development Agency (SIDA) as a thematic expert on Sexual and Reproductive Health Rights projects in Eastern Africa. He worked as a regional advocacy manager for Network of African National Human Rights Institutions (NANHRI) and programme advisor at the Kenya Human Rights Commission (KHRC) under the Equality and Non-Discrimination programme.

Ashwanee Budoo-Scholtz is the programme manager of the Master's in Human Rights and Democratization in Africa at the Centre for Human Rights, Faculty of Law, University of Pretoria, where she completed her LLD in 2016. She holds a LLB (UOM), LLM, and LLD (Pretoria). Her research, teaching, and training area is the African human rights system. She has co-edited the following books: *The Impact of the Maputo Protocol in Selected African States*; *COVID-19 and Women's Intersectionalities in Africa*; and the two-volume series on *Violence against Women and Criminal Justice in Africa*.

Ebenezer Durojaye is a professor of law at the Centre for Human Rights, University of Pretoria, South Africa. His areas of research include human rights, socio-economic rights, sexual and reproductive health and rights, gender, and constitutionalism. He has written extensively in these areas.

Ayeranga Godfrey holds a Bachelor of Laws (LLB) (Hons) degree from Uganda Christian University; a Master of Laws (LLM) degree in Human Rights and Democratization from the Centre for Human Rights, University of Pretoria, and a Post Graduate Diploma in Legal Practice from the Kenya School of Law, Kenya. His research interests are in the field(s) of prisoners' rights, maternal healthcare rights, socio-economic rights, human rights, social justice, international law, criminal justice, and international criminal law. He currently works as a lecturer at the Faculty of Law, Cavendish University Uganda.

Godfrey Kangaude earned his Doctor of Laws from the University of Pretoria in 2020 and conducted postdoctoral research with the Critical Studies in Sexualities and Reproduction (CSSR) Program at the University of Rhodes in 2022. An activist and legal scholar, he focuses on sexual and reproductive justice. He is the founding executive director of Nyale Institute, an NGO in Malawi. His work delves into adolescent sexualities, reproductive justice, and their intersections with colonial legacies, cultural norms, public law, and justice systems. A current project is to facilitate reproductive justice and health access for child survivors of sexual violence.

Soila Kigera is an advocate of the High Court of Kenya and practises as in-house lawyer in an international oil company. She is a corporate legal counsel with 10 years' experience. She holds an LLM in Sexual and Reproductive Health Rights in Africa from the University of Pretoria and is a qualified company secretary. Soila is also a member of the Law Society of Kenya (LSK), the Institute of Certified Secretaries (ICS), and the Federation of Women Lawyers in Kenya (FIDA).

Catriona Macleod is a distinguished professor of psychology and South African Research Chairs Initiative (SARChI) chair of Critical Studies in Sexualities and Reproduction at Rhodes University, South Africa. Prof. Macleod's major scholastic contributions have been in two main areas: sexual and reproductive health and feminist theory in psychology. She has written extensively in national and international journals in relation to teenage pregnancy, abortion, sex education, feminist psychology, and postcolonialism. She is the sole author of the book titled *'Adolescence', Pregnancy and Abortion: Constructing a Threat of Degeneration* (published by Routledge), which was awarded the Distinguished Publication Award by the Association for Women in Psychology.

Bhavna Mahadew is a law lecturer at the University of Technology, Mauritius. She is currently enrolled as an LLD candidate at the University of Western Cape, where she is researching on the right to health. She has published a number of journal articles and book chapters on diverse areas of law in a multidisciplinary manner.

Roopanand Mahadew is an associate professor in law based at the Department of Law, University of Mauritius. He holds an LLB (Hons) from the University of Mauritius, an LLM in Human Rights and Democratization in Africa from the University of Pretoria and an LLD from the University of Western Cape. His research and teaching interests are in international human rights law, public international law, and legal research methodology. He was the former head of the Department of Law at the University of Mauritius from 2017 to 2019.

Simangele Mavundla is a graduate research fellow at the School of Law and Management Studies, University of KwaZulu Natal, where her PhD in law studies was completed in 2021. Mavundla is now the coordinator for law at the Institute for Distance Education at the University of Eswatini. She holds a PhD Law (UKZN), LLM (Pretoria), and LLB (Eswatini). Her areas of interest in teaching and research include international human rights law, gender and law, disability rights, and youth policies. She has contributed chapters to the following books: *Sexual Harassment, Law and Human Rights in Africa: The Impact of the Maputo Protocol in Selected African States* and *Violence Against Women and Criminal Justice in Africa*.

Mansha Mohee is a research consultant with the Governance and Shareholder Relations Section of the Office of the Secretary General of the African Development Bank Group. She holds an LLM in International Law from University College London; an LLM in Human Rights and Democratization in Africa from the Centre for Human Rights, University of Pretoria; and an LLB in Law with French Law from the University of Birmingham. Her primary research interests lie in international human rights law and international development law in Africa and the Global South.

Obiajulu Nnamuchi, LLB (Awka), LLM (Notre Dame), LLM (Toronto), LLM (Lund), MA (Louisville), SJD (Loyola, Chicago), is a professor of law and bioethics, *former* Head, Department of Public Law at the University of

Nigeria, where he teaches at the Faculty of Law and College of Medicine. He is the founder of the Centre for Health, Bioethics and Human Rights (CHBHR) and director of its section on Bioethics. Prof. Nnamuchi's scholarly interests are centred on the intersection of law and medicine, human rights, global health, bioethics, and health governance and financing – areas on which he has written extensively.

Paul O. Ogendi is the coordinator/senior lecturer at the Faculty of Law, University of Nairobi Kisumu Campus, Kenya. His teaching focuses on medical law and ethics, commercial law, international trade/economic law, evidence law, human rights, advocate of the High Court of Kenya, and other courses. Dr. Ogendi is also a postdoctoral fellow and an honorary research fellow and part-time lecturer with the Chinese University in Hong Kong (CUHK) and University of KwaZulu-Natal (UKZN), respectively. His research interests include intellectual property, human rights and access to medicines, post-COVID-19 sustainable vaccines law and policy, data governance for health innovation, and artificial intelligence.

Aisosa Jennifer Omoruyi obtained her LLB degree in 2012 from the University of Benin, Nigeria; LLM in International Human rights Law in 2016; and PhD in 2021, both from the University of the Western Cape, Cape Town, South Africa. Her research interests include the right to health, the right to food, sexual and reproductive health, and rights of women and intersectional discrimination. As a postdoctoral researcher with the Dullah Omar Institute, she has been involved in research on the legal frameworks for the prevention of diet-related non-communicable diseases in South Africa.

Miyienda Pauline is a lawyer with bias in human rights, an author, and a lecturer. She holds a Master of Arts degree in Human Rights and Development and a Bachelor of Laws degree. She has co-authored published articles, and she is enthusiastic about research in general. She is an advocate for children's rights. Her interest is in maternal health rights, women's rights and prisoners' rights, and social justice. She currently works as a lecturer at the Faculty of Law, Cavendish University Uganda.

Keikantse Phele is a human rights lawyer and researcher. She holds a Bachelor of Laws degree from the University of Botswana and a Master of Laws (LLM) in Sexual and Reproductive Rights in Africa from the University of Pretoria. She is currently a PhD candidate at the University of Cape Town. She is a co-founder and curator of the Gaborone Book Festival. Keikantse is a 2018 alumna of the prestigious Mandela Washington Fellowship (YALI) under the Civic Leadership Track and was based at the Rutgers University Brunswick Campus. Her areas of expertise include sexual and reproductive rights, women's rights, diversity, inclusion and belonging, public interest litigation, LGBTIQA+ rights, and indigenous minority rights. She is currently based in Gaborone, Botswana.

Muwanguzi M. Robert holds an LLB (MUK), LLM (UWC/HUB), MA HRTS (MUK), and LLD (UWC/HUB). His research interests are in issues arising from the intersections of natural resources law, human rights, and public international law. He is a senior lecturer at Cavendish University Uganda.

Ann Strode is a professor at the University of KwaZulu-Natal – BA.LLB. LLM. PhD (UKZN) South Africa. Strode is a well-established author who has produced more than 50 peer-reviewed publications. She has a keen research interest in HIV as a human rights issue. She has published widely on the ethical–legal complexities of adolescent HIV prevention research. She is a member of the Social Sciences and Health Research Ethics Committee, University of KwaZulu Natal.

FOREWORD

When the World Health Organization (WHO) first declared the COVID-19 pandemic in March of 2020, it was already obvious that this was indeed a health crisis with a truly global reach and ramifications. What was only beginning to be obvious, however, were the very unequal ways in which the pandemic would impact different regions, countries, and individuals.

One of the most, and least, surprising things about the pandemic is just how unsurprising the inequity of its impacts has been. While the virus does not discriminate, it has laid bare just how much human beings, and the societies we have constructed, do. Thus, along traditional lines of inequality, we have tended to see more far-reaching, life-altering impacts on the already impoverished, marginalized, disenfranchised, and discriminated sectors of both individual societies and our shared global world.

The disproportionate negative impacts on already vulnerable populations have been not just in terms of the direct impact of the virus itself, but, and equally so, also in terms of the human responses. Government assistance, vaccine availability, media attention, and even shared global concern have, in many cases, only served to further exacerbate existing inequalities. Sentiments of being 'all in this together' quickly evaporated in the face of limited resources and even more so once solutions were found.

For all of the above reasons, and many more, this volume is a must read for anyone concerned about the unequal impact of the pandemic and, more importantly, about how to remedy existing, and future, inequality. With a focus on Africa, one of the most impoverished and often overlooked regions of the world, this volume helps bring voice to the voiceless and is a critical contribution to a must-have battle for social equality.

J. Michael Ryan
Series Editor, *The COVID-19 Pandemic Series*
October 2023

PART I

Conceptual issues

1

INTRODUCTION

Ebenezer Durojaye and Roopanand Mahadew

1.1 Introduction

The COVID-19 pandemic has exposed the weaknesses of health systems in many African countries, particularly in sub-Saharan Africa. The disease has a potentially devastating impact on health systems. This is because of its high risk of transmission and inherent challenges in testing or isolating patients as early as possible due to their atypical or asymptomatic presentation. With the adoption of measures such as lockdowns by many African states, essential health services were either completely unavailable or reduced to a minimum because of the lack of staff and medical supplies. For instance, maternal and child health services were affected as well as essential services for other groups of patients.[1] According to Dr Shobha Suri from the Observer Research Foundation, an Indian policy institute, in May 2021 a modelling study indicated an increase in deaths up to 10%, 20%, and 36% due to HIV, tuberculosis (TB), and malaria, respectively, during the pandemic in low- and middle-income countries, which are by large African countries.[2] She further highlighted that a study from Kenya indicated long-lasting TB burden – about 25,000 additional cases due to lockdown disruptions.[3] The pandemic has led to disturbance in the provision of HIV services in sub-Saharan Africa, adding to the HIV death burden with the number hovering around 500,000.[4] Other health-related services, particularly sexual and reproductive health services, equally suffered some setbacks as a result of the pandemic. Studies have shown that as a result of the pandemic, maternal healthcare services, family planning services, and abortion services were all negatively impacted, resulting in avoidable deaths and morbidities.[5] In other situations, vulnerable and marginalized groups such as adolescent girls, persons with disabilities, and

DOI: 10.4324/9781032671437-2

refugees and asylum seekers encountered difficulties in accessing healthcare services as result of the pandemic.

While a majority of the studies have viewed and critiqued the pandemic as a violation of, *inter alia*, the human right to health and proposed solutions of different dimensions such as medical, legal, financial, social, and political, very little focus has been laid on whether the human right to health and its attendant obligations can be a normative framework on the basis of which pandemics such as COVID-19, and, unfortunately, similar future ones, can be dealt with.

1.2 Rationale

This book focuses on the potential of using the right to health as a normative framework in responding to the devastating consequences of future pandemics such as the COVID-19 pandemic. While there is ample literature on the right to health in general, there is a lack of academic literature on the impact of the COVID-19 pandemic on the right to health and its framework of availability, accessibility, acceptability, and quality. The importance of such an endeavour is further highlighted by the relative failures of states, irrespective of their economic capability to combat the pandemic and its effects. Many states, particularly African states, have faced challenges in ensuring the availability and accessibility of the pandemic-related health coverages, resulting in shortages in life-saving medical care and services, including diagnostic tests, ventilators, and oxygen cylinders, and in personal protective equipment for healthcare workers and other frontline staff.[6] Austerity measures, adjustment programmes, and fees have rendered essential and life-saving services inaccessible for certain vulnerable and marginalized populations.

The implementation of the right to health through healthcare systems demands that treatments are based on medical evidence; that testing and care are not denied on the basis of disability, age, or inability to pay; and that states allocate the maximum available resources to health. The COVID-19 pandemic has further brought to fore the challenges regarding allocation of resources to the health sector in Africa. Beyond exposing the lack of preparedness of many African countries to combating the pandemic, there was also the perennial problem of underfunding of the health sector. Successive African governments have failed to adequately allocate resources to the health sector to address the lack of infrastructure and shortages of skilled healthcare personnel. This, in turn, has led to what is termed 'medical tourism', a situation where many Africans, especially the leaders, have resorted to jetting out of the continent for the treatment of minor health challenges.

Sadly, during the pandemic, many of the politicians and well-to-do who got infected could not travel out due to the lockdowns, thereby resulting in their death. Many government health institutions lacked the basic facilities to save or treat those infected and save lives.[7] Healthcare facilities, including quarantine centres, were overburdened and overstretched due to poor allocation of resources and inadequate healthcare providers. The situation was dire for millions of disadvantaged Africans who could not afford to go to private hospitals due to high cost of treatment.[8] Thus, this book attempts to capture the impact of the pandemic on the realization of the right to health of specific groups. More importantly, it highlights the importance of a rights-based approach to addressing these challenges.

The gross underfunding of the healthcare systems in many African countries exacerbated the impact of the pandemic as many deaths, including those of notable politicians, could have been avoided. In addition, many of the healthcare providers were unduly exposed to the pandemic, and some indeed lost their lives due to poor working conditions and lack of protective gadgets. It is therefore clear that the right to health ought to be regarded as a basis for informing states' responses to the pandemic.

1.2.1 Objectives

Against this backdrop, this book seeks to address the following issues:

1) To explore how the COVID-19 pandemic impacted the enjoyment of the right to health in Africa
2) To discuss the relevance of the right to health approach as an appropriate response to addressing a public health emergency such as COVID-19
3) To examine the roles of regional institutions and national institutions/bodies in addressing the health rights-related consequences of the COVID-19 pandemic in Africa
4) To explore opportunities that exist for African governments towards addressing the impact of COVID-19 on the health systems in the region and preparing for future pandemics.

1.3 Conceptual framework for the book

This book adopts the right to health as a framework with a focus on inequality and discrimination in light of the COVID-19 pandemic. The key aspects of the right to health, as would be discussed later, form the basis upon which the arguments in the various chapters of the book have been articulated. Access to health care and the construction of hospitals are commonly linked to the right to health. While this may be true, there are still other aspects of the right to health. It consists of a wide range of elements or factors that can support healthy living. These are referred to as the 'underlying determinants of health' by the Committee on Economic, Social, and Cultural Rights (CESCR).[9] These determinants are safe food, safe drinking water, adequate sanitation, adequate nutrition and housing, healthy working and environmental conditions, health-related education and information, and gender inequality.[10] During the pandemic, these social determinants became very relevant in curtailing the pandemic. For many in disadvantaged communities, access to these social determinants became difficult, further exacerbating the impact of the pandemic in those communities.[11]

The right to health is also associated with certain freedoms including the right to be free from torture and other cruel, barbaric, or humiliating treatment or punishment, as well as the right to be free from forced sterilization and other non-consensual medical procedures.[12] There are equally certain entitlements associated with the right to health, such as the right to a healthcare system that gives everyone an equal chance to achieve the best possible level of health; the right to prevention, treatment, and control of diseases; access to essential medicines; maternal, child, and reproductive health; equal and timely access to basic health services; the provision of health-related education and information; and participation of the population in health-related decision-making at the national and community levels.[13] All people must have access to equal health services, products, and facilities. A fundamental human rights value that is essential to the exercise of the right to the best achievable level of health is non-discrimination. All facilities, services, and medical facilities must be readily available, accessible, acceptable, and of decent quality.[14] A state must have enough functional public health and healthcare facilities, as well as related supplies and services.

They must be financially feasible, non-discriminatory, and physically accessible to all segments of the population, notably children, teenagers, older people, people with disabilities, and other groups that are vulnerable. Additionally, accessibility implies the right to request, receive, and disseminate health information in a manner that is accessible (for everyone, including people with disabilities), but it does not restrict the right to have private health information handled with care. Additionally, the facilities, products, and services should adhere to medical ethics and be gender- and culturally sensitive. They should therefore be acceptable from both a medical and a cultural perspective. They must also be of high quality and appropriate in terms of science and medicine. In particular, this calls for skilled medical personnel, medications that have been scientifically approved and are still valid, hospital supplies, proper sanitation, and clean water.[15]

The notion of non-discrimination and equality is primordial in attempting to assess the impact of the pandemic on the healthcare system in African countries covered in this book. Any distinction, exclusion, or restriction made on the basis of different reasons that have the effect or goal of undermining or preventing the recognition, enjoyment, or exercise of human rights and basic freedoms is referred to as discrimination. It is associated with the marginalization of particular population groups and, more often than not, lies at the heart of underlying structural injustices in society.[16] These groups may therefore become more susceptible to poverty and illness as a result. It should come as no surprise that historically oppressed and underprivileged communities frequently suffer an unfairly disproportionate number of health issues.[17] For instance, studies have demonstrated that in certain societies, ethnic minority groups, people in informal settlements, and indigenous peoples are unable to have access to adequate housing and safe drinking water, and their children are prone to die young and experience severe starvation than the general population.[18] They also get fewer health services and information about health issues.

When someone experiences double or many forms of discrimination, such as discrimination based on sex and ethnicity, nationality, or age, particularly in the context of public health emergencies such as COVID-19, the effects are exacerbated. For instance, indigenous women and women in disadvantaged communities are more susceptible to physical and sexual abuse than the general population and often receive fewer health and reproductive treatments and information.[19] Equal opportunity and non-discrimination are the core tenets of human rights and essential elements of the right to health. The ensuing non-exhaustive grounds of discrimination are listed in the International Covenant on Economic, Social, and Cultural Rights (Article 2 (2)) and the Convention on the Rights of the Child (Article 2 (1)): race, colour, sex, language, religion, political opinion, national or social origin, property, disability, birth, or other status. The CESCR states that 'other status' can refer to sexual orientation or health status (such as HIV/AIDS).[20] States have a duty to prohibit and end all forms of discrimination, ensure that everyone has equal access to health care, and address the root causes of diseases. Additionally, the Convention on the Elimination of All Forms of Racial Discrimination (Article 5) emphasizes the need for states to outlaw and abolish racial discrimination and to protect everyone's right to access public health and medical treatment.[21]

Furthermore, non-discrimination and equality indicate that states must take into account the unique characteristics and requirements of groups who typically experience special health issues, such as greater mortality rates or susceptibility to particular diseases. Specific health standards must be applied to certain demographic groups, such as women, children, or people with disabilities, in order to ensure that there is no discrimination. When some groups of people have consistently faced discrimination from either private actors or state parties, positive measures of protection are especially required. In a similar vein, the CESCR has emphasized that there is no excuse for vulnerable members of society not being protected against health-related discrimination, whether in practice or under the law. Therefore, even in difficult circumstances such as the COVID-19 period, society's most vulnerable members must be protected, perhaps by implementing relatively affordable focused programmes.[22] During the pandemic, many African countries failed to give priority to the health needs of vulnerable and marginalized groups.

States have the primary obligations to promote and protect human rights. International human rights treaties, which have been ratified by states, impose obligations on states to implement the provisions of these treaties. Furthermore, state parties have a duty to give effect to these rights within their territories through ratifying human rights treaties. Article 2 (1) of the International Covenant on Economic, Social, and Cultural Rights emphasizes that states have a duty to gradually realize all of the rights guaranteed by the covenant.[23] This is an underlying admission that states have resource limitations and that implementing treaty obligations requires time. As a result, several covenant-protected rights, including the right to health, are thought to be subject to gradual realization. While not all aspects of the rights guaranteed by the covenant can or will be fulfilled immediately, states must, at the very least, demonstrate that they are doing everything in their power to ensure the realization of the rights guaranteed by the covenant.[24] Resources that are available include both those that are present inside a state and those that are accessible from the international community through international cooperation and aid, as stated in Article 2 (1).

Other documents such as the United Nations Charter, the Universal Declaration of Human Rights, and the Convention on the Rights of the Child also emphasize the importance of international cooperation and aid.[25] It does not replace domestic commitments, but it is particularly relevant when a state needs support from other states in order to implement economic, social, and cultural rights because it is unable to do so on its own. States that are in a position to help others in this way are especially obligated to cooperate internationally. Therefore, states should actively pursue international collaboration and aid, as well as offer economic and technical support, to help other states fulfil their commitments under international agreements in connection to the right to health in a non-discriminatory and equal manner.[26]

Sadly, during the COVID-19 pandemic, developed countries did not provide the needed support to the poorer countries to ensure access to health facilities as well as goods and services. In particular, with regard to vaccines, some developed countries where these vaccines are produced blocked access to these vaccines by insisting on patent rights. This made it difficult for those in poor countries to secure access to these vaccines. These challenges are captured in Chapters 4–6 of this book.

All of the covenant's rights are subject to the idea of progressive realization, but some obligations have an immediate impact. These include the commitment to ensure that all rights are exercised without discrimination and the duty to take steps – concrete, deliberate, and targeted steps – towards the realization of all rights, including the right to health.[27] Retrogressive actions are not permitted in this regard unless a state can show that it has used all reasonable efforts to fulfil its responsibilities.[28] A range of actions are needed to realize the right to health. International treaties do not provide a set of guidelines for implementing the right to health because the most practical steps will differ from state to state. Article 2 (1) of the International Covenant on Economic, Social, and Cultural Rights only specifies that 'all appropriate means, including, in particular, the adoption of legislative measures', must be used to ensure the full implementation of the rights guaranteed by the treaty.

The CESCR has emphasized that states should, at the very least, create a national plan based on human rights principles that specifies the goals of that strategy in order to ensure that everyone enjoys the right to health.[29] The creation and execution of such a strategy will depend on the indicators and benchmarks that are set. The expectations of a state will change over time because the right to health is one that is subject to gradual realization.[30] Therefore, a state needs a tool to track and assess these mutable aspects of the right to health. Indicators, particularly when broken down, offer helpful information on how the right to health is implemented in a specific nation. For these indicators, Office of the High Commissioner for Human Rights (OHCHR) is creating a conceptual and methodological framework. Such indicators will be very useful to monitor state responses to public health emergencies such as the COVID-19 pandemic.

The CESCR has also emphasized that states have a fundamental responsibility to ensure that each of the rights guaranteed by the covenant is met at a minimum acceptable level.[31] Although these fundamental levels are somewhat resource-dependent, the state should prioritize them in its efforts to fully implement the covenant's rights. Regarding the right to health, the committee has emphasized that states must guarantee the right of access to health facilities, goods, and services on a non-discriminatory basis, particularly for vulnerable or marginalized groups; access to the bare minimum of nutrient-adequate and safe food; access to shelter, housing, and sanitation; an adequate supply of safe drinking water; and the provision of essential drugs: equitable distribution of all health services, facilities, and products.[32]

Furthermore, states' obligations pertaining to the right to health normally fall within three categories: respect, protect, and fulfil. States must refrain from obstructing the right to health directly or indirectly in order to uphold the requirement of respect. States should refrain from, among other things, denying or restricting access to healthcare services; marketing dangerous drugs; enforcing discriminatory practices regarding women's health status and needs; restricting access to contraceptives and other methods of maintaining sexual and reproductive health; hiding, censoring, or incorrectly interpreting and representing health information; and violating the right to privacy (e.g. of those who are HIV/AIDS positive).[33] The CESCR further emphasized in its general comment number 14 that states parties must respect the right to health as it is practised in other nations.

States should pass legislation or take other steps to make sure that private providers of healthcare or other services (such as regulating the ingredients in food items) abide by human rights norms; prevent privatization from endangering the availability, accessibility, acceptability, and quality of healthcare organizations, goods, and services; and shield people from actions by third parties that might be detrimental to their right to health.[34] The CESCR in its General Comment No. 14 has emphasized that state parties should prohibit third parties from infringing on other states' rights to health. It additionally said that state parties should take precautions to ensure that their agreements do not negatively affect the right to health while negotiating international or multilateral accords.[35] In the context of COVID-19, states would be expected to ensure that trade agreements such as the Trade-Related Aspects of Intellectual Property Rights (TRIPS) Agreement[36] do not hinder access to vaccines.

In order to fully implement and fulfil the right to health, states are obligated to adopt proper legislative, administrative, budgetary, judicial, promotional, and other measures. States must, for example, develop a national health strategy or plan that covers both the public and private sectors.[37] They must also ensure that health care is provided, including programmes to vaccinate against infectious diseases and services to lessen and prevent additional disabilities. Also, states must guarantee that everyone has equal access to fundamental health determinants like wholesome food, sanitary conditions, and clean water, and ensure that public health infrastructures offer services for sexual and reproductive health and that the number of doctors and other medical personnel is adequate and they are properly trained.[38] They are required by law to offer guidance and information on health-related topics like the right to the best possible level of health depends on efficient and integrated health systems that cover both medical services and the fundamental factors that influence health.

1.4 Overview of chapters

The book is divided into three main parts as follows.

1.4.1 Part I – Conceptual issues

Chapter 1 by Durojaye and Mahadew provides an overview of the book detailing its objective and rationale. It further provides the theoretical framework of the book and the summary of each chapter.

In Chapter 2, Kigera examines discriminatory practices against women during the pandemic. She notes that the COVID-19 pandemic has laid bare the multilayered dimensions of discrimination that women face in accessing health care. Using Kenya as a case study, she observes that delivery of healthcare services is premised on the right to health, which is a fundamental human right provided in the constitution and international law. In her view even in the face of public health emergencies, such as COVID-19, states are still expected to meet certain core obligations and carry out subsequent concrete steps to realize the right to access to healthcare services immediately.

Chapter 3 by Mahadew and Mahadew focuses on the interrelatedness, indivisibility, and interdependence of human rights in the context of COVID-19. While the authors note that during the pandemic the human right that is directly relevant is the right to health and, rightly so, focus has been on this right, they contend that other rights are equally important in the context of the pandemic. This chapter argues that a potential violation of the right to health can lead to violation of other rights such as the right to life, the right to freedom of movement, the right to work, and the right to protection from discrimination. In particular, the authors argue that the interrelatedness of human rights in the context of COVID-19 compels states to take a broader approach in terms of the protection and promotion of all human rights and not merely the right to health.

1.4.2 Part II – The impact of COVID-19 on access to health goods and services

In Chapter 4, Ogendi evaluates the situation of vaccine inequity in developing countries with a special focus on Africa. Special attention is given to the role of intellectual property or pharmaceutical patents, which is bedrock of the current market approach to vaccines access. Arguably, the right to health and the right to enjoy the benefits of scientific progress require access to vaccines for all, but this appears to be largely ignored because of the current inequities.

Chapter 5 by Nnamuchi deals with the issue of vaccine mandate. He argues that while some favour attaining herd immunity through natural infection, others prefer the route of vaccines. According to him, a key proponent of the latter is the World Health Organization (WHO). But although WHO advocates vaccination as an avenue to achieving herd immunity, it frowns upon the natural infection approach and compulsory vaccination. Yet, several nations, most remarkably the United States, are proceeding to impose vaccine mandates on their people, even those with religious or other objections. He notes that this coercive exercise of power raises a number of questions, some of which have profound significance to the enjoyment of the right to health, particularly in Africa. Should Africa join the bandwagon? In other words, is it appropriate for countries in the region to impose vaccine mandates? These are some of the questions the chapter hopes to answer.

In Chapter 6, Omoruyi notes that the absence of viewing how the COVID-19 pandemic intersects with pre-existing inequalities, rather than a blanket attribution of the nature of vulnerability or marginalization, can lead to a failure in the response. The chapter adapts the theory of intersectionality as a framework to emphasize the need to have a contextual understanding of the impact of the pandemic on various groups and design responses accordingly. With respect to ensuring access to vaccines for vulnerable and marginalized groups, it requires strategies that are based on their peculiar circumstances or barriers to access in a bid to ensure that the vaccines reach them and uptake is encouraged.

Budoo-Scholtz, in Chapter 7, discusses the importance of budgetary allocation in addressing the pandemic. According to her, a human rights approach to budgetary allocation has been considered as an important aspect for the realization of rights such as the right to health. She discusses whether allocation of extra resources during the COVID-19 pandemic had adopted a human rights approach or whether most of the budget was for personnel and overheads, which is the case for many African budgets. The chapter takes a rights-based approach to budgetary allocation to ensure realization of rights and examine whether budgetary allocations during the COVID-19 pandemic adopted a human rights approach.

1.4.3 Part III – The impact of COVID-19 on the right to health of disadvantaged and marginalized groups

In Chapter 8, Robert et al. discuss the impact of COVID-19-related restrictions on access to maternal healthcare services for rural women. It articulates the key lessons that African governments like Kenya and Uganda should take from this health crisis in order to curb the re-occurrence of similar abuses in the future. In both countries, the governments adopted a number of restrictions/measures in the form of lockdowns and curfews in a bid to contain the spread of the virus. These measures hindered women in rural Kenya and Uganda from accessing essential maternal healthcare-related services, thereby leading to numerous preventable deaths, injuries, and losses.

Chapter 9 by Mavundla and Strode focuses on the impact of the pandemic on the sexual and reproductive health and rights of women. The authors note that many countries, including Eswatini, found themselves having to shift their focus and resources from other pressing priorities to deal with the aftermath of COVID-19 effectively. According to them, COVID-19 has been a health concern that has seriously stressed many health systems of many countries worldwide, both developed and developing countries. The authors highlight Eswatini's commitments to sexual and reproductive health and rights (SRHR), noting some of the constraints and impact of COVID-19 on SRHR in the country. Furthermore, using Eswatini as a case study, the chapter explores how international law obligations are assisting in the creation of a legal framework for SRHRs but has a limited impact on implementation.

Mohee in Chapter 10 examines the protection of health of minorities and vulnerable and marginalized groups during the pandemic. Drawing from an analysis of state duties on the protection of the right to heath amid pandemics, the chapter argues that states have a minimum core obligation to ensure non-discriminatory and equitable access to health services, especially for vulnerable and marginalized groups. It, however, notes that specific guidance on relevant normative parameters has been wanting. The author argues that in Africa, vulnerable groups, notably poor communities and women and girls as well as sexual minorities have been among the most disproportionately affected by national containment measures and the socio-economic impacts of the pandemic. It recommends, among others, robust data systems for better planning and monitoring of assistance, a stronger role of the regional human rights organs in guiding state duties in this regard, prioritization of health in national budget allocations, more compelling mobilization in the face of global health inequities, and the recognition of health risks in conflict-affected and fragile areas in responses.

The focus of Chapter 11 by Kangaude and Macleod is on the nexus between CVOID-19 and the SRHR of adolescents. The chapter discusses the experience of adolescents during the pandemic, especially the dysfunction that contributed to sexual and reproductive health challenges for adolescents such as loss of access of services to prevent pregnancy and sexually transmitted infections, experience of sexual violence and abuse, and mental health challenges. It further engages the notion of home and how the responsiveness of home to the needs and the rights of adolescents in times of pandemic containment measures could be improved. It engages how home and the institution of the family interact with systems of support and protection for adolescents from the perspective of the rights of the child and the obligations of states to realize the rights of the child to sexual and reproductive health in pandemic times.

Chapter 12 by Adebanjo discusses the problems of Africa's health sector as exacerbated by COVID-19 and examines the effect that this has had on the rights and well-being of healthcare workers in the region. The author examines the situation in select countries within the region and juxtaposes it with the impact of the pandemic on healthcare workers in select countries in the Global North. The chapter then proposes ways of mitigating the impact of COVID-19 on healthcare workers in Africa and protecting their rights in the face of the pandemic.

Atonga in Chapter 13 examines the impact of COVID-19 on access to sexual and reproductive health care, particularly family planning and abortion services. According to the author, in addition to the lockdowns and restrictions in movement, there was also a scale-down of essential healthcare intervention and withdrawal of critical reproductive health services. The worst hit services included HIV/AIDS care and treatment, access to contraceptives, and abortion. The author contends that with the limited access to abortion care having been withdrawn, women retorted to unsafe and clandestine abortions.

In Chapter 14, Durojaye examines the role of regional human rights bodies and national courts in addressing human rights violations in the context of the COVID-19 pandemic. The author assesses the role played by the Commission during previous public health emergencies and during the COVID-19 pandemic and argues that the Commission could have done better than it did in setting norms and standards to protect the human rights of vulnerable and marginalized groups in the region. The chapter further discusses the role of national courts in protecting human rights in the wake of imposition of lockdowns to curb the spread of COVID-19 in African countries.

Phele in Chapter 15 contends that what was evident globally in the past two years is that gender-based violence cuts across all nations with similar trends, and that there are various efforts made by countries to reduce it. As per the author, the escalation of gender-based violence (GBV) across sub-Saharan Africa particularly among women, girls, key, and vulnerable populations was reported in 2022. Thus, apart from the burden of COVID-19 on healthcare systems, a sharp rise in GBV cases added to the existing vulnerabilities of those who are on the margins of society. Her chapter therefore focuses on the nexus of COVID-19 and gender-based violence in Botswana with a comparative analysis of Kenya and Nigeria during COVID-19. It highlights selected regional experiences in tackling gender-based violence.

Notes

1 T Ahmed, AE Rahman, TG Amole et al 'The effect of COVID-19 on maternal newborn and child health (MNCH) services in Bangladesh, Nigeria and South Africa: Call for a contextualised pandemic response in LMICs' (2021) 20(77) *International Journal for Equity in Health* available at https://doi.org/10.1186/s12939-021-01414-5.

2 S Suri 'COVID19's impact on Africa, why it goes beyond healthcare' (2021) available at www.orfonline.org/expert-speak/covid19s-impact-on-africa-why-it-goes-beyond-healthcare/ (accessed 30 June 2021).

3 As above.

4 As above.

5 See, for instance, O Mackett 'The effects of COVID-19 on women in South Africa: An analysis using the Social Provisioning Framework' (2020) 18 *Social and Health Sciences*.

6 See WHO 'Act now, act together – 2020–2021 impact report' (2021) available at https://www.who.int/publications/m/item/act-now-act-together-2020-2021-impact-report

7 GA Tessema, Y Kinfu, BA Dachew et al 'The COVID-19 pandemic and healthcare systems in Africa: A scoping review of preparedness, impact and response' (2021) *BMJ Global Health* available at https://doi.org/10.1136/bmjgh-2021-00717.

8 As above.

9 See UN Committee on Economic, Social and Cultural Rights (CESCR) *General comment no. 14: The right to the highest attainable standard of health (art. 12 of the covenant)*, 11 August 2000, E/C.12/2000/4.

10 OHCHR 'The right to health – Fact Sheet No 31' available at www.ohchr.org/sites/default/files/Documents/Publications/Factsheet31.pdf (accessed 27 September 2023) 3.

11 See, for instance, R Nanima & E Durojaye *Socio-economic rights impact of COVID-19 in selected informal settlements in Cape Town* (2020)

12 As above.
13 UN Committee on Economic, Social and Cultural Rights (CESCR) (n 9 above).
14 See IFHHRO Medical Human Rights Network 'AAAQ framework' available at www.ifhhro.org/topics/aaaq-framework/ (accessed 27 September 2023).
15 UNICEF 'Availability, accessibility, acceptability and quality framework' available at https://gbvguidelines.org/wp/wp-content/uploads/2019/11/AAAQ-framework-Nov-2019-WEB.pdf (accessed 27 September 2023).
16 AE Yamin *When misfortune becomes injustice: Evolving human rights struggles for health and social equality* (2020).
17 See P Farmer *Pathologies of power: Health human rights and the new war on the poor* (2003).
18 See UN 'Equality and discrimination' available at www.un.org/ruleoflaw/thematic-areas/human-rights/equality-and-non-discrimination/ (accessed 27 September 2023).
19 See, for instance, B Ngcamu & E Mantzaris 'The effects of COVID-19 on vulnerable groups: A reflection on South African informal urban settlements' (2021) 9 *African Public Service Delivery and Performance Review* 2021.
20 See General Comment 20 of the CESCR on Non-discrimination in the enjoyment of socio-economic rights.
21 UN General Assembly *International convention on the elimination of all forms of racial discrimination*, 21 December 1965, United Nations, Treaty Series, vol. 660, p. 195.
22 See CESCR 'General comment no 14: The right to the highest attainable standard of health' UN Doc E/C.12/2000/4 para 18.
23 International Covenant on Economic, Social and Cultural Rights, adopted December 16, 1966, preamble, G.A. Res. 2200A (XXI), U.N. GAOR, Supp. No. 16, U.N. Doc A/6316 (1966) (entered into force 2 September 1990).
24 UN Committee on Economic, Social and Cultural Rights (CESCR) General Comment No. 3 (1990) on the nature of state parties' obligations.
25 See Articles 1, 55, and 56 of the UN Charter; Articles 22 and 28 of the Universal Declaration of Human Rights; and Articles 4 and 24 of the Convention on the Rights of the Child.
26 CESCR 'General Comment No 3 (1990) on the nature of state parties' obligations; see also CESCR 'General Comment No 14: The Right to the Highest Attainable Standard of Health' paras 38–42.
27 See General Comment 14 (n 22 above).
28 L Montel et al 'How should implementation of the human right to health be assessed? A scoping review of the public health literature from 2000 to 2021' (2022) 139 *International Journal for Equity in Health*.
29 CESCR General Comment 14 (n 22 above).
30 See as above, para 53–62.
31 See as above, para 43.
32 See OHCHR Fact Sheet No 13 (n 7 above) 25.
33 See CESCR general Comment 14 (n 22 above), and CEDAW General Recommendation 24
34 CESCR General Comment 14, see also Committee on the Rights of the Child General Comment 15 on article 24 on the right to health.
35 As above.
36 TRIPS: Agreement on Trade-Related Aspects of Intellectual Property Rights, 15 April 1994, Marrakesh Agreement Establishing the World Trade Organization, Annex 1C, 1869 U.N.T.S. 1197 (1994) [hereinafter TRIPS Agreement].01
37 CESCR General Comment 14 (n 22 above).
38 As above.

2

DISCRIMINATORY PRACTICES AGAINST WOMEN IN ACCESS TO HEALTH CARE IN KENYA IN THE CONTEXT OF THE COVID-19 PANDEMIC

Soila Kigera

2.1 Introduction

The Severe Acute Respiratory Syndrome Coronavirus 2 (SARS-CoV-2), which was first reported in Wuhan, China, caused a pandemic of acute respiratory disease named 'coronavirus disease of 2019' (COVID-19), which threatened the health and lives of humans across the globe.[1] COVID-19 was first reported in Kenya in March 2020 and eventually spread across the 47 autonomous counties. According to the World Health Organization (WHO), at the end of March 2022, there were 323,423 reported cases of COVID-19 and 5,648 deaths resulting from the virus in Kenya.[2] Although the loss of lives in Kenya was not as nearly as great as compared to other countries, the indirect impact of the pandemic exacerbated the already existing social and economic issues surrounding access of healthcare services.

As a result of the pandemic, the government of Kenya put in place a lot of stringent measures to curb the spread of the virus, some of which had severe economic and humanitarian consequences and brought about high incidences of violation of human rights.[3] Major organizations and businesses were forced to close, especially in the informal sector, which accounts for the majority of the work force.[4] The closing down of schools and other institutions of learning also brought about sexual and reproductive health crisis, with 100,000 teenage pregnancies being reported during the lockdown period.[5]

In addition, the dusk-to-dawn curfews triggered by the loss of jobs saw a hike in sexual and domestic violence against women. To crown it all, between the months of June and August 2020, there was a nationwide strike of nurses and doctors across the 47 counties on account of poor working conditions, which led to a disruption of health services.[6]

DOI: 10.4324/9781032671437-3

The response to the COVID-19 virus by the state inadvertently shifted from a health crisis to a security crisis.[7] The right of health and access to healthcare services was positioned in isolation to other rights.[8] However, the right of health and access to healthcare services cannot be enjoyed without addressing other rights.[9] The underlying social determinants of health are based on other social, economic, and even political rights.[10] The right to food, housing, work, education, human dignity, and non-discrimination are just among the rights that are integral components of the right to health.[11]

Access of healthcare services is premised on the right to health, which is a fundamental human right provided in both regional and international treaties and the Constitution of Kenya. These human rights instruments place on states obligations to facilitate, provide, and promote administrative, budgetary, judicial, promotional, and other measures for the realization of the right to health and ultimately the access to healthcare services.[12] These instruments inherently address the different elements of access and their co-relation to the two dominant proponents of access, that is, the health system and the population. Access cannot be confined to the presence of health facilities, but there must be actual utilization of the services and a proper fit between the population and the health system.[13] Utilization of these services goes beyond the provision of preventive, curative, or palliative health care but also extends to the underlying social determinants of health.[14]

Women, including also girls, have unique health needs, and studies have shown that during times of crisis, conflicts, or epidemics, women face a greater challenge in accessing healthcare services due to the pre-existing multiple and intersecting facets of inequality and discrimination.[15] The right to health cannot be recognized in a bubble but can only be fulfilled when other rights that advance the right to health are protected and respected as well.[16] It is therefore imperative that all human rights failings which lead to social exclusion, humiliation, stigmatization, and essentially discrimination against women in accessing healthcare services are addressed.[17]

The effects of the pandemic and subsequent government restrictions led to severe economic and humanitarian consequences, job losses, and lack of access to health services, especially sexual and reproductive health services.[18] Even among struggling economies with limited resources, there are certain core obligations and subsequent concrete steps that each state must realize immediately.[19] Measures adopted by the states to curb the spread of the pandemic or flatten the curve of infections must be time limited, reasonable, proportionate, non-discriminatory, and grounded in law to ensure that all human rights are protected.[20]

2.1.1 The right to health

The right to health was first articulated in the constitution of WHO in 1946[21] and later mentioned in the Universal Declaration of Human Rights (UDH) in

1948 as part of the right to adequate standard of living.[22] The right to health is now expressly provided under the African human rights and the international system. The International Covenant on Economic, Social, and Cultural Rights (ICESCR),[23] the Convention on the Rights of the Child (CRC),[24] Article 12 of the International Convention on the Elimination of all forms of Discrimination Against Women (CEDAW),[25] Article 16 of the African Charter on Human and Peoples' Rights (African Charter),[26] and the African Charter on the Rights and Welfare of the Child[27] provide for the 'right to enjoy the best attainable state of physical and mental health'. The Protocol to the African Charter on Human and Peoples' Rights on the Rights of Women (Maputo Protocol) in Africa defines the right to health to include sexual and reproductive health.[28]

Apart from the international covenants, the Beijing Declaration and the Platform of Action of the Fourth World Conference on Women (the Beijing Platform)[29] and the Programme of Action of the International Conference on Population and Development (the Cairo Programme)[30] have come to be regarded as authoritative frameworks to address civil, political, social, economic, and cultural inequalities and in particular the right to health with regard to women.[31]

Kenya has ratified both regional and international conventions that provide for the right to health. Additionally, the constitution provides every person with the right to the highest standard of health, which also includes access to healthcare services.[32] The constitution further places an obligation on the state to take legislative, policy, and other measures, including the setting of standards, to achieve the progressive realization of this right.[33] The realization of this right also places an obligation on all state organs and public officers to address the needs of vulnerable groups. Women are categorized as one of the vulnerable groups.[34]

Apart from the constitution, Kenya has enacted various statutes and policies related to the administration of healthcare services.

The Committee on Economic, Social and Cultural Rights (CESCR) being the primary body tasked with overseeing the implementation of Article 12 has interpreted the right to health to encompass both freedoms and entitlements.[35] The former entitles people the right to make decisions concerning their health without interference, while the latter provides the right to enjoy access to equal opportunity and quality health care.[36] The right, however, is not construed as a guarantee to be healthy as there are many factors that would affect the health of an individual, such as genetic conditions that are above the control of the state.[37]

2.1.2 Access

Access plays a predominant role in the right to health.[38] Although there are many theories conceptualizing the definition of access, two proponents always emerge – the health system and the population. Access therefore entails the ability of the population to reach and obtain appropriate health services when needed. This definition encompasses the health system factors, which comprise the structures, resources, procedures, regulations, and institutions in which services are delivered.[39] It also takes into account the underlying social determinants which affect the populations' ability to obtain and utilize health services and ultimately attain the highest standard of health to live a dignified life.

The CESCR has defined the right to health in all its forms to contain four essential, interrelated, elements, that is, availability, acceptability, accessibility, and quality (AAAQ), which all address the characteristics that encompass access.[40] Availability connotes the presence of functioning public health facilities, goods, and services.[41] The element of acceptability ensures that the goods and services are delivered in a culturally appropriate manner and respecting the aspect of confidentiality of each individual.[42] Quality ensures that the goods and services provided are scientifically and medically appropriate and of good quality.[43]

The CESCR places an obligation on state parties to ensure that every person has access to health facilities, goods, and services within their jurisdiction without discrimination.[44] However, the presence of health facilities alone does not itself imply access, but there must be actual utilization of the services and a proper fit between the population and the health system.[45] Utilization of these services goes beyond the provision of preventive, curative, or palliative health care but also extends to the underlying social determinants.[46]

Poverty, income inequality, and marginalization are some of the factors that affect access to health services.[47] These factors are manifested through laws and policies that shape the economic environment.[48] It is becoming more and more acceptable that the right to health cannot solely be pegged on the provision of healthcare services, but it is also an outcome of socio-economic development.[49] Socio-economic factors promote conditions that allow people to access health care and lead a healthy life. Access to food and nutrition, housing, and safe and clean drinking water, and a healthy occupational environment are all underlying determinants that shape an individual's health status.[50]

Therefore, for the right to access healthcare services to be actualized, there must be a determination by the state to eradicate or reduce poverty and institute policies that ensure more equitable distribution of wealth so as to raise the living standards of its citizens.[51] The African Commission on Human and Peoples' Rights (African Commission) advocated for the right to health to be incorporated in development plans and for states to put in place national poverty reduction strategies for the right to be realized.[52]

2.1.2.1 Economic accessibility (affordability)

For health care to be accessible, health facilities, goods, and services, including medicine, must be affordable to all.[53] Most patients in Africa pay for health services out of pocket, and this affects their household income.[54] The report of the Special Rapporteur on health with regard to access to medicine stated that two-thirds of expenditures on medicines were financed through out-of-pocket payments.[55] In Kenya, the number of people covered by health insurance as of 2018 was 19.9% of the population.[56] In addition, 29% of the total expenditure of the Kenyan health system is funded by out-of-pocket payments. These payments have been increasing gradually over the years from USD 15 per capita in 1995 to USD 38 in 2014.[57] The increasing cost of healthcare services pushes 11 million Africans into poverty every year.[58]

Affordability is based on two interacting factors, that is, the ability to pay and healthcare costs.[59] Healthcare costs are a result of direct and indirect costs of essential medicines, goods, and services.[60] These costs are influenced by the competitiveness of the market, availability of suppliers, transportation costs, and government policies.[61] The state must, therefore, play a crucial role in ensuring that the pricing is fair and equitable to avoid the disproportionate burdening of poorer households.[62] In 2020, a research that was conducted in the slums of Kenya revealed an increase in the cost of many health-related items like face masks, hand sanitizers, and disinfectants in private facilities and pharmacies.[63] Due to the shortages of drugs and other goods in public facilities, many people were forced to buy from private pharmacies.[64]

The cost of treating COVID-19 has also been exponentially high. In 2020, research was undertaken in Kenya's public health facilities to determine the unit cost per patient for completing COVID-19 treatment and the daily cost of COVID-19 management.[65] The research revealed that the cost of treating patients who were asymptomatic and with mild to moderate symptoms was Kshs 1993.01 (USD 18.89) and Kshs 1995.17 (USD 18.991) per day, respectively.[66] The unit costs for these two groups of patients were only based on home-based care management adopted by the state. In the event that these patients were admitted in a general ward, the unit costs would increase to Kshs 6717 (USD 63.68) and Kshs 6719.90 (USD 63.70) for patients who are asymptomatic and with mild to moderate symptoms, respectively.[67] As for the unit cost of case management for patients with COVID-19 who were serious and critical, the daily cost was estimated at Kshs 13,137 (USD 124.50) and Kshs 63,243.11 (USD 599.51), respectively.[68] The biggest cost drivers were personal protective equipment (PPE) and pharmaceuticals.[69] Considering that most patients in Kenya pay for health services out of pocket, it would be safe to state that only a small percentage would have the ability to sustain such payments.

Equity is another key in economic accessibility.[70] Equity dictates that healthcare services and medicines should be made economically accessible to all sectors of the population.[71]

The true effect of inequity has been experienced during the ongoing pandemic. The global inequalities between high-income countries and low-income countries played a major role in the access of vaccines.[72] As of 2021, 1.5 billion vaccine doses had been administered in the world, with 75% of those doses being supplied to only 10 countries.[73] Unfortunately, only fewer than 25 million doses were administered in Africa.[74] This is in the backdrop of the United Nations Secretary General terming vaccines as 'global public goods'.[75] There has been a tug of three different competing interests[76]: The pharmaceutical industries protecting their patent-based exclusive rights, high-income nation states wanting to secure the vaccines so as to speed up national recovery, and humanitarian, global political, economic interests.[77] The high-income countries opted to enter into Advance Purchase Agreements with manufacturers of vaccines to secure priority to future vaccines.[78] Such bilateral agreements erode collaboration between countries in a path to securing global health security.[79] They particularly disadvantage low-income countries who do not have the economic capacity to make financial bargains that may entice pharmaceutical companies to enter into these bilateral agreements.[80] Although international institutions offered solutions to African countries by offering emergency credit, these short-term solutions only increased the indebtedness of some of the hardest-hit economies.[81] The result was the exacerbation of the growing global inequalities.

As of March 2022, Kenya had only received 17.4 million doses of vaccines.[82] Using these vaccines, only 8.1 million people are fully vaccinated, which is 15.2% of the population.[83] Inequity perpetuated by imbalances of power and wealth has an impact on the protection and fulfilments of the rights to health. It locks out segments of population from accessing a fundamental right.

2.1.2.2 Availability

The CESCR in its General Comment 14 describes availability as access to functioning healthcare facilities, goods, and services in sufficient quantity by all sections of the population, including the marginalized people, indigenous and minority groups, women and children, adolescents, persons living with HIV/AIDS, and older persons.[84] It also entails creating conditions that allow people to timely access preventive, curative, and rehabilitative services.[85] It also includes ensuring that medicine is made available in sufficient quantities to meet the needs of the people and giving priority to select essential medicines as prescribed by WHO.[86] The African Commission sets the availability of essential medicines listed in the WHO Action Programme on Essential Drugs as one of the minimum core obligations for each state.[87] WHO acknowledged that one of the greatest challenges in Africa in combatting COVID-19 was the lack of essential equipment and human resources.[88]

With a population of approximately 47 million, Kenya has 64,181 beds across both private and public hospitals.[89] A research undertaken in 2020 reported that only 58% of these beds were in hospitals with access to oxygen supply.[90] Out of that number, only 537 qualified as ICU beds equipped to manage patients who were critically ill.[91] Additionally, the research also showed that of the 537 ICU beds only 281 had accompanying ventilators.[92] The availability of equipment for initial and continued medical care of suspected and confirmed patients formed part of the checklist by WHO for isolation and case management as one of the indicators of hospitals' preparedness in response to the COVID-19 pandemic.[93] Although the guidelines provided by the government of Kenya for the management of COVID-19, made provision for oxygen therapy and mechanical ventilation to be administered to critically ill patients there was a deficiency of the essential medical equipment.[94]

Availability also entails meeting the underlying determinants of health, which entails that health facilities must contain equipment, medical supplies, essential drugs, and the presence of sufficiently skilled and experienced staff.[95] It is also essential that the staff are well trained and receive competitive salaries.

Reports have indicated that clinical staff play a huge role in the management of the COVID-19 disease.[96] Kenya has 58,000 registered nurses and 12,000 registered doctors over a population of 47 million people.[97] In June 2020, 18,000 nurses employed in public health facilities went on strike, followed shortly by doctors in August 2020.[98] They lamented on the state's failure to provide PPE, and where it was provided, it was of poor quality.[99] This accounted for the infection rates among health workers, which constituted 2.6% of all infections in the country.[100] There was also a shortage of trained health workers, which led to the overburdening and overworking of the existing human resource.[101] The health workers demanded the government to provide them with comprehensive health insurance, better remuneration and for it to be paid on time, and exemptions for doctors who had pre-existing conditions or were pregnant.[102] The strike by doctors was eventually called off in December 2020, while nurses resumed in February 2021.[103] This had a huge impact on the public health system, with many resorting to more costly private facilities and self-medication.

The location of health facilities is key to people who require the services achieving this dimension of access.[104] Additionally, there must be a degree of fit between the community and the health facility.[105] This takes into consideration that the hours of operation are amenable and there is timely access for emergency services.[106] During the pandemic, government restrictions like lockdowns disrupted the administration of essential services.[107] WHO urged states to prioritize certain high-risk categories like preventing and treating communicable diseases, averting child morbidity and mortality, maintaining treatment regimens for chronic diseases, continuity of critical inpatient care, and managing emergency care.[108]

2.1.2.3 Information accessibility

The right to health is an all-inclusive right which encompasses access to information and health-related education.[109] Access to information is one of the entitlements of the right to health.[110] The CESCR defines it as the right to seek, receive, and impart information concerning health issues.[111] This right can only be realizable if the community is literate. Therefore, the right to education is indispensable in realizing other rights like the right to health.[112] Education plays a vital role in promoting human rights and enlightening the minds of people to give them freedom to make knowledgeable decisions concerning their health.[113] The African Commission also stressed on the importance of health-related information and education.[114]

Health-related information should be available, accessible, acceptable, and reliable.[115] It should also be available in different languages and in a form accessible even by those with disabilities.[116] The purpose of information is to create awareness to the public.[117] This can only be achievable through effective communication between the health system and the public.[118]

The outbreak of COVID-19 saw the proliferation of misinformation, termed as 'infodemic'.[119] The Internet has become a dominant source for health-related information due to the availability of affordable Internet and a huge number of mobile devices.[120] Misinformation appeared in different forms like conspiracy theories and misaligned religious beliefs.[121] Misinformation plays a huge role in vaccine hesitancy, which poses a great threat especially to vulnerable groups like pregnant women.[122] Research also reveals that false information is a significant predictor of how individuals will respond to COVID-19.[123]

Misinformation is also a key driver of stigma and fear.[124] The many unknowns of the virus created a fertile ground for misconceptions.[125] Effective information also plays a significant role in promoting acceptability of health services.[126] The information needs to address patients' worries and quell any unwarranted beliefs that they may have in relation to a medical service or goods.[127] A survey carried out by the Ministry of Health in collaboration with the Kenya Medical Research Institute (KEMRI) and the African Institute for Development Policy (AFIDEP) between June and July 2020 in a bid to control the spread of the virus revealed that 62% of the respondents had basic knowledge of COVID-19 but wanted more information on the prevention and treatment of COVID-19.[128] The survey also revealed that the stigma connected with the virus was high, with 71% of the respondents stating that they were not comfortable being in the same office or school with someone who had contracted the virus.[129]

Enforcement of the Ministry of Health's regulations on the burying of people who had succumbed to the virus also fuelled stigma in the community. In particular, there was a public outcry when one citizen's burial was conducted at night and in a shallow grave by public health officials. A statement released by the Kenya Human Rights Commission urged the state to uphold human dignity and to conduct funerals with respect to the family and community.[130] They advised the state that the stigma and discrimination surrounding the burial of persons who succumbed to COVID-19 would only discourage the public from coming forward to seek help.[131]

The African Union (AU) in partnership with the Africa CDC; United Nations Educational, Scientific and Cultural Organization (UNESCO); United Nations Children's Fund (UNICEF); United States Centers for Disease Control and Prevention (US CDC); United Nations Global Pulse; and WHO launched the Africa Infodemic Response Alliance (AIRA) to combat the threat of infodemic.[132] This network was tasked with identifying gaps and misinformation, simplifying technical knowledge, amplifying correct information, and quantifying the impact of the infodemic.[133]

2.2 Discriminatory practices against women in accessing health care

The right to non-discrimination emanates from equality and dignity of human beings, which are provided for in the Charter of the United Nations[134] and the UDH.[135] The International Covenant on Civil and Political Rights (ICCPR) states that all persons are equal before the law and are therefore entitled to equal treatment before the law without discrimination.[136] The same is provided for in the Convention on the Rights of Persons with Disabilities.[137] However, the convention goes further to prohibit discrimination particularly on the ground of discrimination and obligates state parties to ensure that reasonable accommodation is provided.[138] The CEDAW[139] and the International Convention on the Elimination of All Forms of Racial Discrimination[140] expanded the meaning of discrimination by highlighting three markers, that is, distinction, exclusion, or restriction, that impair or nullify the recognition or enjoyment of a right. The Human Rights Committee (HRC) has also used these three markers to expound on discrimination that touches on civil and political rights.[141] This right of discrimination is not only limited to first-generation rights. The CESCR has also interpreted this right to include the prohibition of discrimination in the enjoyment of economic, social, and cultural rights including the right to health.[142]

At the regional level, the African Charter is a unique instrument as it recognizes all generations of rights, and in addition social economic rights are justiciable.[143] Under the charter, all people are therefore entitled to enjoyment of all generations of rights without discrimination.[144] This duty of enjoyment of rights is placed not only on the state but also on individuals.[145] Likewise, the Maputo Protocol also provides for both civil and political rights; economic, social, and cultural rights; and group rights, but it also goes a step further to provide for sexual and reproductive rights.[146] The protocol recognizes that discrimination may be manifested in different forms.[147] It also particularly recognizes widows, elderly women, and women with disabilities as people who are at risk of suffering multiple forms of discrimination.[148]

The Kenyan Constitution recognizes that every person is equal before the law and is therefore entitled to equal protection and benefit of the law.[149] It expounds on the right of equality to mean equal treatment of both men and women in all spheres and the full enjoyment of all rights and freedoms.[150] The constitution also recognizes that discrimination may be manifested directly and indirectly against persons.[151]

Discrimination undermines the fulfilment and enjoyment of economic, social, and cultural rights, which includes the right to health and inherently the right to access to health care.[152] The Special Rapporteur, Dainius Puras, in his final report stated that the COVID-19 pandemic could not only be solved by public health measures.[153] It required states to address human rights issues also.[154] His report highlighted on the interrelatedness and indivisibility of the socio-economic rights like employment rights to the right to health.[155] The right to health cannot be recognized in a bubble but can only be fulfilled when other rights that advance the right to health are protected and respected as well.[156] It is therefore imperative that all human rights failings that lead to social exclusion, humiliation, stigmatization, and essentially non-discrimination are addressed.[157]

2.2.1 Gender inequality

The report of the Special Rapporteur on health recognized that women are among the groups of people who face inequality and discrimination during times of crisis.[158] The report reiterated that inequality and discrimination are the major contributors to poor health outcomes.[159] Gender inequality towards women during the pandemic has particularly manifested in the area of health and well-being.[160]

Gender inequality is perpetuated when there is a failure to respect women's right and in particular the right to sexual and reproductive health.[161] States therefore have an obligation to provide reasonable accommodation to health aspects that are unique to women and girls.[162] The CEDAW provides that in order to eliminate discrimination, particularly in the field of health care, a state party must ensure the provision of services relating to pregnancy and the post-natal period and family planning services.[163] Gender equity as relates to the provision of healthcare services recognizes the biological and the sociocultural difference that influence the health of women in order to remedy inequalities.[164] The CESCR stated that one of the major goals for every state in realizing the right to health is reducing maternal mortality and morbidity and protecting women from gender-based violence (GBV).[165]

Before the pandemic, Kenya had unacceptably high maternal and neonatal mortality rates at 342 out of every 100,000 and 19 out of every 100,000 live births, respectively.[166] The risk for maternal mortality was even higher in younger adolescents.[167] The main reason for such high deaths was the lack of high-quality healthcare services.[168] A scarcity of resources resulting from the pandemic increased maternal mortality and morbidity, adolescent pregnancy, and HIV and sexually transmitted infections (STIs) among women and girls.[169]

During the pandemic, there was a diversion of resources to meet the needs of the general public ignoring the unique vulnerabilities faced by adolescent girls, pregnant women, and newborns.[170] This resulted to the exacerbation of maternal mortality and morbidity, increased rates of teenage pregnancies, and increase in HIV and sexually transmitted diseases.[171] According to various reports, 100,000 teenage girls were reported to be pregnant during the pandemic lockdown.[172] This resulted in the president setting up a taskforce in July 2020 to investigate teenage defilement and pregnancy.[173]

Discrimination may also be manifested in the laws and policies of a state that may appear neutral but have a disproportionate impact.[174] Stringent restrictions on movement have jeopardized the physical and reproductive health of women.[175] They have shut arenas of escape and access to health care, safe shelters, education, employment, and economic life.[176] The Kenyan Ministry of Health acknowledged that although the interventions made by the government slowed down the infection rate of the virus, it brought about new challenges. There was a drop in outpatient services and an increase in reported cases of maternal and children's death during the curfew hours. There was also a disruption of routine immunization, family planning and antenatal care, and the routine management of people living with non-communicable diseases like cancer, diabetes, mental health, hypertension, and heart diseases.

The report of the Special Rapporteur stated that government restrictions that are passed to promote public health but curtail freedoms must be closely monitored.[177] These restrictions have the propensity to impoverish vulnerable communities and prevent access to basic necessities and healthcare services.[178] In addition, these measures adopted by states must also be in agreement with the Siracusa Principles on the Limitation and Derogation Provisions in the ICCPR.[179] These principles provide that the measures put in place to combat the pandemic must be time-limited, reasonable, proportionate, non-discriminatory, and grounded in law to ensure protection of all human rights.[180]

2.2.2 Health inequities

The CESCR has defined the right to health to also include a wide range of socio-economic factors that enable people to lead a healthy life.[181] These include underlying determinants of health like clean and portable water, a healthy environment, food and nutrition, and housing.[182] One of the recommendations made by WHO in remedying health inequities was improving the quality of the daily life of people.[183] This encompasses safe, secure, and fairly paid work; quality education; quality housing; clean water; and sanitation.[184] Africa is still grappling with high rates of unemployment and poverty, which are all underlying factors that impact the enjoyment of the right to health.[185] Even in the 21st century, securing clean drinking water, sanitation, and housing still remains a tremendous challenge.[186] The healthcare system and the economy are also burdened with the cost of treating HIV/AIDS, tuberculosis, and injuries as a result of rampant road traffic accidents.[187]

It is becoming more and more acceptable that the right to health cannot solely be pegged on the provision of healthcare services only, but it is also an outcome of socio-economic development.[188] A total of 740 million women around the world work in the informal economy, which was significantly affected during the pandemic.[189] In Kenya, although there was reduction of income for both genders, the number of women who lost their income was double that of men.[190] This plunged a lot of women into poverty, preventing them from accessing healthcare services and the underlying determinants of health.[191] In order to cope with economic burdens, many women entered into transactional sex to meet their daily needs.[192]

Although the rate of infection in Africa was comparatively lower than that in countries in Europe, Asia, and the Americas, the COVID-19 pandemic exacerbated the already struggling economies of many African countries.[193] Containment measures to stop the spread of the virus like complete lockdowns and movement restrictions had a huge social and economic impact.[194] The burden of these containment measures was especially felt by low-income houses and a big majority of people who work in the informal sector.[195] These led to the loss of livelihoods, especially of many daily wage earners.[196] In 2020, when the state issued directives for the cancellation of international flights, flower farms were forced to dispose produce worth millions of dollars.[197] Consequently, 30,000 temporary workers lost their jobs, and 40,000 permanent workers were sent home on paid leave.[198] In addition, there was also a significant slowdown in trade, tourism, and government spending, which led to the loss of many jobs in the private sector.[199] No income meant no access to basic commodities like food, housing, and clean drinking water that are integral in sustaining livelihoods.[200] A survey undertaken during the pandemic indicated more women reported to have skipped meals and foregone healthcare services because of no income.

Distribution of power, money, and resources also plays a big part in propagating health inequities.[201] Different government policies and the allocation of government resources may either improve or worsen health care.[202] In Kenya, women constitute a significant percentage of the health sector workforce. As a result, women were more exposed to infection in the line of duty. In June 2020, 18,000 nurses employed in public health facilities went on strike.[203] They lamented on the state's failure to provide PPE, and where it was provided, it was of poor quality.[204] There was a shortage of trained health workers, which led to the overburdening and overworking of the existing human resource.[205] They demanded for the government to provide them with comprehensive health insurance and better remuneration and for it to be paid on time.[206]

2.2.3 Gender-based violence

CEDAW in its definition of discrimination includes GBV because this is violence that is targeted towards women based on their sex.[207] GBV includes physical and sexual abuse, threats, coercion, and deprivation of liberty. The CESCR in its General Comment 14 on the right to health forbids any discrimination in the access of healthcare services on the basis of sex.[208] Both the CEDAW and CESCR Committees agree that GBV, which is a form of discrimination, nullifies women's enjoyment of human rights.[209]

The COVID-19 pandemic laid bare the multilayered dimensions of discrimination that women face. The isolation directives therefore exacerbated the pre-existing social and gender inequalities faced by women. Before the outbreak of the pandemic, 243 million women globally between the ages of 18–49 years were subjected to sexual or physical violence perpetrated by intimate partners and data shows the number intensified during the pandemic.[210] In March 2020, the government of Kenya started implementing restrictive policies such as the closure of schools and all-night curfews.[211] In a month of the imposition of the curfews, Liverpool VCT Care and Treatment (LVCT) received significantly more cases of women and adolescent girls reporting violence as compared to that in the pre-COVID-19 season.[212] As per the report by the State Department for Gender, between the months of June and September 2020, 1,195 cases of violence against women and girls were reported.[213] This period coincided with the toughest COVID-19 containment measures.[214]

During the pandemic, adolescent girls were also particularly vulnerable, especially after the closure of schools, and the result was an increase in the cases of female genital mutilation (FGM) and pregnancies.[215]

The reports showed that the cases of GBV were primarily perpetuated by intimate partners and family members.[216] The CEDAW terms family violence as one of the most insidious forms of violence against women. The economic impact of the pandemic has forced many women to stay in these violent relationships.[217]

GBV is a weapon that keeps women in lower levels of education and in subordinate roles at home and work.[218] It therefore limits the capabilities of women in attaining the underlying determinants of health, which are essential components to the right to access healthcare services.[219]

Before the outbreak of the pandemic, GBV services were not considered essential services in Kenya. It is only after a public outcry over the increase in the reported cases of GBV during the pandemic did the state put in place a community engagement health strategy and term GBV services as essential.[220] This strategy, however, did not fully capture the comprehensive services and programmes for GBV survivors.[221] The containment measures by the state only made access to GBV services harder to attain because of the curfew hours. The police also remain the primary gatekeepers of reporting on GBV, and during the pandemic, more focus was placed on enforcement of curfews.[222] There were also reports of mismanagement of GBV cases and corrupt practices to the detriment of women.[223]

2.3 Opportunities that exist for the Kenyan government towards addressing the impact of COVID-19 on the health systems in the region

Although Kenya had lower numbers of infection than other countries in Europe, the Americas, and Asia, the impact of the pandemic has had severe socio-economic consequences. Subsequent control measures by the state have led to high incidents of violation of human rights and humanitarian crises.[224] Kenya has recognized the right to health in its domestic legislation and the treaties it has ratified. Even among struggling economies with limited resources, there are certain core obligations and subsequent concrete steps that each state must realize immediately.[225]

In 1993, the Vienna Declaration and Programme of Action proclaimed that human rights are the birth right of every human being.[226] Therefore, there can never be a situation that warrants the suspension of human rights, including a pandemic. The universal nature of human rights underlines that all human beings have a claim to a dignified existence no matter their race or socio-economic status.[227]

2.3.1 Containment measures

On 28 February 2020, the president issued Executive Order No. 2 of 2020 for the constitution of a National Emergency Committee on Coronavirus.[228] Thereafter, the state through the Ministry of Health came up with more than 100 guidelines or policies on combatting and managing the spread of the virus.

However, measures adopted by the state to curb the spread of the pandemic or flatten the curve of infections must be in line with the Siracusa Principles on the Limitation and Derogation Provisions in ICCPR.[229] These measures must be time-limited, reasonable, proportionate, non-discriminatory, and grounded in law to ensure that all human rights are protected.[230] The ambit on non-discrimination entails that these measures should also take into consideration the needs of vulnerable people like women who are at a higher risk of facing inequality and discrimination. The states should not implement blanket containment measures but should tailor-make measures that are least intrusive to protect public health.[231] Reasonable accommodation measures should also be put in place to protect people with high risk of contracting the virus.[232]

In addition, the guidelines and processes used to administer vaccines should be fair and transparent, and the criteria used to determine the priority of vaccination should be based on non-discriminatory principles.[233]

Additionally, the state should ensure that the public receives accurate, regular, accessible science-based information on the threat of COVID-19, precautionary measures to be adopted, and their impact.[234] Accessibility also entails that the information is in different languages and in a format accessible also by persons with disabilities.[235] Information plays a great role in diffusing stigma and consequently an outbreak of violence. It also demystifies the administration of the vaccine and quells any fears or hesitancy the public may have in taking it up.[236] On the other hand, vaccination passports and certificates should not be used a means to curtail the rights and freedoms of those who choose not to take up the vaccine.

The state also has a role to ensure that all healthcare workers have all the requisite PPE and that hospitals have sufficient medical equipment and supplies to combat the virus.[237] In addition, they should ensure that healthcare workers have conducive working conditions and additional compensation for overtime hours.[238]

Ability to pay is a huge impediment to accessing medical services, and the state has an obligation to ensure people are not disproportionately burdened by healthcare costs. One of the mechanisms in achieving this would be to put in measures to refrain or subsidize taxes on essential medicines and medical supplies to make them affordable.[239] This is because taxes constitute the third largest component in prices of medicine and medical supplies.[240]

As states take all measures to curb the spread of the virus, resources should also be allocated to preventive, curative, and rehabilitative health care.[241] Mechanisms for safe access to healthcare services for non-COVID-19-related problems should also be implemented in all public and private facilities.[242]

The state should also be cognizant that accessibility to health care also requires that the underlying social determinants to health are addressed. Consequently, the state should ensure that there is access to safe and portable water and make arrangements to increase localized water dispensers to people living in informal settlements.[243]

Measures should also be put in place for social and economic empowerment measures to mitigate the economic effects of the pandemic.[244] This includes a rollout of an economic stimulus package through supplementary budget in both national and county governments to cushion women from the impact of the pandemic. Additionally, the state should put in social mechanisms to support vulnerable women in the community, like the elderly, orphans, persons living with disabilities, refugees, and marginalized communities who were greatly impacted by the pandemic.

2.3.2 Addressing GBV

Stringent restrictions on movement and isolation measures have unintentionally granted people greater freedom to act without restrictions.[245] Cases of domestic and intimate partner violence have been on the rise.[246] Women have been trapped in self-isolation with violent partners with no means of escape.[247] There has also been an increase in violence against healthcare workers.[248] The stigma against persons who have been diagnosed with the virus has also caused an outbreak of violence. The state therefore has an obligation to enhance community structures of reporting GBV.[249]

The state has taken commendable steps in addressing GBV cases by setting up a toll-free hotline for victims of GBV to report incidences.[250] The line is manned by trained police officers who help survivors locate a police station closest to them.[251] The survivors are also directed on where they could access psychological, medical, and other essential services.[252] In addition, the state through the Ministry of Health also termed GBV as one of the essential services.[253] Additionally, a service called 'Policare' was set up to give GBV survivors access to multisectoral services within 48 hours.[254]

Nevertheless, the state needs to ensure that GBV services are available in all health facilities and with sufficient well-trained health workers. The services should also include psychosocial services and post-care rape kits and medicines. Over and above, the state should ensure that there are sufficient shelters in every county for women to seek cover. A survey by the State Department for Gender revealed that the country had very few shelters.

Additionally, they should also put in place reporting technology or helplines to make reporting accessible, especially for victims of abuse, that are accessible 24 hours a day.[255] The GBV hotline was reportedly only operational for few hours of the day to allow the staff to meet the curfew hours. Reporting technology should also be simple and accessible to ensure that the service is accessible even for marginalized groups of women. Police officers should also be trained on how to treat incidences of GBV, and a gender desk should be set up in every police post as they are usually the first point of contact of a survivor of GBV.

The state should also prioritize the investigation and prosecution of cases relating to sexual and physical violence. There have been delays in obtaining protection orders and the prosecution of GBV cases in court.

It is also important that healthcare workers, police, and judicial officers are trained in handling cases on sexual and physical violence. The public should also be sensitized to influence behavioural change to curb harmful practices like child marriage and FGM.[256] Sensitization also creates awareness to survivors of GBV on where to seek help.[257]

2.3.3 Legislation and enforcement

Enforcement is only possible based on existing legislation, policies, and directives. Kenya has numerous statutes, policies that address issues surrounding access to healthcare services including GBV, FGM, and sexual offences. The state is also a signatory to many commitments like Sustainable Development Goal (SDG) 3, with overarching goals on health issues. The state therefore has an obligation to oversee the implementation and enforcement of these commitments not only at the national level but also across the 47 semi-autonomous counties.

The state also has a duty to ensure there are clear enforceable laws on the protection of marginalized groups, fiscal policies to mitigate the socio-economic impact of COVID-19, and health policies to address the issues in the health system, among others.[258] The legislative and decision-making process should incorporate community-based organizations (CSOs), women groups, and civil society organizations to ensure the guarantee of protection of women's rights.[259]

The pandemic has also brought to light the issues of data protection with regard to contact tracing and surveillance.[260] The state should adopt clear, enforceable guidelines on contact tracing and surveillance of people within the ambit of human rights[261] in addition to enacting penal laws on misinformation.[262]

2.3.4 Accountability

Corruption has been titled the second pandemic. The African Commission issued a statement condemning the misuse of emergency relief funds and corrupt practices in the procurement and supply of medical supplies.[263] The Special Rapporteur on health also reiterated on the negative effect that corruption has on good governance, rule of law, development, and equitable enjoyment of human rights.[264] It is therefore imperative that the state implement anti-corruption measures and put in place transparent and accountable processes in the administration of emergency funds.[265]

The African Commission also acknowledged the role that governance plays in the administration of critical and scarce resources by member states and how their utilization would have an impact on the health of individuals.[266] It urged members to uphold their obligations under the African Union Convention on Prevention and Combating Corruption.[267] In addition, member states were also urged to respect the rule of law and implement anti-corruption measures and accountable processes for the administration of emergency relief funds.[268]

In May 2020, the International Monetary Fund issued Kenya with 739 million dollars in the form of an interest-free loan under the Rapid Credit Facility so as to overcome the initial shock of the pandemic.[269] As of August 2020, Kenya has secured over two billion dollars from the international community.[270] There have been numerous allegations of the misuse of the emergency funds, theft of medical equipment, and flouting of public procurement laws.[271]

Accountability also entails implementing policies that ensure checks and balances mechanisms, oversight requirements, and conflict-of-interest provisions in the administration of emergency funds.[272] Additionally, decisions made on the administration of emergency funds should also be done transparently and in consultation with other key players and public participation. There has been no transparency and public participation from key stakeholders in the administration of the funds. Public participation is based on the Constitution of Kenya, which bestows on the people authority in the implementation of the constitution.[273]

Accountability also entails that the state respect the rule of law and ensure the protection of journalists who expose corruption incidents. The respect of the rule law also bestows on the state a duty to investigate and prosecute persons involved in corruption scandals.[274]

2.3.5 Data and information collection and protection

Collection of data is a critical function in helping states identify the effects of the pandemic, generate indicators that will be used in monitoring mechanisms, enable them implement appropriate measures, carry out mapping, and share good practices.[275]

However, states have to ensure that all invasive use of technologies that were used as part of the containment measures of COVID-19 such as contact tracing are in line with human rights provisions, especially on privacy and patient confidentiality.[276]

2.3.6 Protection and promotion of human rights

In his report, the Special Rapporteur on health urged states that coronavirus cannot be solved only by public health and emergency measures.[277] It also requires that human rights are addressed.[278] It is not possible to enjoy the right to health without addressing human rights failings. Human rights cannot be applied selectively even in times of crisis.[279] The prevention and management measures of the pandemic must be cognizant that the right to health can only be fulfilled when other rights are also respected and protected.[280]

The Kenyan Constitution places on the state and every state organ the duty to observe, respect, protect, and fulfil the rights provided under the

Bill of Rights.[281] This duty is not limited only to Kenyan laws but also to the enactment and implementation of international and regional instruments.[282] This requires the state to take legislative and other measures to ensure the realization of every person's right to access healthcare services.[283] These measures should also consider and address the needs of vulnerable persons in the community.[284]

The issue of financial constraints is not sufficient reason for the state to fail to meet its obligation under the right to health.[285] The state must prove before a court or tribunal that the resources are not available and that in their allocation of resources, they gave priority to ensuring the widest possible enjoyment of the right to access healthcare services.[286] Nevertheless, the CESCR maintains that there are certain immediate obligations in relation to the right to health.[287] For instance, the right to health must be realized without discrimination of any kind, and the state must take deliberate and concrete steps in realizing the right to access healthcare services.[288]

The right to health like other rights imposes on the state three levels of obligations.[289] The state and all its organs must therefore take these concrete steps to ensure realization of the right.

i) Respect

The state must ensure that the containment measures taken, like the dusk-to-dawn curfews, do not limit women's access to essential services like post-rape care, emergency operations, GBV services, childbirth services, and psychosocial care.

The state should also refrain from issuing directives and policies that limit the rights of people for lack of vaccination passports. As of 24 March 2022, only 15.2% of the population had been vaccinated due to unavailability of vaccines.[290] It would therefore be a violation of the rights of people to refrain their liberties and freedoms where vaccines are not readily available.

ii) Protect

The state should ensure that there is equal access and distribution of vaccines to all people. In addition, women should have access to essential, palliative, and preventive services and routine management of non-communicable diseases.

The state should also ensure that healthcare services and medicines are economically accessible to all sectors of the population. It also includes ensuring that health facilities contain equipment, medical supplies, essential drugs, and the presence of sufficiently skilled and experienced staff.

The duty of protection also ensures that harmful practices like GBV and FGM do not interfere with women's access to healthcare services.

iii) Fulfil

The state needs to formulate a detailed health plan to ensure access of healthcare services even during the pandemic. This includes budgetary allocations by both national and county governments that give priority to ensure the widest possible enjoyment of the right to access healthcare services. In addition, they must also ensure access to underlying determinants of health like nutritiously safe food and potable drinking water, basic sanitation, and adequate housing and living conditions.

2.4 Future pandemics

The COVID-19 pandemic exposed the inequities of access to health care in Africa. This is partly due to the fact that African nations heavily depend on external suppliers for their medical requirements.[291] Vaccine nationalism saw African states fall last in the queue to acquire vaccines for their citizens. Africa must take time to reflect and learn from the past epidemics that have plagued the continent and the period it took to access life-saving vaccines. It is estimated that between 1997 and 2007, approximately 12 million Africans died due to lack of access to antiretroviral drugs to treat HIV because of the high price that made them out of reach.[292] Supply of vaccines to the African continent must not be left to the mercy of UN agencies. To adequately prepare in case of any eventuality of emerging pandemics, African nations must proactively develop their capacity to manufacture vaccines within the continent.

The African continent holds 17% of the global population and spends approximately 1.3 billion dollars on vaccines, but only 1% of these vaccines are manufactured in Africa.[293] Only seven countries in Africa have companies that manufacture vaccines.[294] Out of those seven, even fewer operate across the value chain from manufacturing, fill, to finish to distribution. Senegal is the only country that exports WHO pre-qualified vaccines.[295]

In 2016, African states endorsed the declaration on Universal Access to Immunization as a cornerstone for health and development in Africa and collectively committed to allocate funds and make domestic and innovative finance investments to meet the costs of vaccines.[296] Some of the persistent barriers that have impeded the manufacture of vaccines within the African region are the cost of vaccines and the initial investment capital, the bottlenecks within the international value chain, non-uniformity of national and regional regulations, approvals by international organizations like WHO, and vaccine hesitancy.[297]

The AU in collaboration with member states should therefore take the lead in coming up with a regional vaccine-manufacturing strategy to address these barriers. The strategy would not focus on reinventing the wheel but on empowering the already existing structures like the African CDC and mRNA Vaccine Technology Hub to collate information, enhance the technical expertise within the continent, and develop plans to strengthen the value chain in sourcing for raw materials, production, storage, and distribution.[298]

A study carried out by the African Vaccine Manufacturing Initiative (AVMI), WHO, and United Nations Industrial Development Organization (UNIDO) showed that the cost of building a vaccine manufacturing plant in Africa would be 60–130 million dollars.[299] Such a commitment would require the collaboration of African governments, private sector companies, and African development banks to come up with a continent-wide industrial strategy to make it advantageous for each nation to take up such an investment.[300] Such investments can only attract investors if there is certainty of demand for the vaccines within the African market. There has been a preference for internationally imported vaccines because of their competitive prices.[301] In 2021, the South Africa-based company Aspen Pharmacare entered into a partnership agreement with Johnson & Johnson to manufacture 400 million doses of COVID-19 vaccine. Unfortunately, there was no uptake from African nations.[302] Market certainty can be cured by initiating engagements with the current big buyers of vaccines and by having distribution agreements between the African governments and the African manufacturing companies.[303]

Additionally, in order to build trust among the African nations to encourage the uptake of locally made vaccines, public education campaigns must be undertaken to educate, demystify, and correct the myriad of information around vaccines.

2.5 Conclusion

Both regional and international treaties have repeatedly pronounced themselves on the importance of the right to health and its interdependence on other non-derogable and fundamental rights like the right to life and human dignity. The Universal Declaration of Human Rights is generally agreed to be the foundation and inspiration of many treaties and declarations. It represents that all human beings, whatever the nationality, residence, or colour, are born free and equal in rights and dignity.[304] These rights are inalienable whether in times of conflict or repression in the society.[305] They are commitments made to remind and prevent the repetition of the atrocities that had been witnessed over the years against human beings.

The pronouncements in these treaties have always been used to keep states accountable to each other. However, at the outbreak of the pandemic, it was clear that power, money, and resources outweighed the right to health and indefinitely the right to life. The asymmetries in power played a big part in the distribution and allocation of drugs, information, and technology that could have been used to save the lives of many Africans.

It is not enough to prohibit discrimination. States must actually ensure that all their laws embody the principle of equality and they end intentionally discriminatory actions and structures and take concrete, practical steps to minimize health inequities, which are obstacles to realizing the right to health. Even in the midst of a pandemic with limited resources, there are certain core obligations and subsequent concrete steps that each state must realize immediately to uphold the sanctity of life.

Notes

1 Ministry of Health *Interim guidance on continuity of essential health services during COVID-19 pandemic* (2020) 6.
2 https://covid19.who.int/region/afro/country/ke (accessed 13 April 2022).
3 N John et al 'COVID-19 and gender-based violence (GBV): Hard to reach women and girls, services and programmes in Kenya' (2021) 29 *Gender & Development* 57.
4 Kenya Human Rights Commission 'Wanton impunity and exclusion: A report based on human rights violations amid COVID-19 in Kenya' (2020) x available at https://www.khrc.or.ke/index.php/publications/223-wanton-impunity-and-exclusion-a-report-based-on-human-rights-violations-amid-covid-19-in-kenya-april-august-2020/file (accessed 28 January 2021).
5 As above.
6 www.hrw.org/news/2021/10/21/kenya-pandemic-health-workers-lack-protection (accessed 13 April 2020).
7 Kenya Human Rights Commission (n 4 above) 1.
8 As above.
9 General Assembly 'Final report of the special rapporteur on the right of everyone to the enjoyment of the highest attainable standard of physical and mental health' Dainius Puras, UN Doc A/75/163, 16 July 2020, para 4.
10 As above, para 18.
11 Committee on ESCR, General Comment No 14 *The right to the highest attainable standard of health* (art 12 of the Covenant) (22nd session, 2000) [UN Doc E/C 12/ 2000/4] para 4.
12 As above, para 33.
13 B Cabieses & P Bird 'Glossary of access to health care and related concepts for low – and middle – income countries (LMICs): A critical review of international literature' (2014) 44(4) *International Journal of Health Services* 851.
14 Committee on ESCR, General Comment No 14 (n 11 above) para 34.
15 J Pinchoff et al 'Gendered economic social and health effects of the COVID-19 pandemic and mitigation policies in Kenya: Evidence from a prospective cohort survey in Nairobi informal settlements' (2021) *British Medical Journal* 2.
16 General Assembly (n 9 above) para 17.
17 As above.
18 African Commission Resolution 449 on Human and Peoples' Rights as central pillar of successful response to COVID-19 and recovery from its socio-political impacts -ACHPR/Res. 449(LXVI) adopted at its 44th ordinary session held from 13 July to 7 August 2020 in Banjul, the Gambia.
19 Committee on ESCR, General Comment No 14 (n 11 above) para 30.
20 General Assembly (n 9 above) para 12.
21 Constitution of the World Health Organization, adopted by the International Health Conference on 22 July 1946, opened for signature on 22 July 1946, and entered into force on 7 April 1948 available at www.who.int/governance/en (accessed 9 January 2022).

22 Art 24.
23 Art 12.
24 Art 24.
25 Art 12.
26 Art 16.
27 Art 14.
28 As above.
29 United Nations *Report of the fourth world conference on women* (1995).
30 United Nations *Report of the international conference on population and development* (1994).
31 C Ngwena & R Cook 'Rights concerning health' in D Brand & C Heyns (eds) *Socio-economic rights in South Africa* (2005) 110.
32 Constitution of Kenya, 2010 art 43(1).
33 As above art 21 (2).
34 As above art 21 (3).
35 C Ngwena & R Cook 'Rights concerning health' in Brand & Heyns (eds) (n 31 above) 116.
36 As above.
37 Committee on ESCR, General Comment No 14 (n 11 above) para 8.
38 MS Giorgi *The human right to equal access to healthcare* (2012) 3.
39 J Levesque et al 'Patient-centered access to health care: Conceptualising access at the interface of health systems and populations' (2013) 12 *International Journal for Equity in Health* 2.
40 Committee on ESCR, General Comment No 14 (n 11 above) para 12.
41 As above.
42 As above, para 12 (a).
43 Committee on ESCR, General Comment No 14 (n 11 above) para 12 (d).
44 As above, para 12 (b).
45 Cabieses & Bird (n 13 above) 851.
46 Committee on ESCR, General Comment No 14 (n 11 above) para 4.
47 As above, para 38.
48 Cabieses & Bird (n 13 above) 852.
49 C Ngwena 'The recognition of access to health care as a human right in South Africa: Is it enough?' (2000) 5(1) *Health and Human Rights* 37.
50 Committee on ESCR, General Comment No 14 (n 11 above) para 4.
51 Ngwena (n 49 above) 38.
52 African Commission Resolution on Access to Health and needed Medicines in Africa ACHPR/Res. 141(XXXXIIII)08 adopted at its 44th ordinary session held from 10 to 24 November 2008 in Abuja, Nigeria.
53 F Amimo et al 'A review of prospective pathways and impacts of COVID -19 on the accessibility, safety, quality and affordability of essential medicines and vaccines for universal health coverage in Africa' (2021) *Globalization and Health* 8.
54 World Bank, World Health Organization, JICA, The Global Fund to Fight AIDS, Tuberculosis and Malaria, and the African Development Bank *UHC in Africa: A framework for action* (2016) 4.
55 UN Human Rights Council (HRC) 'On access to medicines' Report of the Special Rapporteur, Anand Grover UN Doc A/HRC/23/42, 1 May 2005.
56 Ministry of Health 'Kenya health sector strategic plan: Transforming health systems; achieving universal coverage by 2022' (2018) 113 available at https://extranet.who.int/countryplanningcycles/sites/default/files/public_file_rep/KEN_Kenya_Health-Sector-Strategic-Plan-2018-2023.pdf (accessed 28 January 2021).
57 World Bank et al (n 54 above) 6.
58 As above.
59 M Thiede, P Akweongo & D McIntyre 'Exploring the dimensions of access' in D. McIntyre & G. Mooney (eds) *The economics of health equity* (2007) 109.

60 As above.
61 Amimo et al (n 53 above) 7.
62 UN Human Rights Council (HRC) (n 55 above) para 20.
63 SAK Ahmed et al 'Impact of societal response to COVID-19 on access to healthcare for non-COVID-19 health issues in the slum communities of Bangladesh, Kenya, Nigeria and Pakistan: Results of pre-COVID and COVID-19 lockdown stakeholder agreements' (2020) 5 *BMJ Global Health* 9.
64 Ahmed et al (n 63 above) 10.
65 E Barasa et al 'Examining unit costs for COVID-19 case management in Kenya' (2021) 6 *BMJ Global Health* 3.
66 As above.
67 As above, 5.
68 As above, 6.
69 As above.
70 UN Human Rights Council (HRC) (n 55 above) para 20.
71 Committee on ESCR, General Comment No 14 (n 11 above) 12 (b).
72 W Hein & A Paschke 'Access to COVID-19 vaccines and medicines: A global public good' (2020) *German Institute of Global and Area Studies* 7.
73 E Torreele & JJ Amon 'Equitable COVID-19 vaccine access' (2021) 23(1) *Health & Human Rights Journal* 273.
74 As above.
75 www.un.org/press/en/2021/sgsm20620.doc.htm (accessed 28 January 2021)
76 Hein & Paschke (n 72 above) 7.
77 As above.
78 AL Phelan et al 'Legal Agreements: Barriers and enablers to global equitable COVID-19 vaccine access' (2020) 396 *The Lancet* 1.
79 As above.
80 As above.
81 Hein & Paschke (n 72 above) 4.
82 www.health.go.ke/sites/default/files/2023-05/ministry-of-health-kenya-covid-19-immunization-status-report-12th-may-2022.pdf (accessed 13 April 2022)
83 As above.
84 Committee on ESCR, General Comment No 14 (n 11 above) para 12 (b).
85 As above.
86 UN Human Rights Council (HRC) (n 55 above) para 4.
87 African Commission Resolution (n 52 above).
88 World Health Organization 'The Corona virus disease 2019 (COVID-19): Strategic preparedness and response plan for the WHO African region' (2021) 5 available at https://www.afro.who.int/sites/default/files/2021-04/WHO%20AFR%20Covid-19%202021%20SRP_Final_16042021.pdf (accessed 09 January 2024).
89 EW Barasa et al 'Assessing the hospital surge capacity of the Kenyan health system in the face of COVID-19 pandemic' (2020) *PLOS One* 5.
90 As above, 5.
91 As above, 5.
92 As above, 5.
93 World Health Organization 'Hospital readiness checklist for COVID-19'(2020) 6 available at https://www.emro.who.int/images/stories/coronavirus/documents/hospital_readiness_checklist_for_covid_19.pdf?ua=1 (accessed 09 January 2024).
94 Ministry of Health 'Guidelines on case management of COVID-19 in Kenya' (2021) 23 available at https://healthsciences.uonbi.ac.ke/sites/default/files/2021-10/Final%20GUIDELINES%20ON%20THE%20MANAGEMENT%2001-09-21.pdf (accessed 09 January 2024).
95 Cabieses & Bird (n 13 above) 851.
96 OB Da'ar & F Kalmey 'The level of countries preparedness to health risks during COVID-19 and pre-pandemic: The differential response to health systems

building blocks and socioeconomic indicators' (2023) 13(16) *Health Economics Review* 7.
97 www.hrw.org/news/2021/10/21/kenya-pandemic-health-workers-lack-protection (accessed 13 April 2022)
98 As above.
99 As above.
100 TK Ng'ang'a 'Impact of COVID-19 measures on Kenya's health system' (2021) available at https://publication.aercafricalibrary.org/server/api/core/bitstreams/1ea295fb-2c4a-4fac-87c7-d9abc2691cd2/content (accessed 09 January 2024).
101 www.hrw.org (n 97 above).
102 www.nytimes.com/2020/08/21/world/africa/kenya-doctors-strike-coronavirus.html
103 www.hrw.org (n 97 above).
104 Thiede et al (n 59 above) 109.
105 As above, 108.
106 As above.
107 AM Lusambili et al ' "We have a lot of home deliveries": A qualitative study on the impact of COVID-19 on access to and utilisation of reproductive, maternal, new-born and child healthcare among refugee women in urban Eastleigh, Kenya' (2020) *Journal of Migration & Health* 4.
108 World Health Organization (n 88 above) 21.
109 Committee on ESCR, General Comment No 14 (n 11 above) para 11.
110 As above.
111 As above, para 12 (b).
112 Committee on ESCR, General Comment No 13, *The right to education* (art 13 of the Covenant) (21st session, 1999) [UN Doc E/C.12/1999/10)] para 1.
113 As above, 1.
114 African Commission Resolution on 14.1 (a), (b), (c) and (f) and Article 14. 2 (a) and (c) of the Protocol to the African Charter on Human and Peoples' Rights on the Rights of Women in Africa.
115 As above, para 28 (b).
116 As above, para 28 (d).
117 Thiede et al (n 59 above) 111.
118 E Saurman 'Improving access: Modifying Penchansky and Thomas's theory of access'(2016) 21(1) *Journal of Health Services Research Policy* 38.
119 F Ennab et al 'Implications of social media misinformation on COVID-19 vaccine confidence among pregnant women in Africa' (2022) 14 *Clinical Epidemiology and Global Health* 1.
120 Z Barua et al 'Effects of misinformation on COVID-19 individual responses and recommendations for resilience of disastrous consequences of misinformation' (2020) 8 *Progress in Disaster Science* 1.
121 Barua et al (n 120 above) 2.
122 Ennab et al (n 119 above) 1.
123 Barua et al (n 120 above) 5.
124 Ennab et al (n 119 above) 2.
125 K Roelen et al 'COVID-19 in LMICs: The need to place stigma front and centre to its response' (2020) 32 *European Journal of Development Research* 6.
126 Saurman (n 118 above) 38.
127 As above.
128 Ministry of Health 'An assessment of knowledge, attitudes, perception and practice about COVID-19 among Kenyan population' (2020) 3 available at https://www.kemri.go.ke/wp-content/uploads/2021/07/Covid-19-KAPP-Study-Policy-Brief-27-8-2020-2.pdf (accessed 9 January 2024).
129 As above.

130 www.khrc.or.ke/2015-03-04-10-37-01/press-releases/713-let-s-maintain-dignity-of-the-dead-during-the-covid-19-crisis.html (accessed 13 April 2022)
131 As above.
132 www.afro.who.int/aira (accessed 31 January 2022).
133 As above.
134 United Nations *Charter of the United Nations*, 24 October 1945, 1 UNTS XVI.
135 Art 24 (n 22 above) art 1.
136 UN General Assembly *International covenant on civil and political rights*, 16 December 1966, United Nations, Treaty Series, vol. 999, p. 171 art 26.
137 UN General Assembly Convention on the Rights of Persons with Disabilities, 24 January 2007, A/RES/61/106 art 5(1).
138 As above, art 5 (2) & (3).
139 Art 16 (n 26 above) art 1.
140 UN General Assembly *International convention on the elimination of all forms of racial discrimination*, 21 December 1965, United Nations, Treaty Series, vol. 660, p. 195, art 1.
141 UN Human Rights Committee (HRC) *CCPR general comment no. 18: Non-discrimination*, 10 November 1989, para 7.
142 UN Committee on Economic, Social and Cultural Rights (CESCR) *General comment no. 20: Non-discrimination in economic, social and cultural rights (art. 2, para. 2, of the International covenant on economic, social and cultural rights)*, 2 July 2009, E/C.12/GC/20, para 3.
143 Centre for Human Rights *A guide to the African human rights system* (2016) 5.
144 Art 16 (n 26 above) art 2.
145 As above, preamble.
146 Centre for Human Rights (n 143 above) 6.
147 Art 14 (n 28 above) art 2.
148 As above, arts 19, 22 & 23.
149 Constitution of Kenya (n 32 above) art 27(1).
150 As above, art 27(2) & 27(3).
151 As above, art 27(4).
152 Art 16 (n 26 above) art 1.
153 General Assembly (n 9 above) para 17.
154 As above, para 17.
155 As above, para 28.
156 As above, para 17.
157 As above.
158 As above.
159 As above, para 7.
160 AN Fisher & MK Ryan 'Gender inequalities during COVID-19' (2021) 24(2) *Group Processes & Intergroup Relations* 237.
161 General Assembly (n 9 above) para 19.
162 Art 12 (n 25 above) art 2.
163 As above, para 12.
164 Committee on ESCR, General Comment No 14 (n 11 above) para 20.
165 As above, para 21.
166 RW Kimani et al 'Maternal and new-born care during COVID-19 pandemic in Kenya: Re-contextualising the community midwifery model' (2020) *Human Resources for Health* 2.
167 www.who.int/news-room/fact-sheets/detail/maternal-mortality (accessed 31 January 2022).
168 As above.
169 MM Morse & G Anderson *The shadow pandemic: How COVID-19 crisis is exacerbating gender inequality* (2020).
170 Kimani et al (n 166 above) 1.

171 As above.
172 Kenya Human Rights Commission (n 4 above) x.
173 John et al (n 3 above) 15.
174 UN Committee on Economic, Social and Cultural Rights (CESCR) (n 142 above) para 10 (b).
175 General Assembly (n 9 above) para 22.
176 C Bradbury-Jones & L Isham 'The pandemic paradox: The course of COVID-19 on domestic violence' (2020) *Journal of Clinical Nursing* 2047.
177 General Assembly (n 9 above) para 33.
178 As above, para 22.
179 UN Commission on Human Rights *The Siracusa principles on the limitation and derogation provisions in the international covenant on civil and political rights*, 28 September 1984, E/CN.4/1985/4. Lusambili et al (n 107 above) para 12.
180 General Assembly (n 9 above) para 12.
181 Committee on ESCR, General Comment No 14 (n 11 above) para 4.
182 As above.
183 World Health Organization & Commission on Social Determinants of Health 'Closing the gap in a generation: Health equity through action on the social determinants of health' (2008) 1 available at https://iris.who.int/bitstream/handle/10665/69832/WHO_IER_CSDH_08.1_eng.pdf?sequence=1 (accessed 9 January 2024).
184 As above, 10.
185 Ngwena (n 49 above) 37
186 As above.
187 As above.
188 As above.
189 Morse & Anderson (n 169 above).
190 United Nations (n 100 above) 38.
191 As above.
192 John et al (n 3 above) 10.
193 S Bilal et al 'Saving Africa's private sector jobs during the Corona virus pandemic' (2020) 2 available at https://www.tralac.org/documents/resources/covid-19/3292-saving-africa-s-private-sector-jobs-during-the-coronavirus-pandemic-april-2020/file.html (accessed 09 January 2024).
194 United Nations Conference on Trade Development *Assessing the impact of COVID-19 on Africa's economic development* UNCTAD/ALDC/MISC/2020/3 6.
195 As above.
196 As above, 14.
197 Kenya Human Rights Commission (n 4 above) 22.
198 As Above.
199 United Nations Conference on Trade Development (n 194 above) 3.
200 As above, 6.
201 World Health Organization & Commission on Social Determinants of Health (n 183 above) 18.
202 As above.
203 www.hrw.org/news/2021/10/21/kenya-pandemic-health-workers-lack-protection (accessed 13 April 2022).
204 As above.
205 As above.
206 As above.
207 UN Committee on the Elimination of Discrimination Against Women (CEDAW) *CEDAW general recommendation no. 19: Violence against women* (1992) para 6.
208 Committee on ESCR, General Comment No 14 (n 11 above) para 18.

209 UN Committee on the Elimination of Discrimination Against Women (CEDAW) (n 207 above) para 7 & Committee on ESCR, General Comment No 14 (n 11 above) para 18.
210 United Nations 'Policy brief: The impact of COVID-19 on women' (2020) 19 available at https://www.unwomen.org/sites/default/files/Headquarters/Attachments/Sections/Library/Publications/2020/Policy-brief-The-impact-of-COVID-19-on-women-en.pdf (accessed 9 January 2024).
211 John et al (n 3 above) 57.
212 As above.
213 SDG Kenya Forum 'Gender statistics: Covid-19 and violence against women in Kenya' available at www.planning.go.ke/wp-content/uploads/2021/05/GENDER-STATISTICS_COVID_VAWG_KOMBA.pdf (accessed 18 October 2023).
214 As above, 9.
215 United Nations (n 100 above) 60.
216 As above, 61.
217 UN Committee on the Elimination of Discrimination Against Women (CEDAW) (n 207 above) para 23.
218 As above, para 11.
219 As above, para 14.
220 John et al (n 3 above) 57.
221 As above.
222 As above, 58.
223 As above.
224 African Commission Resolution 449 (n 18 above).
225 Committee on ESCR, General Comment No 14 (n 11 above) para 30.
226 UN General Assembly, Vienna Declaration and Programme of Action, 12 July 1993, A/CONF.157/23.
227 F Viljoen *International human rights law in Africa* (2012) 9.
228 John et al (n 3 above) 58.
229 UN Commission on Human Rights (n 179 above).
230 General Assembly (n 9 above) para 12.
231 UN Commission on Human Rights 'Statement on COVID-19 and the human rights of persons with disabilities' (2020) available at www.ohchr.org/EN/News Events/Pages/DisplayNews.aspx?NewsID=25942 (accessed 31 January 2022).
232 As above.
233 General Assembly (n 9 above) para 55.
234 African Commission on Human and Peoples' Rights 'Press release by the special rapporteur on freedom of expression and access to information in Africa on the importance of access to the internet in responding to the COVID-19 pandemic' (2020) available at https://achpr.au.int/en/news/press-releases/2020-04-08/press-release-special-rapporteur-freedom-expression.
235 As above.
236 www.afro.who.int/aira (accessed 31 January 2022).
237 African Commission Resolution 449 (n 18 above).
238 As above.
239 UN Human Rights Council (HRC) (n 55 above) para 34.
240 As above.
241 African Commission Resolution 449 (n 18 above).
242 As above.
243 United Nations Human Rights & African Union *7 possible actions: Women's rights and COVID-19* (2020) 5.
244 United Nations Human Rights & African Union (n 243 above) 2.
245 Bradbury-Jones & Isham (n 176 above) 2047.
246 United Nations (n 210 above) 17.

247 As above.
248 As above.
249 United Nations Human Rights & African Union (n 243 above) 3.
250 John et al (n 3 above) 64.
251 As above.
252 As above.
253 As above.
254 As above.
255 United Nations Human Rights & African Union (n 243 above) 3. United Nations (n 100 above) 68. John et al (n 3 above) 65.
256 United Nations (n 100 above) 68. United Nations Human Rights & African Union (n 243 above) 3.
257 United Nations (n 100 above) 68.
258 As above.
259 United Nations Human Rights & African Union (n 243 above) 4.
260 General Assembly (n 9 above) para 85 & 86.
261 As above.
262 African Commission on Human and Peoples' Rights (n 234 above).
263 African Commission on Human and Peoples' Rights 'Statement of the African commission on human and peoples' rights and the African Union advisory board on corruption on corruption and COVID-19' (2020) available at https://achpr.au.int/index.php/sw/node/217.
264 As above.
265 As above.
266 As above.
267 African Union *African Union convention on preventing and combating corruption* (2003 July 11).
268 Art 14 (n 148 above).
269 www.imf.org/en/News/Articles/2021/03/17/na031721-imf-loan-to-support-economic-recovery-in-kenya (accessed 13 April 2022).
270 www.aa.com.tr/en/africa/kenya-to-probe-alleged-fraud-in-coronavirus-funds/1954113 (accessed 13 April 2022).
271 www.one.org/africa/blog/corruption-undermining-kenya-covid19-response/ (accessed 13 April 2022).
272 General Assembly (n 9 above) para 39.
273 Constitution of Kenya (n 32 above) arts 1& 2.
274 African Commission on Human and Peoples' Rights (n 263 above).
275 United Nations Human Rights & African Union (n 243 above) 8.
276 General Assembly (n 9 above) para 85 & 86.
277 As above, para 5.
278 As above, para 5.
279 As above, para 17.
280 As above, para 17.
281 Constitution of Kenya (n 32 above) art 21(1).
282 As above, art 21(4).
283 As above, art 21(2).
284 As above.
285 As above, art 20(5).
286 As above, art 20(5) (a) & (b).
287 Committee on ESCR, General Comment No 14 (n 11 above) para 30.
288 As above, para 31.
289 As above, para 33.
290 www.health.go.ke (n 82 above).

291 T Abiodun et al 'Vaccine manufacturing in Africa: What it takes and why it matters' (2021) *Tony Blair Institute for Global Change* 5.
292 J Nkengasong et al 'COVID-19 vaccines: How to ensure Africa has access' (2020) 586 *Nature Journal* 198.
293 Abiodun et al (n 291 above) 6.
294 As above.
295 As above.
296 African Union Assembly 'Declaration on universal access to immunization as a cornerstone for health and development in Africa' 30–31 January 2017, Assembly/AU/Dec.624(XXVIII).
297 Abiodun et al (n 291 above) 13 & 14.
298 As above, 16.
299 E Lamptey et al 'COVID-19 vaccines development in Africa: A review of current situation and existing challenges of vaccine production' (2022) 11 *Clinical and Experimental Vaccine Research* 86.
300 Abiodun et al (n 291 above) 16.
301 Lamptey et al (n 302 above) 85.
302 P Adepoju 'Africa CDC warns COVID-19 vaccination production could cease' (2022) 399 *the Lancet*.
303 Abiodun et al (n 291 above) 16.
304 UN General Assembly (n 140 above) art 1.
305 As above.

3

INDIVISIBILITY AND INTERDEPENDENCE OF HUMAN RIGHTS IN THE CONTEXT OF COVID-19

Bhavna Mahadew and Roopanand Mahadew

3.1 Introduction

Human rights are crucial in determining how to respond to pandemics – both for the immediate public health crisis and for the longer-term effects on people's lives and means of subsistence. Human rights prioritize persons. Better results in controlling the pandemic, providing universal access to health care, and safeguarding human dignity emerge from responses that are shaped by and respect human rights. But they also draw our attention to the most affected individuals, their circumstances, and available solutions. In order to emerge from this catastrophe with more just and sustainable society, progress, and peace, they are laying the foundation now. The current problem facing the planet is unprecedented. A global response is necessary to this crisis because it is fundamentally a global public health emergency on a magnitude that has not been witnessed in a century.

Countries are forced to take extraordinary steps in light of the unusual situation and to protect life. Widespread lockdowns, implemented to prevent virus propagation, inevitably restrict freedom of movement and, as a result, freedom to exercise many other human rights. Such actions may unintentionally have an impact on people's lives; security; access to health care, food, water, and sanitation; employment; education; and leisure. To lessen any such unwanted effects, steps must be taken. Human rights are a potent collection of tools that the international community has at its disposal that enable states to respond to threats and crises in a way that prioritizes individuals. Emphasis is laid on how the crisis is hurting people on the ground, especially the most vulnerable ones, and what can be done about it right away and in the long run when viewing the crisis and its effects through a human rights lens.

DOI: 10.4324/9781032671437-4

Each and every state on the planet faces a unique difficulty in ensuring that all individuals have access to human rights. The public health crisis is quickly combining with the economic, social, and political situations of societies. The COVID-19 situation has made those in society who are least protected even more vulnerable. Deep economic and social disparities, inferior healthcare systems, and inadequate social safety nets are being brought to light and demand immediate attention as part of the public health response. Women, men, children, teenagers, and elderly persons; immigrants and refugees; the impoverished; individuals with disabilities; people who are detained; members of certain minority groups; and LGBTI people, among others, are all affected in different ways.

In view of stopping the pandemic's spread and safeguarding lives, state authorities must use all available means. Decisions are being taken quickly, and while most are well-intentioned, some may unintentionally have negative effects. To maintain the trust that must exist between the populace and their government, especially during a crisis, responses must be proportionate to the outbreak. Human rights serve as a guide for how states should utilize their authority so that it is used for the good of the people and not for their detriment. Human rights can assist states in recalibrating their response strategies in the current crisis to optimize their efficacy in battling the disease and minimize unfavourable effects. One important interrogation is whether this recalibration goes through the prism of indivisibility of human rights.

Indivisibility is a phrase used to describe how the main types of rights are essentially complementary to one another.[1] They are very suitable for a shared existence, which has the effect of strengthening and reinforcing them through a process of 'synergy' and symbiosis, rather than clashing or exhibiting conflict.[2] The terms 'corresponding', 'interlocking', 'interconnected', 'overlapping', 'mutually reinforcing', and 'enriching' can also be used to characterize rights. Complementarists frequently find that a single human rights claim violates both the civil and political rights (CPR) and the socio-economic rights (ESCR). For example, this draws attention to the decision of the United Nations (UN) Committee Against Torture that racializes violence on Roma people, and the demolishing of their dwellings constitutes a breach of both the right to housing (ESCR) and the freedom from torture (CPR).[3] According to Novogrodsky, ESCR and CPR are 'deeply intertwined' for those at risk.[4] Indivisibilists give several examples of how CPR and ESCR benefit from each other's accomplishments and, conversely, are undermined by each right that is denied. However, it seems that there comes a point where pursuing one right at the expense of another has diminishing results. Thus, according to Eide, rights can interact 'positively, negatively, and through balancing' in at least three different ways.[5] Nevertheless, this fails to account for circumstances where the exercise of one right directly precludes the exercise of another, such as when a government is chosen democratically but its policies are anti-welfare.

In light of the above, this chapter focuses on the indivisibility and interdependence of human rights in the context of the COVID-19 pandemic. This chapter shows how human rights are interconnected and how a potential violation of one right, like the right to health, can result in violations of other rights, such the right to life, the right to freedom of movement, the right to employment, and the right to be protected from discrimination. It makes the case that the universality of human rights within the COVID-19 framework requires states to preserve and advance all human rights, not only the right to health. It also evaluates how international organizations, such the African Union and the UN, have accounted for this interconnectedness in their strategies and tactics for fighting the virus.

3.2 The context

Human Rights Day, observed on December 10 every year, commemorates the adoption of the Universal Declaration of Human Rights (UDHR) by the UN General Assembly on that day in 1948. Nearly 75 years after it was passed, the UDHR is still a shining example of the principle of the indivisibility of rights, which holds that each right depends on the others' fulfilment and that the denial of one right prevents the enjoyment of all the others. It is crucial to reiterate this idea in the post-COVID era. For example, the World Health Organization (WHO) had just finished evaluating the novel Omicron variant when the US and some European nations used emergency powers to impose restrictions on freedom of movement for the sake of public health.[6] Instead of acting on recommendations from WHO and others to vaccinate everyone on the globe, politicians in wealthier nations have moved towards briefings, borders, and boosters.[7]

The subsequent argument over sealing off borders or curtailing freedom in the name of public health disguised what was actually needed to effectively contain COVID-19. One of the South African scientists who discovered the Omicron variant pleaded with wealthier nations to aid South Africa financially and scientifically, stating that the population there 'cannot be in lockdown without financial support'.[8] To put it another way, providing individuals with the various tools they require to stop the spread of Omicron locally was deemed as the most efficient approach to stop it from spreading internationally. This brings to mind the early stages of the pandemic when governments all over the world rushed to enact well-known measures to protect economic and social rights, such as paid sick leave, money transfers, and unemployment benefits, in an effort to incentivize people to stay indoors and prevent COVID infection.[9] According to the World Bank, from April to December 2020, nations spent at least $800 billion on more than 1,400 social protection programmes, benefiting more than a billion people.[10] This was not just some random act of kindness; it was a laudable expansion of the social safety net that prevented deaths while allaying people's concerns about the government restricting their freedoms.[11]

These actions were classic illustrations of the interdependence of rights. It illustrated that the rights to social safety and a reasonable standard of living are inextricably linked to the rights to life and liberty. Indeed, the UDHR does not establish a hierarchy between the rights to life, liberty, and security of the person and guarantees each of these rights in a separate article. These rights were not divided until after the UDHR was adopted, during the negotiations of separate treaties on civil and political rights and economic, social, and cultural rights. Jensen has even argued that the notions of three generations of human rights has no 'solid historical or analytical basis and it obscures rather than clarifies the relationship between rights'.[12] It should be underlined that the first convention created at the end of the Cold War, the Convention on the Rights of the Child, brought these issues back together by combining, for instance, the rights to life, survival, and development into a single right.

It was a great miscalculation to divide these inalienable rights, and the following pandemics would show why. The HIV/AIDS epidemic, for instance, showed that ensuring access to HIV treatment not only satisfies the right to health but also makes it possible to exercise other rights including the right to employment, education, and political engagement. Similarly, COVID-19 has served as a reminder that everyone must have access to a variety of social and economic assistance in order to adhere to policies that shield them from illness and death. The same reasoning can be used to argue against vaccine requirements. Unvaccinated people are prone to live in poverty, be susceptible to eviction or food insecurity, or be employed in jobs that subject them to infection. Lack of health coverage was the most effective predictor of who in the US remained unvaccinated, according to Kaiser Family Foundation (KFF).[13] This implies that providing people with a certain level of economic and social stability may also lessen the need for coercive measures to safeguard the public's health.

One of the great ironies of COVID-19 is that the world engages in a discussion between individual freedom and community security simply and only when it is essential to emphasize most on the unity of human rights. The very way COVID-19 is framed – as merely a 'public health emergency' – ignores the fact that the pandemic is also an economic catastrophe, a crisis of human survival that exposes individuals to novel diseases as well as deprivation. The interconnectedness of human rights must be affirmed, and these conflicts must be combined. The rights to life, health, information, economic security, survival and development, and non-discrimination transcend these false dichotomies. These are the rights that COVID-19 most directly implicates. The more this is ignored, the more the epidemic evolves and spreads.

3.3 Is human rights central to COVID-19 (and similar pandemic) response?

Human rights are universal, interconnected, and supportive of one another. According to the UN, the global response to COVID-19 must include measures at the national and community levels as well. The latest UN report on human rights, which was made public by the Secretary-General, claims that the freedom of movement, the right to health and access to care, and the duty to preserve human life are 'frontline in the current pandemic'. A new WHO guidance note on human rights and COVID-19 adds, 'embracing human rights as an integral part of our public health response will not only provide ethical guidance during these challenging times but also lay the groundwork for how the world responds to public health crises going forward'.[14] For instance, WHO's recently established COVID-19 Solidarity Response Fund is supporting national initiatives that 'assist vulnerable and at-risk countries, especially those with weak health systems, to step up their preparedness to prevent COVID-19, enhance their abilities to detect and test for the virus, and bolster their ability to respond to the spread'.[15]

The committees of experts entrusted with the implementation of international human rights conventions globally and the chairs of the ten UN human rights treaty bodies have also reacted to the pandemic. 'No one should be denied health care because of stigma or because they belong to a group that may be marginalised', the group said in a joint press release.[16] Furthermore, prejudice is inadmissible in the use of life-saving treatments in response to the virus, according to more than 60 UN special procedures mandate-holders, particularly the UN Independent Expert on Sexual Orientation and Gender Identity. It was also stated by the group that 'everyone has the right to health'.[17] Discrimination has been explicitly forbidden in the UN's response to COVID-19. According to the UN Secretary-General, 'it is shameful to see increasing acts of racial discrimination and prejudice as we fight the COVID19 pandemic – a crisis that affects us all'.[18] E. Tendayi Achiume, the head of the UN independent anti-racism monitor, added that 'political rhetoric and policy that stokes fear and diminishes the equality of all people is counterproductive'.[19] In other words, when everyone works together, society is best positioned to react.

The UN Secretary-General has now launched a new report that calls on 'political leaders and other actors, including religious leaders, to speak out and take action against discrimination, hate speech, ageism, xenophobia, racism, or violence arising from this pandemic, and promote inclusion and unity'.[20] Additionally, it demands that national and local recovery plans take into account COVID-19's disproportionate effects on immigrants, refugees, people who have been forcibly displaced, people who lack access to adequate housing or water, people who are disabled, women, older people, LGBTI people, children, and people who are in detention or institutions.[21]

In reaction to COVID-19, governments and cities throughout the world have made unprecedented efforts. This includes measures that order the people of a country to remain indoors, travel bans, and limitations on public gatherings. A number of UN independent human rights experts, notably the UN Special Rapporteur on the right to freedom of assembly, admitted in a joint statement that it might be necessary to take some emergency measures. The group does, however, advise that any emergency measures taken by authorities 'be narrowly tailored and should be the least intrusive means to protect public health and should not be used simply to quash dissent'.[22] According to their experts, implementing a rights-based strategy that includes laws safeguarding minorities will 'facilitate the emergence of healthy societies with rule of law and human rights protections'.[23]

As the Internet is a vital source of information on the pandemic, David Kaye, the UN Special Rapporteur on freedom of expression, has also cautioned against measures that might hinder it.[24] In addition, it is said in the latest report issued by the Secretary-General that 'people need agency and voice in a crisis and this is a time when, perhaps more than ever, authorities need to be honest and open, receptive, and answerable to the people they are trying to protect'.[25] It suggests that emergency measures be declared formally and that they be non-discriminatory, time-bound, proportionate, and compliant with international law.[26]

The international community has also been reminded by the Secretary-General that 'we are only as strong as the weakest health system in our interconnected world'.[27] To reverse the trend on COVID-19, strong and inclusive public institutions are necessary. As an illustration, the UN Special Rapporteur on the rights of persons with disabilities, Catalina Devandas, has suggested that information bulletins and national public campaigns be made accessible 'to the public in sign language and accessible means, modes and formats, including accessible digital technology, captioning, relay services, text messages, easy-to-read and plain language'.[28] 'The primary line of defence against the coronavirus is now housing and home has rarely been more of a life or death situation', according to the UN Special Rapporteur on the right to adequate housing.[29] The situation at home has never been more dire. Increasing social safety nets will also make it easier for entire civilizations to recover. According to the most recent UN report on human rights and COVID-19, 'strengthening economic and social rights strengthens resilience for the long haul'.[30] Suspension of home evictions, offering or extending sick leave to employees, and providing child care for important workers are a few examples of best practices in the report.

UN representatives have made it clear that it is essential to take into account how COVID-19 measures may affect particular communities, especially women and girls. For instance, UN Women has provided a 10-point checklist for decision-makers in governments, municipalities, parliaments, and other groups to ensure that women and girls are included in pandemic responses.[31] A technical brief on COVID-19 responses and sexual and reproductive health and rights was also produced by the UN Population Fund (UNFPA). It is advised by UNFPA that age- and sex-specific data be gathered accurately and completely, that reporting avenues for gender-based violence (GBV) cases be expanded to include more people, and that COVID-19 responses not reinforce unfavourable standards or inequalities.[32] In addition, the Secretary-General's assessment urges combating domestic violence and domestic GBV and ensuring fair and equitable representation in COVID-19 rehabilitation efforts in order to lessen the pandemic's negative effects on women.[33]

In response to COVID-19, on 9 April 2020, the UN Human Rights Council convened a first-ever virtual information session. A human rights-based strategy to the crisis was demanded during the web session by dozens of nations from each major world area, the High Commissioner for Human Rights, and civil society organizations. The extensive discussion covered a wide range of subjects, including the pressing need to safeguard journalists, the possibility of making exceptions for humanitarian reasons, and specific economic sanctions.[34] 'COVID-19 is about human rights; it has an impact on all human rights in their interdependence and indivisible nature. We ought to treat each other with respect and dignity at this point in time because it is about who we are as people. Therefore, it's really about human rights', the delegation from South Africa remarked.[35] The delegation from the Kingdom of the Netherlands added, 'The UN's human rights voice needs to be loud and clear in this global crisis'. On 30 April, the UN Human Rights Council is anticipated to electronically reconvene to discuss the pandemic. Not only is it the moral thing to do, but it is also essential for the effectiveness of the global COVID-19 reaction. As stated by Michelle Bachelet, the UN High Commissioner for Human Rights, 'COVID-19 is a test for our societies, [and] human dignity and rights need to be front and centre in that effort, not an afterthought'.[36]

3.4 The indivisibility and interdependence principle: A background

One of the foundational elements of international human rights law is the indivisibility principle.[37] This principle did not exist at the time of the creation of the UDHR; it only appeared subsequently. In particular, the Teheran Proclamation of 1968 contains the first mention of the indivisible nature of human rights.[38] According to paragraph 13 of the document, it is impossible for civil and political rights to be fully realized without also enjoying economic, social, and cultural rights.[39] This declaration placed more emphasis on the separation between civil and political rights and economic, social, and cultural rights rather than on the idea that all human rights are inseparable when taken collectively.

Thus, the idea of indivisibility appears to have developed to bridge the political gap between two distinct categories of human rights. The international human rights legal framework had always been characterized by this human rights duality. For instance, socio-economic rights were added to the original draft of the Covenant on Human Rights. The International Covenant on Civil and Political Rights (ICCPR) and the International Covenant on Economic, Social, and Cultural Rights (ICESCR) were two separate international human rights law treaties that were adopted in 1966 as a result of this proposal's rejection. Two years thereafter, the Teheran Proclamation adopted the indivisibility principle in this setting.[40] The idea goes that a tool to guarantee a strong and consistent application of both types of human rights was necessary for the worldwide community of human rights law.[41]

This viewpoint has continued to be reflected in additional human rights law publications. The General Assembly Resolution 32/130 from 1977, for instance, states that 'all human rights and fundamental freedoms are indivisible and interdependent; equal attention and urgent consideration should be given to the implementation, promotion, and protection of both civil and political, as well as economic, social, and cultural rights'.[42] The right to sexual and reproductive health is stressed as being indivisible from other civil, political, economic, social, and cultural rights in the Declaration on the Right to Development and General Comment No. 22 on the matter.[43] Regional treaties have also used the indivisibility concept as a rhetorical device to erode the boundary across two categories of human rights. When declaring that 'the satisfaction of economic, social, and cultural rights is a guarantee for the enjoyment of civil and political rights', the African Charter on Human and Peoples' Rights takes an analogous position.[44]

Over time, the indivisibility principle has come to encompass more aspects to it.[45] As an example, the indivisible characteristics of human rights began to be proclaimed as an ideal in order to encourage the adoption of a systemic perspective on human rights.[46] This conceptual change in emphasis was greatly aided by post-Cold War documents, most notably the 1993 Vienna Declaration, which describes all human rights as, among other things, indivisible. New developments in international human rights legislation helped broaden the indivisibility principle's application. By indiscriminately including examples from both groups of rights, some human rights conventions such as the Convention on the Elimination of All Forms of Discrimination Against Women and the Convention on the Rights of the Child have particularly compromised the difference between the two groups of rights and, in turn, helped provide fresh perspectives through which to view the indivisibility principle.[47] The EU's Charter of Fundamental Rights of the European Union, which includes both civil-political freedoms and what it alludes to as solidarity rights (socio-economic rights), among other rights, is an example of a regional endeavour to codify human rights.[48]

Distinctions between different rights categories have become even more blurred as a result of the 'mainstreaming' of human rights. For example, the Committee on Economic, Social, and Cultural Rights has repeatedly 'read' participatory rights 'into' socio-economic rights through the prism of due diligence responsibilities, despite the fact that they are expressly recognized in the ICCPR.[49] As a result, certain rights, including the right to housing, food, water, and employment, may be violated in certain situations due to participation failures. Such mainstreaming activities have been referred to as 'the representation par excellence of the doctrine of the indivisibility of human rights', which is indivisibility in action, in the dearth of an official treaty basis.[50] The literature also indicates that this change in how indivisibility is conceptualized has led to an increase in the uncertainty of its significance to the extent of it becoming 'meaningless sloganeering'.[51] Despite this criticism, the UN has never clarified the precise meaning of the indivisibility concept.

The elusive definition of the indivisibility principle and the improbable consequences that might follow have since piqued experts' interest.[52] In reality, the definitional question surrounding its meaning is not simply a philosophical investigation but also a pertinent query intimately related to its application.[53] The theoretical and practical debate over whether the fulfilment of some human rights may be chosen over others is complicated by the idea that human rights are indivisible.[54] This topic becomes extremely pertinent, especially when the UN passes human rights legislation that may demand that human rights be prioritized. The International Covenant on Economic, Social, and Cultural Rights' (ICESCR's) provision requiring states to realize economic, social, and cultural rights gradually and in accordance with the actual resources at their disposal is a noteworthy example.[55] The Maastricht Guidelines (no. 10) and the Limburg Principles (nos. 25 and 72) are additional instruments on differing implementation. By stating that some subsistence rights should be upheld irrespective of the effective availability of resources, these instruments subtly acknowledge that as soon as the minimum core obligations are met, states have some latitude on how they implement human rights.[56] As a result, theories about what indivisibility implies in human rights law started to be put out by academics. The majority of scholars concur that the mutually reinforcing nature of human rights is implied by their indivisibility.[57] The question whether indivisibility ought to be applied to all human rights (so-called system-wide indivisibility) or only a select few (so-called widespread indivisibility) is frequently debated.[58]

The interdependence and indivisibility of human rights has traditionally been used to support the idea that economic and social rights must be judicialized since only through their complete protection and enforcement can civil and political rights be fully exercised. But the current crisis demonstrates more than just how basic political and civic rights, like the right to assemble, are essentially postponed in order to defend the social right to health. Additionally, it demonstrates that the full protection of civil and political rights is a precondition for the full guarantee of economic, social, and cultural rights (ESCR), underscoring the fact that the interdependence and indivisibility of human rights can also be used in the opposite direction.

The interdependence and indivisibility of human rights is used invertedly under the presumption that ensuring ESCER also entails preserving civil and political rights. The actions necessary to stop the coronavirus pandemic are consistent with this view. These must guarantee civil and political rights as well if they are to fully implement ESCER rights. For instance, COVID-19 has a significant impact on the right to health, which is interconnected with other human rights like the right to life, human dignity, the prohibition against cruel or inhumane treatment, and the right to unrestricted access to information. The actions performed in response to the virus also demonstrate how crucial it is for the civil right to freedom of movement to be upheld in order for the right to labour, which is often categorized as an economic right, to exist. As a result, it is crucial to use all available measures to battle this pandemic and its effects, especially in view of recent developments in the strengthening of a vision for the comprehensive and collaborative protection of human rights. Regarding the interdependence, universality, indivisibility, intersectionality, and transversality of human rights, all actions must be taken with complete observance of international human rights norms.

Therefore, the pro persona principle must be followed along with the norms of proportionality, reasonability, and temporality when determining any restrictions that the states apply during a state of emergency. Additionally, they must adhere to the principles of non-discrimination, public health objectives, and not disproportionately harming the right to privacy and personal data protection. There is little doubt that this virus pandemic will change everything and endure a long time, necessitating adaptability and reinvention. It is to be hoped that it will ultimately result in a better, more comprehensive, and integral approach to the protection of human rights as the crisis demonstrates unequivocally that such protection does not consist of picking and choosing which rights to uphold but rather that the full protection of all human rights is necessary for the exercise of each individual right.

3.5 A reinterpretation of indivisibility and interdependence of human rights in the context of COVID-19 and future pandemics

The COVID-19 outbreak highlights the necessity to strengthen the holistic approach to human rights. The safeguard of socio-economic rights and civil and political rights is determined by interdependence and indivisibility. In order to help individuals and groups who are vulnerable, this protection must be strengthened. For illustration, it was reaffirmed, as discussed earlier, in the context of COVID-19 that the fundamental right to health is also reliant on the right to information as a vital component of the right to free speech. Therefore, it is crucial to take into account the universality, indivisibility, interdependence, and relationship between rights; equality and non-discrimination; the gender perspective, plurality, and intersectionality; the inclusiveness; accountability; appreciation for the state of law; and bolstering interstate cooperation. This suggests that in addition to being in compliance with scientific standards, actions that can impact or hinder the enjoyment and accomplishment of human rights must adhere to the concepts of temporality, legality, rationality, proportionality, and necessity.

In terms of the emergency's urgency, it has been demonstrated that the disease has a distinct effect on historically marginalized and vulnerable groups, which calls for strengthened protection. In this way, the pandemic presents one with three major structural challenges: Socio-economic inequality, past discriminatory behaviours, and institutional democratic issues. Several signs indicate the multifaceted nature of the crises that intensifies these systemic deficiencies and directs attention to such difficulties. The solutions to COVID-19 are failing those living in poverty, according to Philip Alston, former UN Special Rapporteur on extreme poverty and human rights, who made this claim in April 2020.

3.5.1 Regional standards: Africa

The African Commission on Human and Peoples' Rights was the first regional organization to urgently encourage member states to address the health emergency in accordance with human rights and in consideration of their interdependence and indivisibility in the wake of the pandemic. The Declaration of 24 March 2020 underlined 'the Human and Peoples, in particular Article 4 on the right to life, Article 9 on the right to access information, and Article 16 on the right to health'.[59] A press statement regarding the pandemic was released on 28 February 2020.[60] In response to this call from the African Commission, the group of work on ESCR noted the detrimental effects on health, employment, education, food, and social protection, even with the implementation of safety and social welfare actions set up by multiple member states as an element of their national response to the pandemic.[61] The organization calls on states to take action in accordance with regional treaties and international human rights instruments to guarantee the optimal enjoyment of all rights 'during and after the crisis'[62] and draws attention to the plight of disadvantaged and vulnerable people that scarcely have any voice. They have access to housing under usual conditions, but not equally to education, food, work, sanitation, water, education, or health.

In a complementary manner, the relationship between political rights and the right to health, particularly with regard to the right to elections as a cornerstone of democracy, must be protected during times of public health emergency.[63] According to Solomon Ayele Dersso, president of the African Commission, the probable repercussions of the crisis' socio-economic and humanitarian implications may influence peace processes because both are variables that lead to conflict and insecurities. As a result, the dimension of peace is included in addition to the comprehension of the interdependence and indivisibility of human rights in the context of Africa.[64]

3.5.2 Regional standards: Europe

Through numerous initiatives by regional bodies and their delegates, helpful guides and recommendations for states, as well as statements in support of bolstered defence of vulnerable groups, the shift towards adherence to the principles is apparent of interdependence and indivisibility in this rekindled reading. It has been emphasized that all human rights are indivisible, interdependent, universal, and interrelated. According to Josep Borrell, the EU is 'committed to ensuring that our response safeguards the dignity and human rights of all people without discrimination of any kind'.[65] The fight against COVID-19 hinges on human rights, according to Eamon Gilmore, special representative of the European Union for Human Rights. She stated that

> Protecting and preserving life is the main purpose of this fight. Without the right to life, it is impossible to exercise other rights. To protect life, we must demand the right to health. This, in turn, depends not only on access to care medical, but also the right to drinking water and sanitation, to adequate nutrition appropriate and to a safe and healthy environment. It also requires access to information, so that people are empowered to protect their own health and that of others the rest. And in this health crisis, which requires a collective response and cooperation of people everywhere, respect for civil society is more important than ever. All human rights are interdependent and indivisible.[66]

For his part, the secretary general of the Council of Europe launched as a guide to good practice a set of tools, to remind governments across Europe to guarantee respect for human rights and fundamental rights – calling for the protection of the right to education, freedom of expression, privacy and data, vulnerable groups, and against discrimination – and guarantee democracy and the rule of law during the COVID-19 crisis. Regarding the negative impacts of the pandemic on certain groups, it is worth highlighting the note of the special representative of the secretary general on Migration and Refugees of the Council of Europe, together with the Human Rights Agency Fundamentals of the European Union, which insists on the main safeguards of the fundamental rights of refugees, asylum seekers, and migrants applicable at the external borders of their member states. The European Committee of Social Rights also offers guidance through its website dedicated to 'Social rights in times of pandemic: COVID-19 and the European Social Charter' and examines the measures taken by states with respect to their obligations in matters of social rights.

3.5.3 Renewal of the discourse on indivisibility and interdependence: the transformative potential post COVID-19

COVID-19's enormous effects and multifaceted nature have sparked a period of deep change and reinvention that is characterized by pivotal choices. There is going to be a world before COVID-19 and a world after COVID-19. Since more than 70 years ago, there has been a common understanding that all human rights must be protected in order to preserve the dignity of the individual and the community.[67] It is depicted in the pre-COVID-19 world due to its interconnectedness and indivisibility in conventional reading. In several speeches, inclusion is mentioned from the perspective of social justice, particularly to tackle the needs of vulnerable communities and peoples from the viewpoint of practice, specifically with regard to the right to health and the absence of awareness of it in the fullest sense with the other rights[68]; or of the necessity of developing appropriate tools for monitoring for the purpose of better understanding the situation.

The pandemic has demonstrated the necessity to reconsider the application of the principles of indivisibility and interdependence, and it additionally compelled one to reconsider them in the opposite direction and strengthen the protection of individuals and groups in vulnerable circumstances, with a greater focus on equality, addressing structural deficiencies. The current situation can serve as a springboard for creating a structure that is more integrated, resilient, and sustainable, giving priority to the most vulnerable populations. In accordance with the General Assembly's call to 'contribute to respect for all human rights and fundamental freedoms to the achievement of the purposes and defence of the principles of the Charter of the United Nations'[69] issued in July 2020, and how the UN and international human rights laws were created in reaction to the terrible acts of World War II, the responses to the pandemic may indicate a redefining time. Stressing the efficiency of public authority and the imposition of legislative restrictions on government intervention in the exercise of authority are at the heart of the indivisibility of the right to health and other rights, which is more than just a theoretical concern.[70]

It is suitable to consider a refoundation of human rights in this perspective of ideas, pursue strategies that have the ability to revolutionize society, and consider notions such as jus commune and communities of practice for human rights. For discourse in academia to express global, regional, and domestic responses to the pandemic, the acknowledgement of all human rights must be the cornerstone. It should be emphasized that the efficacy of socio-economic rights is undoubtedly conditioned by the effectiveness of civil and political rights, and vice versa. This is especially true in light of the structural difficulties that must be overcome, which are worsened by their impacts on human rights. Morales aptly synthesizes this perspective as follows:

> Three axes are key, namely, the notion of poverty from its multidimensional scope and reject conceptualization in terms of mere income scarcity and more well assume the capability-centered approach as the conceptual bridge between poverty and human rights; A second milestone is to 're-notice' the degree to which the Poverty also affects people's ability to enjoy their rights civilians and politicians because it denies them a political voice, creates obstacles to claim their situation and are deprived of their abilities to enjoy their human rights. And a third milestone comes from supporting a more substantive orientation of the equality that allows the Cortes, as actors of the democratic process, to consider more adequately the links between poverty and discrimination and broaden the spectrum of the concepts of vulnerability and intersectional discrimination.[71]

3.6 The way forward

The COVID-19 epidemic serves as a warning for our society's growing economic and global interdependence. Nation states may respond rashly in self-defence by concentrating on the current economic and health crises within their own borders. In our interdependent society, it is essential to take a more holistic approach to human rights with the goal of protecting the most vulnerable and fostering global resilience. Focus must be placed on important problems, including education, labour rights, and the protection of the most vulnerable while protecting the right to health. States must give the protection of the rights to life and health a special priority by taking prompt action, exercising caution, supporting the state's responsibility to prevent and mitigate harm, and allocating the greatest amount of resources possible to the right to health under a comprehensive concept. The states' initiatives, plans, and public policies must take into account the most recent scientific research. States must compel and monitor businesses to uphold human rights. A stronger duty is required of groups who are in extremely vulnerable circumstances – of governmental protection for the disabled, the LGBTI community, people of African origin, the elderly, individuals deprived of liberty, women, indigenous peoples, migrants, and refugees.

In order to comply with the legitimate goals of protecting public health, states must closely adhere to the norms of legality, proportionality, necessity, and temporality in any restriction of rights and freedoms. The necessity of proper operation of the powers, particularly the procedures and judicial systems suitable for the protection of rights and freedoms, as well as the assurance of the freedoms of expression and information access, which are fundamental pillars of a democratic regime, must be re-emphasized. Digital surveillance should be rigorously limited to upholding basic freedoms, the non-discrimination principle, and stringent protection of individual rights. This epidemic is a wake-up call and a reminder that basic protections need to be strengthened in order for everyone in our communities to have access to them. In order to defend rights in an emergency, one must do so even when there is no emergency. Resources are not a problem in many other nations because there are sufficient amounts to allow civilization to function while maintaining public safety. Therefore, our inability to defend is a result of our disregard for the interconnectedness of human rights, which needs to be fixed.

Notes

1 S Nixon & L Forman 'Exploring synergies between human rights and public health ethics: A whole greater than the sum of its parts' (2008) 8 *BMC International Health and Human Rights* 1–9.
2 See D Anthony 'Indivisibility of human rights: A Theoretical critique' Unpublished thesis, University of Technology, 2010.
3 LA Thio 'The international legal protection of minorities in the twentieth century: A preliminary orientation' in LA Thio (ed) *Managing babel: The international legal protection of minorities in the twentieth century* (2005) 1–25.
4 N Novogrodsky 'The duty of treatment: Human rights and the HIV/AIDS pandemic' (2009) 12 *Yale Human Rights and Development Law Journal* 12.
5 A Eide 'Interdependence and indivisibility of human rights' in Y Donders & V Volodin (eds) *Human rights in education, science and culture: Legal developments and challenges* (2007) 11.
6 G Ortiz-Millan 'COVID-19 health passes: Practical and ethical issues' (2023) 20 *Journal of Bioethical Inquiry* 125–138.
7 United Nations 'Low-income countries have received just 0.2 per cent of all COVID-19 shots given' available at https://news.un.org/en/story/2021/04/1089392 (accessed 30 August 2023).
8 J Cohen & S Gruskin 'This human rights day, the need to affirm the indivisibility of rights has never been greater' Open Global Rights available at www.openglobalrights.org/this-human-rights-day-the-need-to-affirm-the-indivisibility-of-rights-has-never-been-greater/ (accessed 30 August 2023).
9 See International Labour Organisation 'The impact of the COVID-19 pandemic on jobs and incomes in G20 economies' (2020) available at www.ilo.org/wcmsp5/groups/public/–dgreports/–cabinet/documents/publication/wcms_756331.pdf (accessed 30 August 2023).
10 U Gentilini 'A game changer for social protection? Six reflections on COVID-19 and the future of cash transfers' World Bank Blogs (2021) available at https://blogs.worldbank.org/developmenttalk/game-changer-social-protection-six-reflections-covid-19-and-future-cash-transfers (accessed 30 August 2023).
11 Human Rights Watch 'IMF/World Bank: Targeted safety net programs fall short on rights protection' (2022) available at www.hrw.org/news/2022/04/14/imf/world-bank-targeted-safety-net-programs-fall-short-rights-protection (accessed 30 August 2023).

12 S Jensen 'Putting to rest the three generations theory of human rights' Open Global Rights (2017) available at www.openglobalrights.org/putting-to-rest-the-three-generations-theory-of-human-rights/ (accessed 30 August 2023).
13 A Kirzinger et al 'COVID-19 vaccine monitor: The increasing importance of partisanship in predicting COVID-19 vaccination status' (2021) available at www.kff.org/coronavirus-covid-19/poll-finding/importance-of-partisanship-predicting-vaccination-status/ (accessed 30 August 2023).
14 A Guterres 'We are all in this together: Human rights and COVID-19 response and recovery' UN (2020) available at www.un.org/en/un-coronavirus-communications-team/we-are-all-together-human-rights-and-covid-19-response-and (accessed 20 September 2023).
15 R Kaminski & C Kaufmann 'Why human rights are central to COVID-19 response' (2020) available at https://unfoundation.org/blog/post/why-human-rights-central-covid-19-response/ (accessed 20 September 2023).
16 As above.
17 OHCHR 'UN Human Rights Treaty Bodies call for human rights approach in fighting COVID-19' (2020) available at www.ohchr.org/en/press-releases/2020/03/un-human-rights-treaty-bodies-call-human-rights-approach-fighting-covid-19?LangID=E&NewsID=25742 (accessed 20 September 2023.
18 Kaminski & Kaufmann (n 15 above).
19 OHCHR 'States should take action against COVID-19-related expressions of xenophobia, says UN expert' (2020) available at www.ohchr.org/en/press-releases/2020/03/states-should-take-action-against-covid-19-related-expressions-xenophobia?LangID=E&NewsID=25739 (accessed 20 September 2023).
20 Guterres (n 14 above).
21 As above.
22 OHCHR 'COVID-19: States should not abuse emergency measures to suppress human rights – UN experts' available at www.ohchr.org/en/press-releases/2020/03/covid-19-states-should-not-abuse-emergency-measures-suppress-human-rights-un?LangID=E&NewsID=25722 (accessed 20 September 2023).
23 As above.
24 OHCHR 'COVID-19: Governments must promote and protect access to and free flow of information during pandemic – International experts' available at www.ohchr.org/en/press-releases/2020/03/covid-19-governments-must-promote-and-protect-access-and-free-flow?LangID=E&NewsID=25729 (accessed 20 September 2023).
25 Guterres (n 14 above).
26 As above.
27 As above.
28 OHCHR 'COVID-19: Who is protecting the people with disabilities? – UN rights expert' available at www.ohchr.org/en/press-releases/2020/03/covid-19-who-protecting-people-disabilities-un-rights-expert?LangID=E&NewsID=25725 (accessed 20 September 2023).
29 OHCHR 'Housing, the front line defence against the COVID-19 outbreak, says UN expert' available at www.ohchr.org/en/press-releases/2020/03/housing-front-line-defence-against-covid-19-outbreak-says-un-expert?LangID=E&NewsID=25727 (accessed 20 September 2023).
30 Guterres (n 14 above).
31 UN WOMEN 'Checklist for COVID-19 response by UN Women Deputy Executive Director Åsa Regnér' available at www.unwomen.org/en/news/stories/2020/3/news-checklist-for-covid-19-response-by-ded-regner (accessed 20 September 2023).
32 UNFPA Technical Brief 'COVID-19: A gender lens' available at www.unfpa.org/sites/default/files/resource-pdf/COVID-19_A_Gender_Lens_Guidance_Note.pdf (accessible 20 September 2023).
33 Kaminski & Kaufmann (n 15 above).

34 As above.
35 As above.
36 As above.
37 See J Nickel 'Rethinking indivisibility: Towards a theory of supporting relations between human rights' (2008) 30 Human Rights Quarterly 984.
38 UN 'Proclamation of Teheran: Final act of the international conference on human rights' UN Doc. A/CONF.32/41(1968).
39 As above.
40 International Covenant on Civil and Political Rights (1996), 999 UNTS 171; International Covenant on Economic, Social and Cultural Rights (1996) 993 UNTS 3.
41 D Whelan *Indivisible human rights. Global issues series* (2010) 1.
42 UNGA 'Alternative approaches and ways and means within the United Nations system for improving the effective enjoyment of human rights and fundamental freedoms' (1977) General Assembly Resolution 32/130 para 1(a).
43 UNCESCR 'General Comment No 22 on the right to sexual and reproductive health (art. 12)' E/C.12/GC/22 (2016), para 10.
44 OAU 'African charter on human and peoples' rights' OAU Doc. CAB/LEG/67/3 rev. 5, 21 ILM 58 (1982).
45 J Donnelly & D Whelan *International human rights* (2017) 57.
46 As above.
47 De Beco 'The indivisibility of human rights in light of the convention on the rights of persons with disabilities' (2019) 68 *International Comparative Law Quarterly* 141.
48 EU Charter of Fundamental Rights of the European Union (2000) (7 December 2000).
49 J Temperman 'Public participation in times of privatization: A human rights analysis' (2011) 4 *Erasmus Law Review* 43 at 60–66.
50 As above, 61.
51 C Scott 'Reaching beyond (without abandoning) the category of economic, social, and cultural rights' (1999) 21 *Human Rights Quarterly* 633, at 644.
52 J Nickel 'Indivisibility and linkage arguments: A reply to Gilabert' (2010) *Human Rights Quarterly* 439.
53 A Quintavalla & K Heine 'Priorities and human rights' (2019) 23 *International Journal of Human Rights* 679, 681.
54 H Shue *Basic rights: Subsistence, affluence and US foreign policy* (1996) 26.
55 Article 2.
56 P Alston & G Quinn 'The nature and scope of state parties' obligations under the international covenant on economic, social and cultural rights' in M Ssenyonjo (ed) *Economic, social and cultural rights* (1987) 3–76.
57 P Gilabert 'The importance of linkage arguments for the theory and practice of human rights. A response to James Nickel' (2008) 32 *Human Rights Quarterly* 425.
58 As above.
59 ACHPR 'Press statement of the African Commission on human & peoples' rights on the coronavirus (COVID-19)' 28 February 2020 available at https://bit.ly/30hqOl (accessed 20 September 2023).
60 ACHPR 'Press statement on human rights based effective response to the novel COVID-19 virus in Africa' 24 March 2020 available at https://bit.ly/3mW49Vn (accessed 20 September 2023).
61 ACHPR 'Press release on the impact of the COVID-19 pandemic on economic, social and cultural rights in Africa' 4 June 2020 available at https://bit.ly/3kVlEU8 (accessed 20 September 2023).
62 As above.

63 ACHPR 'Statement of the African Commission on human and peoples' rights on elections in Africa during the COVID-19 pandemic' available at https://bit.ly/2G5hNoA (accessed 20 September 2023).
64 Statement of Commissioner Solomon Ayele Dersso, Chairperson of the African Commission on Human and Peoples' Rights at the Africa Dialogue Series organized by the United Nations Office of the Special Advisor on Africa and the African Union under the theme COVID-19 and silencing the guns in Africa: Challenges and opportunities (20–22 May 2020)' 26 May 2020 available at https://bit.ly/34362qE (accessed 20 September 2023).
65 EU 'Declaration of the high representative of the EU Josep Borrell' 5 May 2020 available at https://bit.ly/36hdL7c (accessed 20 September 2023).
66 E Gilmore 'The combat against COVID-19 is a combat for human rights' 17 April 2021 available at https://bit.ly/2FXqdhT (accessed 20 September 2023).
67 L Minkler & S Sweeney 'On the indivisibility and interdependence of basic rights in developing countries' (2011) 33 *Human Rights Quarterly* 351–396.
68 D Pūras 'Challenges in promoting the interdependence of all human rights' (2019) *Health and Human Rights Journal* available at https://bit.ly/3kQ26Ac (accessed 20 September 2023).
69 UN 'Statement on the occasion of the 75th Anniversary of the UN' A/HRC/44/L.17/Rev.1 14 July 2020.
70 N Hostmaelingen & H Bentzen 'How to operationalise human rights for COVID-19 measures' (2020) 5 *BMJ Global Health*.
71 M Morales Antoniazzi 'The IDH court and the inter-Americanization of democratic test frente al COVID-19' by Sergio García Ramírez and César Astudillo (coordinators), La Corte Interamericana de Derechos Humanos: Organización, operation and transmission. Mexico City: IIJ-UNAM, Tirant lo Blanch (2021) (in imprenta).

PART II

Impact of COVID-19 on access to health related goods and services

4

SITUATION OF COVID-19 VACCINE INEQUITY IN DEVELOPING COUNTRIES

Paul O. Ogendi

4.1 Introduction

Statistics collected at the height of COVID-19 pandemic paint a cruel picture in relation to the vaccine inequity issue. In March 2022, global figures showed 485,243,022 confirmed cases of COVID-19; 6,137,553 deaths; and 11,054,362,790 vaccine doses administered (as of 26 March 2022).[1] In contrast, in the 47 African countries reportedly affected by the pandemic, there were 8,203,785 cases of COVID-19 and 170,166 deaths.[2] Even though Africa was not the hardest hit by COVID-19 in terms of cases and deaths compared to other regions, they were marginalized in terms of vaccine access until the needs of the developed nations had been met. As of early 2022, Africa had received 6% or 540 million vaccine doses despite having 17% of the people in the world.[3] In Kenya, 17,439,527 vaccine doses had been administered as of 23 March 2022.[4]

The WHO declared the pandemic over on 5 May 2023. This is a testimony that the situation has greatly improved from what it was, and access to vaccines played a major role. According to the WHO's weekly epidemiological update on COVID-19, today COVID-19 cases have drastically reduced all over the world.[5] As of 9 August 2023, there have been 769,369,823 confirmed cases of COVID-19 and 6,954,336 deaths reported to the WHO. As of 7 August 2023, a total of 13,492,264,486 vaccine doses have been administered.[6] The role of vaccines in combating pandemics cannot be overemphasized.

Emphasis on vaccines makes sense because physical distancing, face masks, and testing and tracing are not enough to restore normal economic and social life unless herd immunity is developed through vaccination of large portions

DOI: 10.4324/9781032671437-6

of the global population to prevent hospitalization and severe ailment.[7] The solution to pandemics depends heavily on vaccines, which need 'to be produced at scale, priced affordably, allocated globally so that they are available where needed, and widely deployed in local communities'.[8]

In this chapter, we explore some of the lessons learnt during COVID-19 in relation to vaccine inequity and reflect on the future in terms of how to sustainably prepare for future pandemics and guarantee vaccine access for all.

4.2 Vaccine equity as a human right

Vaccine equity is a human right, and this requires that COVID-19 vaccines should be accessible to all on a need basis. The WHO recognizes that health is a fundamental human right, and therefore, '[h]ealth equity is achieved when everyone can attain their full potential for health and well-being'.[9] The experience with COVID-19 vaccines did not support this assertion particularly in relation to the African continent.

In early 2022, during the peak of the pandemic, there were 137 vaccine candidates for COVID-19 undergoing clinical trials and another 194 candidates undergoing preclinical development.[10] These vaccines could be categorized into four types, namely whole virus, protein subunit, viral vector, and nucleic acid (RNA and DNA).[11] So far, about a dozen vaccines have been awarded the WHO emergency use listing (EUL), which means that they can be marketed globally without undergoing the complete clinical trial process.[12] The first vaccine, Comirnaty COVID-19 mRNA vaccine, was put on the market in less than 1 year by Pfizer/BioNTech.[13] Moderna and Johnson & Johnson followed suit with their own vaccines being available also in the market following WHO EUL.[14]

The relatively quick manufacturing and release of the vaccines to the market in less than one year rather than the normal 10 years was attributable to various factors. The first one was that the surface of the virus had a favourable spike protein which favoured vaccine design.[15] Other factors included that coronavirus research started earlier than 2020, a decade earlier, which made it easier to adapt the previous proof-of-concept to the COVID-19 pathogen after the Chinese released its sequence.[16] This shows that continuous research of pathogens should be sustained so that the proof-of-concepts for most pathogens can be generated in advance before an outbreak strikes. Using mRNA and adenovirus technologies also contributed to the quick turnaround time 'from elucidating the genomic sequence to making early prototype vaccines'.[17] The manufacturing at risk concept which did not require full vaccine approval before manufacturing also proved to be a great catalyst.[18] Lastly, the national regulatory authorities in the US, Europe, and Britain also contributed immensely by making use of emergency use approval mechanisms by shortening the time period for approving biologic license application (BLA) via undertaking 'extensive measures to approximate full BLA approval both in terms of adequately assessing COVID-19 vaccines for efficacy and safety, and inspection of vaccine manufacturing facilities'.[19]

Once the vaccines were in the market, the issue of inequity arose since poor countries could not vaccinate their vulnerable populations including for healthcare workers while the rich countries hoarded supplies. In June 2021, 10 rich countries had secured 75% of the 1.5 billion vaccine doses that had been administered some 18 months into the pandemic, and Africa (whose population is 1.36 billion) had secured only 25 million vaccine doses.[20] The immorality was exacerbated by the fact that at the time wealthy countries were administering booster shots, 80% of the African people were yet to get their first dose.[21] Michel describes the situation as 'most scandalous and ethically problematic' because while the rich countries were busy vaccinating as many people as possible including children who were low risk, the developing countries were unable to protect healthcare workers and populations most at risk.[22] Even the 'voluntary' donation system championed by the WHO to bring about vaccine equity was undermined because rich countries used their vast resources to first secure all the vaccines they needed in what was described as 'vaccine nationalism'.[23] Even countries that could afford to purchase vaccines using their own resources had to wait for the supplies to become available because rich countries had signed pre-purchase agreements with the pharmaceutical companies holding patents on the vaccines released in the market. This situation is aptly described as 'market failure'.

The monopoly enjoyed by the pharmaceutical companies and the huge profits made during COVID-19 were mainly attributable to intellectual property rights and specifically patents which protect monopolies. The owners of the patents were reluctant to share their patents with the rest of the world. They also strongly opposed the proposal at the World Trade Organization (WTO) to waive intellectual property rights for the sake of saving lives. The WTO finally passed a weak decision allowing for temporary waiver for vaccines only, and attempts to extend this to diagnostics and therapeutics have been stalled at the WTO.[24] The waiver is weak because in actual sense it only allows for the use of compulsory licensing to manufacture and distribute vaccines in a less restricted manner. In actual sense, there was no real waiver achieved at the WTO.

Lastly, the issue of intellectual property and access to vaccines is important to consider. In the context of COVID-19, the development of vaccines had been favoured by various factors, including the favourable spike protein, expedited national regulatory approvals, and WHO's EULs. Despite all these favours, developing countries had to wait longer to access vaccines because the rich countries had pre-purchase agreements, which meant they got absolute priority to get the vaccines manufactured. Other companies could not engage in the manufacturing of vaccines because of the patents effectively making the pharmaceutical companies monopolies during a crisis situation.

4.3 Tackling the problem of access to vaccines: affordability versus voluntarism paradigms

There are at least two approaches to tackling the problem of access to vaccines. At the crux of the issue are two protagonists, namely those advocating for access to medicines from an affordability standpoint and those who believe on voluntarism or donations. Access to vaccines can draw many parallels with access to medicines movement in this regard.

To begin with, the access to medicines movement became prominent and galvanized in the context of the HIV and AIDS crisis in the 1990s and 2000s.[25] At the time, it became morally reprehensible that antiretroviral drugs were available but millions of people were dying from AIDS-related illnesses in poor countries.[26] The main reason for these avoidable deaths was the cost of antiretroviral drugs, which were exorbitant, and only rich countries could afford to buy them on behalf of their sick populations.[27] The cost was dictated by pharmaceutical companies that could rely on the patent system to enjoy monopoly in the market without competition. Those from poor countries therefore could not access the drugs until later when generic versions became widely available to compete with these companies, effectively transforming HIV and AIDS into a manageable chronic disease as opposed to the death sentence it was for many years in poor countries.[28] There is not much difference with the COVID-19 vaccine experience. In COVID-19, the situation was much worse because apart from the monopolies created by patents, the rich countries technically locked out everyone from accessing vaccines by signing pre-purchase agreements with the manufacturers, thereby making vaccines unavailable for some time even if one had money to purchase them.

Buoyed by their success in the HIV and AIDS sector, today, the access to medicines movement played a leading role in pushing for access to COVID-19 vaccines especially in poor countries. At the global stage, the central message of the movement has been to put lives first before profits in what some see as a direct challenge to the global economic order that currently exists.[29] As it were, the amount of money available in the vaccine business today is humongous. The fact that many companies are yet to share their patents with the rest of the world despite the many COVID-related deaths registered globally shows just how far these companies are willing to go to protect their profits rather than save lives.

To be sure, the vaccine business is now lucrative. At the peak of the pandemic, Oxfam estimates that *Pfizer, BioNTech*, and *Moderna* were making $1,000 every second, which translates to US$ 65,000, while the world's poorest countries remained largely unvaccinated.[30] The majority of the sales by these companies were done to rich countries, and if one considers Pfizer and *BioNTech* alone, they had together delivered less than 1% to low-income countries, while *Moderna* had delivered 0.2%, thereby occasioning 98% of people in low-income countries not to be fully vaccinated.[31] Thankfully, the situation has now stabilized, and African countries can now access vaccines for its people.[32]

What may even be more concerning was that some companies got support from public coffers of up to US$100 billion from the US, Germany, and other countries, but in only half an year the companies had made US$26 billion in revenue according to the People's Vaccine Alliance.[33] The People's Vaccine Alliance also claimed that the 'three corporations are overcharging, pricing vaccines by as much as US$41 billion above the estimated cost of production'.[34] There were also claims that the companies in the US were not paying their fair share of taxes since '[i]n the first half of 2021, Moderna paid a 7% US tax rate and Pfizer paid 15% tax rate, well below the US statutory rate of 21%'.[35] These allegations, if true, represent the highest level of immorality by pharmaceutical companies.

Apart from the sad reality that the pharmaceutical companies were more interested in chasing profits as opposed to saving lives, there was also a concerted effort to undermine the access to medicines movement. Instead of addressing the root causes of the flawed system, multilateral economic institutions conspired to maintain the current world economic order without altering it to suit the ideal situation, which is to save lives by making medicines more affordable in poor countries. In this regard, Krikorian and Torreele observe as follows:[36]

> Initial solutions spearheaded by activists and policy makers in developing countries provided a constitutional right to health and challenged monopoly power of pharmaceutical corporations over a country's sovereign right and ability to provide lifesaving generics for its population. While successful at the domestic level, such approaches were often seen to threaten the global world order, in particular global trade, and were gradually overtaken by a more technocratic, less contentious, and more business-friendly approach that relied on voluntarism by donors and the pharmaceutical industry and focused mainly on low-income countries (LICs, a World Bank-invented grouping of countries based on macroeconomic indicators, not peoples' health needs).

From this quote, it is apparent that the access to medicines movement and now the movement pushing for COVID-19 vaccine equity are being undermined not at the national level but at the global front. The important gains that were made in the HIV and AIDS sector in the past are slowly being eroded by the new paradigm of voluntarism. Krikoria and Torreele note that this new approach which focuses on specific gaps is inadequate since it has failed to confront the key problem regarding access, namely the overall pharmaceutical business model.[37]

They further contend that the same approach has also permeated the COVID-19 discussions and approach to equitable access and in relation to the COVAX and other initiatives made so far as follows: '[a] dose charity associated with the traditional market approach risks once again diverting us from the profound moral, political and economic questioning of the way we finance, govern, and ensure the development and use of essential health tools'.[38] Using the TRIPS Agreement, IP protection has been globalized, and with it, the pharmaceutical companies have gained 'unprecedented control over medical R&D priorities and over the resulting health products, for which they could charge monopoly prices. . . . The access inequities it created for people living in less well-off countries were considered as collaterals that could be addressed through ad hoc solutions based on donor goodwill and market shaping'.[39]

To sum up, the problem of vaccine inequity persisted partly because pharmaceutical companies had succeeded in retaining their monopolies protected by patents and refusing to share their technologies. Arguably, by failing to address the root causes of the problems in the pharmaceutical trade sector, these companies have grown even stronger than before. Currently, countries are divided as donors or recipients of aid, and in this framework,

> [t]he donor determine which countries are 'eligible' to benefit from the solutions they created, and under which conditionalities. The voices of 'recipient' countries and the concerned populations are largely absent in the design and governance of the new global health order. The continued demands by developing countries for systemic solutions to address structural inequities and the dominance of the market over health rights and socioeconomic justice remain largely ignored.[40]

The voluntarism or donor paradigm therefore promotes socio-economic injustice, and something needs to be done urgently to guarantee the human right to health and access to vaccines on a need basis to better handle future pandemics.

4.4 The human rights approach to COVID-19 interventions: what does it require?

The COVID-19 pandemic was first and foremost a public health emergency. Stringent public health responses were necessary to curb it; however, the need to integrate the human rights framework in some of the responses was imperative because of the need to safeguard equity.[41] Using a human rights lens, it is possible to appreciate, in theory, that public health interventions are designed to protect the most vulnerable members of the society, but in practice this is usually not the case (and in some cases, public health policies may be hijacked for political reasons).[42] Furthermore, focusing on a utilitarian approach is not enough, and there is need to focus on the short- and long-term impacts of public health interventions on marginalized communities and establish concrete mechanisms for redress and compensation.[43]

The Committee on Economic, Social and Cultural Rights (CESCR) had adopted at least three statements since COVID-19 erupted. These statements can offer an authoritative glimpse of the human rights approach to the issue of vaccine inequity. In its first statement issued on 17 April 2020, the CESCR noted that while states must take steps to prevent or mitigate COVID-19, it is only through using the human rights framework that states can avoid the risk of violating economic, social, and cultural rights including the right to health and increasing the suffering of the most vulnerable groups.[44] Under its paragraph 14 of the statement, the CESCR observed the need to ensure equity even as states mobilize the necessary resources to combat COVID-19 so as to avoid further burdening the marginalized groups economically.[45] With regard to vaccines, the statement observed that 'State parties should also promote flexibilities or other adjustments in applicable intellectual property regimes to allow universal access to the benefits of scientific advances relating to COVID-19 such as diagnostics, medicines and vaccines'.[46] In this statement, there is no express commitment to overlook the intellectual property rights of owners of patents and other rights. However, there is a recognition that universal access to the benefits of science is needed, and using flexibilities or other adjustments in accordance with the regime in place at the local level is encouraged. Intellectual property is therefore implicitly recognized as a barrier to access to vaccines in the statement.

As more vaccines and technologies to fight COVID-19 became available, the CESCR revisited the issue of universal and equitable access to vaccines on 15 December 2020.[47] According to the CESCR statement on this date, the right to health and the right to enjoy the benefits of scientific progress 'imply that every person has a right to have access to a vaccine for COVID-19 that is safe, effective and based on the application of the best scientific developments'.[48] The CESCR noted that vaccines should not just be produced and made available but everyone must have access. Consequently,

> [i]n order to ensure access to COVID-19 vaccines, States must, firstly, *remove any discrimination* based on grounds such as religion, national origin, sex, sexual orientation and gender identity, race and ethnic identity, age, disability, migration status, social origin, poverty or any other relevant status; secondly, guarantee *physical accessibility* to vaccines, especially for marginalized groups and people living in remote areas, using both State-run and private channels and by strengthening the capacity of health systems to deliver vaccines; thirdly, guarantee *affordability or economic accessibility* for all, including by providing vaccines free of charge,

> at least for lower income persons and the poor, and fourthly, guarantee *access to relevant information*, especially through dissemination of accurate scientific information on the safety and effectiveness of different vaccines, and public campaigns protecting people against false, misleading or pseudoscience information concerning vaccines, which is rapidly spreading on the internet and social media.[49] (my emphasis)

This quote reveals that the issue of access is not simplistic and contains at least four elements: removal of discrimination of any form, physical accessibility, affordability or economic accessibility, and access to relevant information. This is in tandem with the General Comment No. 14 framework, which under its paragraph 12 expounds on the normative contents of the right to health as consisting of availability, *accessibility (which has four overlapping dimensions, namely non-discrimination, physical accessibility, economic accessibility (affordability), and information accessibility*), acceptability, and quality.[50] The CESCR specifically addressed the issue of intellectual property and noted that intellectual property is not a human rights but a social product with a social function.[51] Consequently, it is the obligation of the state to prevent intellectual property and specifically patents from undermining the enjoyment of economic, social, and cultural rights by for example making critical public goods such as vaccines and medicines being inaccessible.[52] The CESCR was even more candid when it noted that the TRIPs Agreement flexibilities may not be adequate to face the pandemic, and it went further to support the call by a number of countries for additional measures and especially those related to the waiver of some provisions of the TRIPs Agreement at the WTO.[53]

On business entities and specifically pharmaceutical companies, the CESCR noted that they 'should refrain from invoking intellectual property rights in a manner that is inconsistent with the right of every person to have access to safe and effective vaccine for COVID-19 and with the obligation of State to guarantee, as expeditiously as possible, universal equitable access to such vaccines'.[54] In this regard, 'States should therefore take all measures necessary to ensure that such business entities do not invoke intellectual property law, either in their own territory or abroad, in a manner that is inconsistent with the right of every person to have access to a safe and effective vaccine for COVID-19'.[55]

At the international level, states were urged to strengthen their cooperation so that there is universal and equitable access to vaccines for COVID-19 globally.[56] The statement also noted that competing for vaccines by states was counterproductive in terms of a global health approach since it will make the pandemic lengthy and difficult to control.[57] Lastly, the CESCR supported the WHO-supported COVAX Global Vaccines facility and noted that it will ensure that the prioritization in the global distribution of vaccines is based on medical needs and public health considerations.[58]

4.5 Why was there vaccine inequity in developing countries?

There are many reasons why vaccine inequity is rampant in the poor developing world compared to the rich developed nations. One of the obvious reasons for this is that rich countries signed pre-purchase agreements with vaccine manufacturers even before the vaccine candidates' clinical trials were completed. This ensured that these countries would be at the fore front in accessing the vaccines once production started.[59] Another significant factor is the poor funding of the COVAX facility which was meant to bridge the access gap by making it possible for poor countries to purchase the vaccines with donations from rich countries.[60] Lastly, some developed countries at the peak of the COVID-19 crisis decided to impose export controls on vaccines, raw materials, and equipment, which further proved to be a crippling factor in terms of response.[61] Interestingly, most of these factors are not IP related because the vaccines were not liberally in the market as yet. As more supplies of the vaccines became available, the IP-related barriers kicked in. Most importantly, the fact that the supply was severely limited at the peak of the COVID-19 pandemic is a clear testimony that IP was a major barrier; otherwise, other companies would have stepped in and made productions especially for the poor countries without relying on licensing arrangements that also left out middle-income economies. Notwithstanding, these factors have further been discussed separately below in detail.

4.5.1 Rich countries' pre-purchase agreements

The current global economic order is based on competition. Because of this, rich countries have used their power to invest in large and reputable pharmaceutical companies in order to secure, on a priority basis, a steady supply of vaccines for COVID-19.[62] The fact is that rich countries pumped billions of funds into big pharmaceutical companies, such as AstraZeneca, Europe's largest, and these companies had entered into pre-purchase agreements with the UK, the US, and the Vaccines Alliance, which is composed of France, Germany, Italy, and the Netherlands.[63] Through these pre-purchase agreements for the COVID-19 vaccine, the US bought 100 million candidates for COVID-19 vaccine supplies from BioNTech and Pfizer, while the UK and EU secured stocks from GlaxoSmithKline, Sanofi, AstraZeneca, and Moderna on guarantee that once the candidate vaccines were out they will be entitled to obtain them first.[64] Available statistics indicated that 'high income countries, representing 16% of the global population, [had] struck pre-orders covering at least 4.2 billion doses of COVID-19 vaccines. These countries [had] secured at least 70% of doses available in 2021 of five leading vaccine candidates, on the basis of known deals'.[65] It has been argued that by signing the pre-purchase agreements, the rich countries restricted the right to health of others since their actions were monopolistic.[66] The reason why pre-purchase agreement is risky is that 'fair access to vaccines is not strategically distributed to high-risk populations around the world and that contributes to the violation of the right to health in developing countries'.[67] Vaccine inequity in any part of the world is a violation of the right to health.

4.5.2 Export controls and/or restrictions

Export control or export restrictions were part of the broader vaccine nationalism debate that also included the pre-purchase agreements. Export controls in the US, India, and the European Union (EU) were particularly concerning where there are a few suppliers of the vaccine for COVID-19 including Ireland, Belgium, France, Great Britain, the US, the Netherlands, Italy, India, Germany, and Canada.[68] In the EU, for example, pharmaceutical companies were prohibited from exporting vaccines if it did not honour existing contracts with the EU.[69] The new rule was that a firm will need permission from EU's 27 member states to supply doses outside the EU.[70] However, some 92 exemptions were granted including vaccine donations to the COVAX facility.[71] It appears therefore from this arrangement that the interest of poor countries were taken into consideration. However, this means that these poor countries could only access their vaccine from the EU through the COVAX facility and not directly through purchase contracts.

Unlike the EU, the US did not restrict export of drugs to foreign countries but instead chose to restrict export of raw materials used to manufacture COVID-19 vaccines using the US Defence Production Act (DPA).[72] Accordingly, the restriction arguably undermined the Quad alliance (the US, Japan, Australia, and India) resolution to expand COVID-19 vaccinations globally.[73] Interestingly, the biggest vaccine maker in the world, the Serum Institute of India (SII), expressed its concerns about the ban noting that 'the U.S. ban on exports of materials like filters and bags, keeping them from U.S. companies, could limit production, especially the Novavax shot that it was set to start making [that] next month'.[74] The restriction was however lifted after many complaints and pressure from the public and severe shortage of raw materials such as single-use bioreactor bags and filters in India.[75]

Even after protesting the US export restrictions, India itself had to impose its own export restriction, which had an adverse impact on meeting the targets set under the COVAX facility for African countries.[76] The Indian government was reacting to the rising number of COVID-19 cases and the need to meet local demand even as the SII still maintained it could still supply the COVAX facility amid immense uncertainties.[77] It was however later reported that logistical challenges in African countries were creating surplus, and this was because of the sudden surge of vaccines after months of delays.[78] At the time, Africa had vaccinated only 8% of its population, and India, which has a similar population of about 1.3 billion, had vaccinated 37% of its population.[79] Apart from vaccines, India also decided to restrict export of syringes, which affected many countries who depended on it to inoculate their people.[80] It was expected that a shortfall of 2–4 billion needles would have been created by the end of the previous year and that African countries were to be hit the hardest.[81]

From the above, export controls or restrictions had a huge impact on access to vaccines, and the nature of the restrictions varied from country to country. In the EU, the restriction exempted the COVAX facility, thereby protecting access to vaccines for many poor African countries even though it relied on donations. However, the decision by the US to restrict export of key raw materials, even though eased after a huge outcry, would have had tremendous consequences in COVAX facility supplies. Perhaps the biggest impact was witnessed when India, when faced with a huge surge in COVID-19 cases, decided to impose restrictions not only on vaccines but also on syringes, thereby affecting many parts of the world including Africa.

4.5.3 Limited funding to the COVAX facility

The COVID-19 Vaccine Global Access (COVAX) facility, which is being coordinated jointly with CEPI and GAVI and was established by WHO in April 2020, seeks to avoid a repeat of the H1N1 scenario where 'rich countries bought up most of the global supply of pandemic influenza vaccines, leaving inadequate amounts for resource-poor countries, many of which were among the world's worst affected'.[82] Despite its good intentions, the COVAX facility has several challenges as enumerated below:[83]

> Apart from the cross-country equity concerns raised by a scenario of low-income countries vaccinating 20% of their population after much wider (if not universal) vaccination in high income countries, there is uncertainty about the supply earmarked for COVAX. Many of the doses secured by COVAX are of vaccines that, as of February, 2021 are just completing clinical trials and might not be available for months to come. COVAX might also gain access to vaccines being developed by CEPI-funded companies that are not as far along in trials, and it might negotiate further agreements with other suppliers. Yet overall, COVAX's supply is precarious and depends on what happens to the vaccines in clinical trials, how much of the successful candidates can be produced quickly, and how much of the output is left for COVAX after sales to national governments.

Therefore, in a nutshell, the COVAX facility, even though critical in bridging the equity gap, faces numerous challenges that it is almost impossible for it to achieve its objective. Nevertheless, there are some countries that would be completely left out of the vaccine access race without the facility. There is a need to strengthen the facility and address the gaps. Developed countries must stop dumping vaccines with short lifespans in African countries, and in East Africa for instance, about 40 million vaccine doses were at risk of going bad.[84] The demand for vaccines has been a major problem, and even as more African countries are due to receive millions of vaccines through COVAX and African Vaccine Acquisition Trust, African countries are required to create demand for these vaccines locally to avoid vaccine apathy.[85]

In closing, the COVAX facility is too important to fail if history is anything to go by. In 2004, the highly pathogenic avian influenza virus just proved to the whole world that when push comes to shove, rich countries that promised to donate vaccines under plans sponsored by the WHO and the UN reneged on their commitments at the expense of poor countries, thereby prolonging the 2004 global pandemic.[86] Sustainability of vaccine programmes for future pandemics needs to be sorted outside the charity model.

4.5.4 Inadequate local manufacturing capacity

During the COVID-19 pandemic, Africa was lagging behind in terms of local manufacturing of vaccines since for many years it had not prioritized domestic production for national outbreak preparedness.[87] With a big population of 1.3 billion people, only 1% of the vaccine doses Africa uses are produced locally despite the high prevalence of infectious diseases.[88] In order to address this challenge, bilateral agreements were negotiated as follows: Algeria negotiated with Russia for the purchase of Sputnik V vaccine, South African countries set up a local manufacturing capacity, and Egypt was in an agreement with China to produce two million doses of Sinovac vaccine at the Vacsera facilities by June 2021.[89] In Egypt, for instance, the plan was to produce at least one billion doses annually of the Chinese Sinovac vaccine.[90] Indeed, the partnership between the two countries and the donations being made to countries such as Palestine made Egypt the main hub for Chinese vaccine diplomacy in Africa and the Middle East.[91] Kenya also announced its plans to begin manufacturing vaccines locally after it emerged that about 70% of medical products are imported, eating into a huge portion of its health budget.[92] All in all, the point being made here is that more should be done to increase Africa's manufacturing capacity for vaccines for future sustainability. The COVID-19 experience is a big wakeup call that you cannot always rely on good neighbourliness. There are somethings that you must do on your own, especially when in an emergency.

4.6 What measures were established to address the vaccine inequity issue?

The previous section focused on the causes of vaccine inequity and identified four factors, namely pre-purchase agreements, export controls/restrictions, lack of adequate funding for the COVAX facility, and lack of local manufacturing. In this section, attention is drawn to the measures that were put in place to deal with the issue of vaccine inequity in the context of the COVID-19 pandemic.

4.6.1 Rich countries' donations

US President Joe Biden urged more donations from world leaders to meet the goal of vaccinating 70% of the world by September 2022.[93] The charitable donations approach is, however, not enough to meet the global needs, and increasing manufacturing abroad is inevitable for sustainability.[94] This is critical because many developing countries still lack the technical capacity to produce vaccines locally apart from India, Brazil, and Vietnam that have some capacity to make local productions of vaccines (other countries such as Australia, Singapore, and South Korea possess advanced technology to produce vaccines in cooperation with companies such as *Pfizer* and *Moderna*).[95]

At the height of COVID-19, donations made sense for the reasons stated earlier and the fact that poor countries had no resources to purchase vaccines on their own and, at some point, the vaccines were hoarded by the developed countries for some time before it became available in the market. In June 2021, the Organization for Economic Cooperation and Development (OECD) members supported counting contributions to the [ACT-A Health Systems Connecter] Pillar[96] in full in official development assistance (ODA) given its focus on support to the health systems of developing countries.[97] While this proposal may boost vaccine equity, it is contentious because the issue of price to be tagged to these vaccines remains contentious, with the initial proposal being US$3 per vaccine and the latest proposal was US$ 6.72, and if pledges made by Canada, the EU, the UK, and the US are considered, at this price 'ODA totals could see an increase of US$10.8billion in the next two years – hardly a minor amount'.[98] 'Some rich countries, the most outspoken being the UK, also considered rechanneling a portion of their unused International Monetary Fund (IMF)-recently allocated Special Drawing Rights (SDRs) to meet their ODA targets, which could imply making savings in their aid budgets in the midst of an unprecedented crisis'.[99]

The amount US$6.72 per dose was taken from the weighted average price as determined by GAVI, and it is expected that an updated price will be used for 2022 reporting.[100] The issue of price is particularly nuanced when one considers that '[e]pidemiologically, a vaccine with 60% efficacy is different from one with 90% efficacy. Other characteristics, such as cold chain requirements and dosage (single versus two doses), and ease of reproduction in other regional sites, are important for negotiating price and engaging in market shaping'.[101]

It therefore emerged that applying a standard price of US$6.72 per vaccine dose was not tenable and should be revised to take into consideration the unique circumstances of each vaccine. Otherwise, channelling ODA to vaccine donations was a welcome move, but it should not come at a great expense to other sectors relying on ODA. Secondly, the donations should not be subjected to domestic supply or prepurchase agreements because this will limit access. Countries like the UK should have also not prioritized their own interest by rechannelling a portion of their unused IMF – recently allocated Special Drawing Rights (SDRs) – to meet their ODA targets. Out of the US$650 billion worth of SDRs approved by IMF to help low- and middle-income countries to respond to the COVID-19 crisis, the UK received US$27.5 billion, which is far much more than what all low-income countries were receiving combined.[102] The concern however was that '[t]he likely course of action-on-lending the SDRs back to certain trusts within the IMF, the World Bank, and other multilateral development banks, to in turn loan to low-income countries-risk burdening countries with increased debt, harmful and time-consuming conditionality, and a limiting of development space'.[103] What is more, '[i]f the UK accounted any lending of its new issuance of SDRs as official development assistance (ODA) and kept rigidly to the 0.5% of gross national income (GNI) ODA target, then grants for other programmes could be cut so as not to overshoot this target'.[104]

4.6.2 mRNA technology transfer hub

Since Africa imports 90% of its vaccines, the WHO, South African consortium, and partners from COVAX got busy putting in place 'a technology transfer hub for mRNA vaccines in South Africa to help boost and scale up vaccine production in Africa'.[105] The technology transfer hub was expected to 'teach African manufacturers how to make mRNA vaccines, like the Pfizer and Moderna COVID-19 vaccines, here in Africa'.[106] In the hub, technology will be established at an industrial scale and clinical development performed. In this project, 'WHO and partners will bring in the production know-how, quality control and necessary licenses to single entity to facilitate a broad and rapid technology transfer to multiple recipients around the world'.[107] The success of the hub will, however, rely on the collaboration between the pharmaceutical companies that have the know-how and smaller ones available or to be established in developing countries. The issue of sustainability is also key. The viability of such a venture must make business sense, and if need be, the government should offer appropriate incentives and guarantees to those daring to take this path in line with the applicable rules of trade.

4.6.3 Partnership to Accelerate COVID-19 Testing

One other factor that undermined vaccination is the low capacity in testing. It was therefore encouraging to see Africa CDC launch a Partnership to Accelerate COVID-19 Testing (PACT), where many technicians were trained, and towards the end of 2021, it had so far conducted 14.5 million COVID-19 tests.[108] Under this partnership, test kits were being made in countries like Kenya, Ethiopia, Nigeria, Morocco, Senegal, and South Africa.[109] PACT was anchored on the African Union Joint Continental Strategy for COVID-19 Outbreak and is aimed to 'ultimately help prevent transmission and deaths, and minimize the social and economic harm associated with COVID-19'.[110] The strategy employed by PACT is test, trace, and treat. In relation to treat, 'PACT TREAT aims to ensure that patients experiencing moderate to severe symptoms have access to the supportive care they need, with minimal impact to the existing healthcare services'.[111]

4.6.4 Voluntary licensing

During the COVID-19 pandemic, the most preferred market-based intervention was voluntary licensing. A good example was the Pfizer voluntary license with the Medicines Patent Pool (MPP) concerning its Paxlovid, which is used in COVID-19 treatment.[112] The best part of the deal was that the license granted to MPP was to be sub-licensed to qualified generic medicine manufacturers to supply to 95 countries the medicine subject to national regulatory approvals.[113] The list included '[a]ll low- and lower-middle-income countries and some upper-middle-income countries in sub-Saharan Africa, as well as countries that have transitioned from lower-middle to upper-middle-income status in the past five years. . . '.[114] Pfizer further committed not to receive any royalties from low-income countries, and as long as COVID-19 remained classified as a public health emergency of international concern (PHEIC) by the WHO, it waived royalties on sales in all countries.[115] The move by Pfizer, even though laudable, drew some attention from People's Vaccine Alliance's spokesperson and Oxfam who noted that many developing countries like Iraq and Lebanon were to be left out of the deal.[116] Another issue they raised is the lack of a similar intervention in regard to vaccines, noting that perhaps the move was driven by profits they continue to reap from supplying vaccines.[117] The UN on its part noted that the license was important since it will facilitate equitable and rapid access to new treatments globally.[118] The G-20 leaders however appeared to favour voluntary license without waiver of patents despite the push at the WTO.[119] As already discussed earlier, this is the route that has been taken with regard to vaccines which as of 2021 were being sold at slightly over US$ 6 per dose. The strong stance on vaccines and patents appears to be relaxed in the case of medicines for treating COVID-19 as demonstrated by Pfizer's deal with MPP.

4.6.5 WTO TRIPS waiver and compulsory licensing

Given the reluctance of rich countries in giving up or waiving their patents to increase vaccine production for the benefit of poor countries, the other option allowed in law is compulsory licensing. The compulsory licensing option had been considered as a potential substitute to the TRIPS waiver, with South Africa and India favouring the former and the EU favouring the latter. Without getting into the details of the two, specific studies had reached different conclusions on the approach preferred. For instance, South Centre reached the conclusion that a TRIPS waiver may be more effective since[120]

> The IP waiver has the potential to overcome some of the limitations of the compulsory licensing system. These include the product-by-product requirement of compulsory licensing that restrict the effective and speedy application of this mechanism, as well as the need to spend time on identifying the patents that cover the products in question prior to issuing a compulsory license. . . . In addition, the barrier posed by marketing authorizations would also be eliminated. Moreover, the issue of remuneration would not arise. . . . Moreover, the waiver would also remove the need to comply with the cumbersome procedure of Article 31*bis* TRIPS in the case of exporting COVID-19 vaccines or medicines to other countries with no or limited manufacturing capacity.

Without providing more analysis, compulsory licensing, even though readily available for use in many jurisdictions, has its own unique challenges which may not be appropriate to deal with in the context of the COVID-19 pandemic. It is because of the reasons highlighted earlier that the TRIPS waiver was recommended. The ultimate decision taken by the WTO during its 12th Ministerial Conference in June 2022 was more of a further relaxation of compulsory licensing conditions for a limited period of five years than a 'real' waiver. Paragraph 8 of the decision delayed the inclusion of diagnostics and therapeutics to a later date, which was before 17 December 2022, but this has not yet happened because of lack of consensus.[121]

Suffice to note, as seen in our previous discussions, the rich countries who control the patents had resolved to making donations through the COVAX facility. As a matter of fact, these donations are paid for since they are counted as part of the ODA contribution. In essence what is happening is that poor countries are buying vaccines at market rates even though the GAVI price was the one used.

4.7 Way forward: investment in vaccine research and development?

It is true that in the future sustainability requires 'global-public-health-driven vaccine development and manufacturing based on equitable access to platform technologies, decentralised and localised innovation, and multiple developers and manufacturers, especially in low- and middle-income countries (LMICs)'.[122] The twin issues of vaccine development and manufacturing are therefore critical to address future pandemics. Enough has been said about manufacturing. What remains to be emphasized is the issue of investment in research and development in vaccine development for futuristic epidemics and pandemics.

In this regard, proposals have been made to prioritize basic research that may assist in stockpiling a range of effective vaccines.[123] This proposal borrows heavily from the military architecture, where it has been noted that the global expenditure is about US$2 trillion a year, and the money required for vaccines is a paltry few hundred million dollars to deal with the next pandemic.[124] The plan entails to develop a universal flu vaccine; however, the more realistic option, if possible, is to 'design several vaccine candidates based on potent anti-head antibodies against a limited set of influenza viruses, perhaps organized by flu subtypes'.[125] Consequently,

> The investment per virus from bench to phase 1 trials is likely to be in the range of $100million to $200million over several years. We envisage that these costs would be borne by public-private partnerships between governments, philanthropy and industry. Organizations such as CEPI, the COVAX Facility and GAVI, the Vaccine Alliance could help convene the expertise and initiate the negotiations needed to deliver the types of vaccines we propose.[126]

It is encouraging that the World Bank is considering investing in 50 countries in terms of vaccine projects, the international monetary fund handling private sector, and the WTO dealing with supply chain issues to support the plan.[127]

4.8 Conclusion

The COVID-19 crisis is one of those challenges that require solidarity and humanity. Sadly, the rich countries insisted on the market approaches to address the problem despite the market failures registered. Notably, vaccine inequity stood out because at the peak of the pandemic, many people in rich countries received vaccines due to their economic power, and poor countries were delayed. In the past during the push for HIV and AIDS antiretroviral medications, the access to medicines movement had called for a new global economic order, but this also failed. Their failure to achieve this new paradigm reflected in the lack of vaccines in many parts of the world, and indeed the time may be ripe to revisit this discourse. At the national level, companies have succeeded in protecting their patent monopolies as well as technologies, thereby making it hard for other countries or companies to produce vaccines even where capacity exists. The human rights approach, specifically the right to health and the right to benefit from scientific approach, requires access to vaccines for all. To the extent that this is not happening, then human rights were violated in favour of market dynamics. The causes of vaccine inequity during COVID-19 are well too known and included rich countries' pre-purchase agreements, export controls/restrictions, limited funding for the COVAX facility, and inadequate manufacturing capacity, especially in Africa. The steps considered to remedy the situation included donations/COVAX, establishment of technology transfer hubs, PACT, subject to licenses especially for treatment drugs, and the issue of TRIPS waiver at the WTO versus compulsory licensing. In relation to the last measure, despite the availability of compulsory licensing option as well as the push to waive TRIPS Agreement, there has been limited success. Both options failed to make a meaningful contribution to the problem of vaccine inequity. Lastly, even the donations approach appeared to have been fused with the market approach through the ODA contributions being the main intervention for vaccine access. While this may go a long way to ameliorate the situation, it is not sustainable in the long run, and it is not the best approach for future pandemics such as the present one. Apart from boosting local manufacturing, real investment in research and development by all countries is what will help prepare effectively for the next pandemic.

4.9 Acknowledgment

This research is supported by the Hong Kong RGC Senior Research Fellow Scheme 2022/23 for a project led by Professor Bryan Mercurio entitled 'Access to Vaccines in a Post-COVID-19 World: Sustainable Legal and Policy Options (Project No. SRFS2223–4H01). The views expressed in this publication do not necessarily represent the views of others involved in the project.

Notes

1 'WHO coronavirus (COVID-19) dashboard' available at https://covid19.who.int (accessed 1 April 2022).
2 'Coronavirus (COVID-19)' *WHO | Regional Office for Africa* available at www.afro.who.int/health-topics/coronavirus-covid-19 (accessed 1 April 2022).
3 '"A moral failure": Global vaccine inequity hits Africa hardest' *Partners in Health* available at www.pih.org/article/moral-failure-global-vaccine-inequity-hits-africa-hardest (accessed 1 April 2022)
4 'Kenya: WHO coronavirus disease (COVID-19) dashboard with vaccination data' available at https://covid19.who.int (accessed 1 April 2022). From 3 January 2020 to 31 March 2022 Kenya had 323,402 confirmed cases and 5,648 COVID-19 related deaths.
5 www.who.int/publications/m/item/weekly-epidemiological-update-on-covid-19–10-august-2023#:~:text=As%20of%206%20August%202023,deaths%20have%20been%20reported%20globally.
6 'WHO coronavirus (COVID-19)' Dashboard available at https://covid19.who.int/
7 OJ Wouters et al 'Challenges in ensuring global access to COVID-19 vaccines: Production, affordability, allocation, and deployment | Elsevier enhanced reader' (2021) 1023 available at https://reader.elsevier.com/reader/sd/pii/S01406736

21003068?token=9EEDB18B6158D824167A3B6BD960AE156DFDD072424B447143C56267F88297AAFB7977FCFAE581BD890D63200B47A9EE&originRegion=eu-west-1&originCreation=20220127071747 (accessed 27 January 2022).

8 As above.

9 'Health equity – global' available at www.who.int/westernpacific/health-topics/health-equity (accessed 3 February 2022).

10 'The COVID-19 vaccine race' available at www.gavi.org/vaccineswork/covid-19-vaccine-race (accessed 16 February 2022).

11 'There are four types of COVID-19 vaccines: Here's how they work | Gavi, the vaccine alliance' available at www.gavi.org/vaccineswork/there-are-four-types-covid-19-vaccines-heres-how-they-work (accessed 16 August 2023).

12 'COVID-19 vaccines with WHO emergency use listing' *WHO – Prequalification of Medical Products (IVDs, Medicines, Vaccines and Immunization Devices, Vector Control* 3 November 2021 available at https://extranet.who.int/pqweb/vaccines/vaccinescovid-19-vaccine-eul-issued (accessed 16 August 2023).

13 'WHO issues its first emergency use validation for a COVID-19 vaccine and emphasizes need for equitable global access' available at www.who.int/news/item/31-12-2020-who-issues-its-first-emergency-use-validation-for-a-covid-19-vaccine-and-emphasizes-need-for-equitable-global-access (accessed 2 August 2023).

14 T Lewis 'How the U.S. pandemic response went wrong – and what went right – during a year of COVID' *Scientific American* available at www.scientificamerican.com/article/how-the-u-s-pandemic-response-went-wrong-and-what-went-right-during-a-year-of-covid/ (accessed 27 July 2023).

15 DR Burton & EJ Topol 'Invest in vaccines now to prevent the next pandemic' (2021) 590 *Nature* 386, 386 available at www.proquest.com/docview/2492472660/abstract/67B0FAE0375A4C21PQ/1 (accessed 26 July 2023).

16 P Hotez et al 'Correcting COVID-19 vaccine misinformation: Lancet commission on COVID-19 vaccines and therapeutics task force members*' (2021) 33 *eClinical Medicine* available at www.thelancet.com/journals/eclinm/article/PIIS2589-5370(21)00060-2/fulltext (accessed 25 July 2023).

17 As above.

18 As above.

19 As above.

20 E Torreele & JJ Amon 'Equitable COVID-19 vaccine access' (June 2021) 23(1) *Health and Human Rights* Special Section: Public and Mental Health, Human Rights, and Atrocity Prevention 273–288, at 273.

21 As above.

22 As above.

23 'Vaccine nationalism: Everything you need to know' *Global Citizen* available at www.globalcitizen.org/en/content/what-is-vaccine-nationalism/ (accessed 1 April 2022). According to Public Citizen, '[t]he term has essentially been coined in the wake of dozens of governments in wealthy countries scrambling to sign deals with pharmaceutical companies directly, to secure vaccines for their own populations – limiting the stock available for others.

Dr. Tedros described it as a "me-first approach" when he spoke to an executive board meeting of the WHO in January.

And while "nationalism" is a wide-ranging political concept that can apply to different contexts, it generally relates to putting the interest of a single nation first, above others, for economic or security reasons – so that's why the vaccine approach mentioned above has been described this way.'

24 'Statement on the extension of the TRIPS waiver for diagnostics and therapeutics for COVID-19' 9 January 2023 available at chrome-extension://efaidnbmn

nnibpcajpcglclefindmkaj/www.southcentre.int/wp-content/uploads/2023/01/SC-Statement_TRIPS-waiver-diagnostics-therapeutics.pdf
25 'Access to medicines in depth access campaign | MSF' *Médecins Sans Frontières (MSF) International* available at www.msf.org/access-medicines-depth-access-campaign (accessed 1 April 2022).
26 As above.
27 As above.
28 As above.
29 As above. According to MSF, '[t]his market failure is our next challenge. The challenge however . . . is for governments . . . the pharmaceutical industry and other NGOs to confront this injustice. What we as civil society demand is change, not charity.'
30 'Pfizer, BioNTech and Moderna making $1,000 profit every second while world's poorest countries remain largely unvaccinated' *Oxfam International* 16 November 2021 available at www.oxfam.org/en/press-releases/pfizer-biontech-and-moderna-making-1000-profit-every-second-while-worlds-poorest (accessed 3 February 2022)
31 As above.
32 Statistica 'Number of administered coronavirus (COVID-19) vaccine doses per 100 people in Africa as of March 15, 2023, by country' available at www.statista.com/statistics/1221298/covid-19-vaccination-rate-in-african-countries/ Published by Doris Dokua Sasu.
33 'Pharmaceutical companies reaping immoral profits from covid vaccines yet paying low tax rates' *ActionAid International* available at https://actionaid.org/news/2021/pharmaceutical-companies-reaping-immoral-profits-covid-vaccines-yet-paying-low-tax-rates (accessed 3 February 2022)
34 As above.
35 As above.
36 G Krikorian & E Torreele 'We cannot win the access to medicines struggle using the same thinking that causes the chronic access crisis' (June 2021) 23(1) *Health and Human Rights* 119–128, 120.
37 As above, 121.
38 As above.
39 As above.
40 As above, 123.
41 S Zweig, AJ Zapf, C Beyrer, D Guhasipir & RJ Haar 'Ensuring rights while protecting health: The importance of using a human rights approach in implementing public health responses to COVID-19' (December 2021) 23(2) *Health and Human Rights* 173–186, 183.
42 As above.
43 As above.
44 CESCR 'Statement on the coronavirus disease (COVID-19) pandemic and economic, social and cultural rights' E/C.12/2020/1 (17 April 2020), para 2.
45 As above.
46 As above, para 21.
47 CESCR 'Statement on universal and equitable access to vaccines for the coronavirus disease (COVID-19)' E/C.12/2020/2 (15 December 2020).
48 As above, para 2.
49 As above, para 4.
50 CESCR 'General Comment No. 14 on the right to the highest attainable standard of health' E/C.12/2000/4 (11 August 2000), para 12.
51 CESCR (n 47 above) para 6.
52 As above.
53 As above.

54 As above, para 7.
55 As above, para 8.
56 As above, para 9.
57 As above, para 10.
58 As above, para 11.
59 'Opinion | What's the plan for vaccinating the world?' 22 September 2021 available at www.medpagetoday.com/opinion/second-opinions/94653 (accessed 6 November 2021)
60 As above.
61 As above.
62 JAY Wattimena & MA Matakena 'Pre-purchase agreement on the COVID-19 vaccine and its impact on the right to health' (2021) 27(4) *SASI* 414.
63 As above, 415.
64 As above. The statistics are staggering: 'The United States government has invested US $1.2 billion in the Astrazeneca vaccine named AZD1222 for 300 million doses, as well as the candidate vaccine by BioNTech and Pfizer for US $ 1.95 billion with a pledge of 100 million doses with options of up to 500 million more doses. Similarly, Australia has also pledged $1.5billion dollars for the development of a candidate vaccine by companies Pfizer and Novavax to obtain up to 134 million doses of vaccine. This is also the pattern played by other countries such as Canada, the US and the UK, which have secured at least five guaranteed vaccine supply deals.'
65 As above
66 Wattimena & Matakena (n 62 above) 415.
67 As above, 421.
68 IA Ibrahim 'Overview of export restrictions on COVID-19 vaccines and their components' (1 June 2021) 25(10) *American Society of International Law* 1.
69 'Coronavirus: WHO criticises EU over vaccine export controls' *BBC News* 30 January 2021 available at www.bbc.com/news/world-europe-55860540 (accessed 31 January 2022).
70 As above.
71 As above.
72 'U.S. curbs on raw material exports could dent new quad alliance's vaccine push' *Reuters* 11 March 2021 available at www.reuters.com/article/us-health-coronavirus-vaccines-quad-idUSKBN2B31M1 (accessed 31 January 2022).
73 As above.
74 As above.
75 'US loosens restrictions on export of COVID-19 vaccine raw materials to India' 27 April 2021 available at www.straitstimes.com/asia/south-asia/us-loosens-restrictions-on-export-of-covid-19-vaccine-raw-materials-to-india (accessed 31 January 2022).
76 April 2021 SJ//01, 'Export restrictions in India could stunt Africa's 2021 vaccination goals' *Devex* 1 April 2021 available at www.devex.com/news/sponsored/export-restrictions-in-india-could-stunt-africa-s-2021-vaccination-goals-99567 (accessed 31 January 2022)
77 As above.
78 KN Das 'India stuck with COVID-19 vaccines it can't export' *Reuters* 15 December 2021 available at www.reuters.com/world/india/india-stuck-with-covid-19-vaccines-it-cant-export-2021-12-14/ (accessed 31 January 2022)
79 As above.
80 KD Singh 'As India limits syringe exports, a supply crunch has buyers looking elsewhere' *The New York Times* 18 November 2021 available at www.nytimes.com/2021/11/18/world/asia/covid-syringes-india.html (accessed 31 January 2022)

81 As above.
82 'Challenges in ensuring global access to COVID-19 vaccines: Production, affordability, allocation, and deployment | Elsevier enhanced reader' (13 Mach 2021) vol. 397, 1028 available at https://reader.elsevier.com/reader/sd/pii/S0140673621003068?token=4C0CDEC8B13E4C9FFBDD5712A043C2AA6F041B49DA370135A4C1F92F968221BA292926FB12749C4E8A93A0C72E2E853B&originRegion=eu-west-1&originCreation=20220127095945 (accessed 27 January 2022).
83 As above.
84 'The East African 25th December 2021' *ENewspaper* available at https://vpn.uonbi.ac.ke/proxy/56d8ac15/https/epaper.nationmedia.com/Kenya/TheEastAfrican/issue/103/25122021103630758/01 (accessed 28 December 2021)
85 As above.
86 JN Nkengasong et al 'COVID-19 vaccines: How to ensure Africa has access' (2020) 586 *Nature* 197.
87 M Massinga Loembé & JN Nkengasong 'COVID-19 vaccine access in Africa: Global distribution, vaccine platforms, and challenges ahead' (2021) 54 *Immunity* 1353.
88 As above.
89 As above.
90 'Egypt, Sinovac agree to speed up vaccine-production technology transfer' *Arab News* 8 January 2022 available at https://arab.news/2p4z7 (accessed 1 April 2022)
91 E Olander 'Egypt is now the main hub for Chinese vaccine diplomacy in Africa and the Middle East' *The China Africa Project* available at https://chinaafricaproject.com/2022/02/21/egypt-is-now-the-main-hub-for-chinese-vaccine-diplomacy-in-africa-and-the-middle-east/ (accessed 1 April 2022)
92 'Kenya to manufacture own COVID-19 vaccines by April' *Daily Nation* 21 December 2021.
93 'Perspective | Biden's plan to vaccinate the world won't work. Here's a better one' *Washington Post* available at www.washingtonpost.com/outlook/2021/09/27/biden-vaccines-globe-inequity-donations/ (accessed 6 November 2021)
94 As above.
95 As above.
96 'ACT-A HSRC' available at https://hlh.who.int/act-a-hsrc-connector (accessed 1 February 2022). According to WHO, '[t]he Access to COVID-19 Tools Accelerator (ACT-A) is a global collaboration to accelerate the development, production, and equitable access to COVID-19 tools (diagnostics, therapeutics, and vaccines). The ACT-A comprises four technical partnerships: three vertical pillars (vaccines, therapeutics and diagnostics) and one transversal Health Systems and Response Connector (HSRC). The ACT-A HSRC is a multi-organization partnership that includes diverse stakeholders as its members. The ACT-A HSRC, co-led by the WHO, UNICEF, Global Fund, and World Bank with support from the Global Financing Facility (GFF), coordinates three key workstreams to support partner organizations and countries on critical aspects relating to uptake of COVID-19 tools. Through close collaboration with partners, the ACT-A HSRC aims to enhance uptake of COVID-19 tools by supporting countries identify needs and gaps, coordinating with partners to address identified bottlenecks, and closely monitoring country progress against global targets.'
97 OECD 'Summary record of the informal meeting of the working party on development finance statistics (WP-STAT)' DCD/DAC/STAT/M(2021)2/FINAL (3 September 2021) para 29 available at www.oecd.org/officialdocuments/publicdisplaydocumentpdf/?cote=DCD/DAC/STAT/M(2021)2/FINAL&docLanguage=En.

98 N Craviotto 'Covid-19 vaccine donations from rich countries to Global South must not be counted as aid' *Eurodad* available at www.eurodad.org/covid_19_vaccine_donations_aid (accessed 1 February 2022)
99 As above.
100 OECD 'Valuation of donation of excess COVID-19 doses to developing countries in ODA' DCD/DAC/STAT (2021)29 (8 December 2021) para 4 available at www.oecd.org/officialdocuments/publicdisplaydocumentpdf/?cote=DCD/DAC/STAT(2021)29&docLanguage=En. Suffice to note, the price is applicable to donations of doses in excess from providers' domestic supply, i.e. when purchase agreement with manufacturers have brought about more doses than needed for domestic vaccination purposes and when this surplus is donated to developing countries.
101 Padmashree Gehl Sampath 'Market shaping and market access in the global vaccines market: Approaches for the future' a paper prepared for the GIZ (2 October 2021) 16 available at www.giz.de/en/downloads/market-shaping-and-market-access-in-the-global-vaccines-market.pdf.
102 'Civil society joint statement on UK channelling of its SDRs allocation' *Bretton Woods Project* 23 August 2021 available at www.brettonwoodsproject.org/2021/08/civil-society-joint-statement-on-uk-channelling-of-its-imf-special-drawing-rights-sdrs-allocation/ (accessed 1 February 2022)
103 As above.
104 'The UK, special drawing rights and Fiscal Gimmickry' *ODI: Think Change* available at https://odi.org/en/insights/the-uk-special-drawing-rights-and-fiscal-gimmickry/ (accessed 1 February 2022. Since 2009, 15 of the 20 largest beneficiaries of the 2009 SDR allocation have made loans to the Poverty Reduction and Growth Trust (PRGT), which provides zero-interest loans to lower income countries either using SDRs or equivalent foreign exchange reserves. Where UK differs with the others however is that it is the only country that has chosen to report substantial proportions of these loans as ODA in its submissions to the OECD DAC.
105 'Towards Africa's first MRNA vaccine technology transfer hub' *WHO | Regional Office for Africa* available at www.afro.who.int/news/towards-africas-first-mrna-vaccine-technology-transfer-hub (accessed 28 December 2021)
106 As above.
107 'Technology transfer hub' *MPP* available at https://medicinespatentpool.org/covid-19/technology-transfer-hub (accessed 1 February 2022)
108 WHO (n 105 above)
109 As above.
110 'Partnership to accelerate COVID-19 testing (PACT) in Africa – resources' *Africa CDC* available at https://africacdc.org/download/partnership-to-accelerate-covid-19-testing-pact-in-africa/ (accessed 1 February 2022)
111 As above.
112 'Pfizer and medicines patent pool reach "Ground-breaking" voluntary licensing deal for new COVID-19 treatment pill' *Health Policy Watch* 16 November 2021 available at https://healthpolicy-watch.news/pfizer-and-medicines-patent-pool/ (accessed 2 February 2022)
113 As above.
114 As above.
115 As above.
116 'Reaction to Pfizer's announcement of voluntary licenses of its COVID-19 oral antiviral treatment Paxlovid to the medicines patent pool' *Oxfam International* 17 November 2021 available at www.oxfam.org/en/press-releases/reaction-pfizers-announcement-voluntary-licenses-its-covid-19-oral-antiviral (accessed 2 February 2022)

117 As above.
118 'COVID-19: Licensing agreement for new candidate drug "an important first step"' *UN News* 16 November 2021 available at https://news.un.org/en/story/2021/11/1105862 (accessed 2 February 2022)
119 F Guarascio 'G20 leaders to back COVID-19 vaccine voluntary licensing, no patent waiver' *Reuters* 20 May 2021 available at www.reuters.com/business/healthcare-pharmaceuticals/drugmakers-make-big-low-cost-vaccine-push-poor-nations-eu-official-2021-05-20/ (accessed 2 February 2022)
120 O Gurgula 'Compulsory licensing vs. the IP waiver: What is the best way to end the COVID-19 pandemic?' 5, 10 available at www.southcentre.int/wp-content/uploads/2021/10/PB104_Compulsory-licensing-vs.-the-IP-waiver_EN-2.pdf (accessed 2 February 2022).
121 WTO 'Members continue discussion on TRIPS Decision extension to therapeutics and diagnostics' available at www.wto.org/english/news_e/news23_e/heal_17mar23_e.htm#:~:text=Under%20paragraph%208%20of%20the,the%20exclusive%20effect%20of%20patents
122 National Library of Medicine 'The future of epidemic and pandemic vaccines to serve global public health needs' available at www.ncbi.nlm.nih.gov/pmc/articles/PMC10052681/#:~:text=Key%20to%20future%20epidemic%20and,%2D%20and%20middle%2Dincome%20countries%20
123 Burton & Topol (n 15 above).
124 As above.
125 As above.
126 As above, 388.
127 A new commitment for vaccine equity and defeating the pandemic by Kristalina Georgieva, Tedros Adhanom Ghebreyesus, David Malpass and Ngozi Okonjo-Iweala available at www.wto.org/english/news_e/roadmap_igo_01jun21_e.htm#:~:text=The%20World%20Bank%20will%20have,for%20the%20plan%20to%20succeed.

5

COVID-19 VACCINE MANDATE AND THE RIGHT TO HEALTH IN AFRICA

Should Africa toe the path of the US?

Obiajulu Nnamuchi

5.1 Introduction and preliminary background

Traditionally, the naming of pathogens and diseases follows a carefully crafted procedure. The virus that was first detected in Wuhan, China, in late 2019 and which triggered a global pandemic[1] was to follow the same pattern. The International Committee on Taxonomy of Viruses (ICTV),[2] which is governed by the Virology Division of the International Union of Microbiological Societies, announced 'severe acute respiratory syndrome coronavirus 2 (SARS-CoV-2)' as the name of the new virus on 11 February 2020.[3] This designation was informed by the fact that the novel virus is genetically related to the coronavirus responsible for the SARS outbreak of 2003, although the two viruses differ.[4] On the same date, the World Health Organization (WHO) unveiled 'COVID-19' as the name of this new disease, in accordance with the guidelines previously developed with the World Organisation for Animal Health (OIE) and the Food and Agriculture Organization (FAO)[5] of the United Nations (UN). In other words, COVID-19 or coronavirus disease is an infectious disease that is caused by the SARS-CoV-2 virus.[6]

The disease affects people in different ways.[7] In most cases, infected people will develop mild to moderate illness and recover without being hospitalized.[8] However, some will become seriously ill and require extensive therapeutic intervention. Among the latter are older adults and people with underlying medical conditions such as cardiovascular disease, diabetes, chronic respiratory disease, or cancer. Latest data from the US Centers for Disease Control and Prevention (CDC) indicates that more than 81% of COVID-19 deaths occur in people over age 65 years.[9] In comparative terms, the number of deaths among this demographic is 97 times higher than that in those aged

DOI: 10.4324/9781032671437-7

18–29 years.[10] Remarkably, while a significant body of knowledge on coronavirus diagnosis, prognosis, and treatments has been accumulated, many areas of uncertainties remain. These uncertainties, particularly the absence of data on the long-term impact of COVID-19 vaccine, more than anything else, is responsible for the disparate responses being rolled out in different jurisdictions throughout the world. Among the responses are regulations regarding wearing of face masks, social distancing, washing of hands, and, more recently, vaccination.

On 23 December 2021, the Centre for Disaster Philanthropy (CDP) reported the number of confirmed cases of the disease to be nearly 269 million, out of which approximately 5.3 million people died globally.[11] Worse still, despite the administration of 9,571,502,663 vaccine doses, as of 19 January 2022, there have been 332,617,707 confirmed cases of COVID-19, including 5,551,314 deaths.[12] These are troubling numbers. Never before, at least since the Spanish influenza (H1N1) or flu pandemic of 1918, has the world witnessed a disease outbreak of cataclysmic proportion as that which began in 2019 – the coronavirus disease. Described as the 'most severe pandemic in recent history', the flu pandemic of 1918 infected about 500 million people or one-third of the world's population, with the number of deaths estimated to be at least 50 million worldwide.[13] It is against this background that the current battle against COVID-19 virus is to be understood, as predicated upon not letting history repeat itself.

Because the world is in uncharted waters, it is difficult to predict with any degree of certainty which intervention would work or vice versa. Although there seems to be a consensus that the starting point of any meaningful victory over the virus is attainment of herd immunity (i.e. when a large proportion of a given population becomes immune to the disease), the path to this goal is shrouded in controversy. While some favour attaining herd immunity through natural infection, others prefer the route of vaccines. A noteworthy proponent of the latter is WHO.[14] But although WHO advocates vaccination as an avenue to achieving herd immunity, it disavows the natural infection approach and compulsory vaccination.[15] Yet, several nations, most notably the US, are undeterred in imposing vaccine mandates upon their people, even on those with religious or other objections. This coercive exercise of power raises a number of questions, some of which have a significant bearing on the right to health and Africa. Should Africa join the bandwagon? In other words, is it appropriate for countries in the region to impose vaccine mandates? Responding to these questions is the task of this chapter, a task that is centred on analysing the ethicolegal and pragmatic considerations governing the relationship between the individual and the state in the realm of public health.

This chapter consists of six sections. Following this introduction, Section 5.2 discusses the state of the coronavirus pandemic in Africa – prevalence and response in the nature of vaccine mandates in select countries.

In Section 5.3, the position in the US is examined, namely the controversy regarding the adoption of the compulsory inoculation scheme by the different tiers of authority in the country. This situation is further examined – in Section 5.4 – in light of the seminal case on vaccine mandate, namely, *Jacobson v. Massachusetts*,[16] as well as relevant ethicolegal and pragmatic considerations. Next are two questions that are critical to understanding the thrust of this work. What does the right to health mean in the context of the vaccine mandate? Are governments which elect to respond to COVID-19 challenges via forced inoculation acting in compliance with the obligations imposed by international human rights law? Interrogating these questions is the subject of Section 5.5. The conclusion – Section 5.6 – projects medical freedom (medical decision-making without interference by a third party) as the most critical element of the right to health and therefore dispositive of the vaccine mandate controversy. It urges Africa not to toe the path of forced inoculation.

5.2 Africa, coronavirus infection, and compulsory vaccination

The current reality is that although no country or region of the world is spared the scourge of coronavirus infection, there is no uniformity in incidence and prevalence. For some inexplicable reasons, nations in Africa have not recorded a similar number of cases or deaths as in other regions. There are 408,455,826 cases of COVID-19 globally, with the highest numbers scattered across North and South Americas, Asia, and Europe.[17] As of 12 February 2022, according to data from the Kaiser Family Foundation (KFF), the US shoulders the highest number of cases (77,122, 131), followed by India and the UK, at 45,586,544 and 18,220,515 infections respectively.[18] The figures are much lower in Africa, with the three worst affected countries – South Africa, Ethiopia, and Nigeria – recording 3,637,673; 467,288; and 253,923 cases respectively.[19] The number of COVID-19-related deaths is also lower in Africa versus other parts of the world. At 914,009 deaths, the US leads the rest of the world, followed by Brazil (637,467), India (507,981), and Russia (332, 010).[20] In Africa, the number of deaths resulting from the infection in the three worst affected countries, namely, South Africa, Ethiopia, and Nigeria are 102,595; 7,574; and 3,155, respectively.[21]

Although the data from Africa pales in comparison to other regions, they are, nonetheless, a source of concern. No responsible government would fold its arms in the face of challenges affecting public safety, regardless of the number of victims. Perhaps, as a result, countries in Africa have adopted the WHO COVID-19 safety protocol, including handwashing, social distancing, and wearing of face coverings.[22] Many are even going as far as imposing vaccine mandate despite opposition, noted previously, from WHO.

In November 2021, Egypt began the implementation of a regulation banning public sector employees who were unvaccinated and untested from entering their offices.[23] Students in public universities were also prohibited from campuses if unvaccinated.[24] The ban from entering government offices was extended to members of the public who have not received at least one vaccine dose, effective 1 December 2021,[25] and by the end of the month, vaccine mandate was imposed on all Egyptians above 18 years.[26] The policy in Morocco is even more stringent. The government introduced a COVID-19 vaccine certificate on 26 October 2021.[27] Individuals who cannot provide the certificate were barred from entering public buildings and businesses, including hotels and restaurants.[28] The certificate was also required for intercity transportation. Non-compliance is punishable with up to three months' imprisonment or a fine of up to US$ 143.[29]

Ghana announced its own compulsory inoculation scheme on 28 November 2021, to become effective from 22 January 2022, but only for some segments of the population, namely, public sector and health workers.[30] The new policy under which, according to the country's Minister of Health, 'nobody would be compelled or forced to take the vaccine against their will', would require proof of full vaccination before anyone could enter government offices.[31] While students attending government schools are under no obligation to be vaccinated, those not vaccinated will be denied admission to the classroom,[32] and proof of vaccination will be required for night clubs, beaches, sports stadiums, and restaurants.[33] In Kenya, a proposed law, which will not force everyone to be inoculated but requires proof of vaccination to enter government offices as well as many businesses and restaurants,[34] was yet to take effect.[35]

Similarly, South Africa does not have a population-wide vaccine mandate. However, relying on guidelines from the Department of Labour, several private sector employers have imposed mandate on their workers.[36] Those who refuse inoculation will be denied access to the premises of their employers, and while some employers might fire them, others would not.[37] The right of employers to dismiss workers for refusing to be vaccinated has been upheld by the South African Conciliation, Mediation and Arbitration in *Theresa Mulderji v. Goldrush Group*.[38] Universities in the country are also issuing their own mandates. In one of such universities, staff, contract workers, and students are required to show proof of vaccination or negative COVID-19 result, otherwise, they will be denied access to the universities and their facilities.[39] While unvaccinated students are not barred from registering classes, they will not be permitted to enter the campus unless granted exemption.[40]

In Nigeria, the vaccine mandate is gradually being rolled out. Under the existing policy, employees of the central government are required to provide proof of vaccination or present a negative test result done within 72 hours.[41] Out of 36 federating units, only two – Edo and Ondo – have announced compulsory COVID-19 vaccination, but only for adults.[42] The order banning individuals without proof of vaccination from public places and large gatherings in Edo state[43] has been halted by the court. The rule in Ondo state, on the other hand, will deny people who are not vaccinated admission to churches, mosques, and other public places.[44]

As to the legitimacy or appropriateness of forced vaccination in Africa, opinion is divided – as is the case in other regions. While some applaud the measure as a necessary public health tool, others fault it on ethical, legal, and pragmatic grounds. Not surprisingly, human rights have been invoked on both sides of the aisle. Faisal Shuaib, who is the head of Nigeria's National Primary Healthcare Development Agency (NPHDA), asserts that individuals who refuse to take the vaccine are endangering the lives of those who have been vaccinated and those who are exempted for medical reasons.[45] As far as he is concerned, for unvaccinated individuals, 'we have to apply the basic rule of law, which stipulates that your human right stops where mine begins'.[46] He contends that although 'you have a right to refuse vaccines', it does not follow that you 'have the right to endanger the health of others'.[47] The Nigerian Medical Association (NMA) stakes a different position. The NMA sees no difference between coronavirus vaccine and other therapeutic interventions, a reason it argues that people have a 'right to reject vaccines the same way they could reject medical treatment'.[48]

In Morocco, the union of lawyers have faulted the country's forced inoculation scheme and requirement of vaccination certificate as an infraction of human rights. The situation is not different in other African nations. Following widespread disapproval and subsequent lawsuit against Kenya's compulsory vaccine programme, a high court in that country halted the implementation of the measure.[49] This summation by Human Rights Watch represents the view of many in Africa, '[i]f the government has an obligation to protect its population from serious threats to public health, the measures must be reasonable and proportionate'.[50] Reasonability and proportionality, as will become evident subsequently, is a legal and an ethical prescription.[51] Many believe that the COVID-19 mandate is neither reasonable nor proportionate to the goal of winning the battle against the pandemic – a subject that the rest of this chapter grapples with.

5.3 COVID-19 vaccine mandate in the US and extant regulations

Similar to other thorny issues in the US, responses to the pandemic in various jurisdictions across the country as well as by the central government mirror the political and ideological bent in each of the units of the government. The 'issue has become so politicised in the United States', intones legal scholar Debbie Kaminer, '[i]t's so tied in with people's political views that it is much more difficult to change someone's mind'.[52] Coercive enforcement measures such as wearing of face masks and vaccination, which are zealously promoted by the left-leaning administration at the centre, are more likely to be replicated in states and local authorities controlled by Democrats than in Republican states. This is also reflected in individual responses to the measures, as evident in a study which shows that of the unvaccinated Americans, the vast majority identify themselves as Republicans, at 60%, compared to 17% respectively of Democrats and Independents.[53]

This wide gulf between the right and left of the political spectrum in the US needs to be accentuated. At the core of the ideological chasm between Republicans and Democrats is the relationship between the individual and the government. Whereas the former is committed to ensuring a limited role for the state in the affairs of men, the latter holds differently. The idea of limited government, which finds expression in libertarian concepts such as individual autonomy[54] or personal liberty, sums up their political belief, explaining why Georgia's Republican Governor Brian Kemp describes the vaccine mandate as an 'unlawful and dangerous overreach' on the part of the Biden administration.[55] Democrats, on the other hand, are generally more accommodating of the paternalistic excesses of the government, as subsequent analysis clearly demonstrates.

5.3.1 Federal government vaccine mandate

The starting point of any meaningful discussion of a vaccine mandate in the US is to note that that there is no unit of government in the country that has decreed a vaccine mandate for all persons, at least not explicitly. Typically, as in the case of the federal government, an identified category of individuals (employees of the federal government, for instance) is specified as required to be vaccinated. Thus, one of the first acts of President Joseph Biden upon assumption of office was the issuance of an executive order requiring the Secretary of Labour, acting through the Assistant Secretary of Labour for Occupational Safety and Health (OSHA), to 'issue, within 2 weeks of the date of this order . . . revised guidance to employers on workplace safety during the COVID pandemic'.[56] The Labour Secretary was further directed to 'consider whether any emergency temporary standards [ETS] on COVID-19 . . . are necessary, and if such standards are determined to be necessary, issue them by March 15, 2021'.[57]

Having concluded that ETS (Rule) regarding coronavirus is needed in the workplace, OSHA issued a standard titled 'COVID-19 Vaccination and Testing ETS', which became effective on 5 November 2021.[58] Applicable to employers with 100 or more employees and designed to protect unvaccinated employees of large corporations from the risk of coronavirus infection in the workplace,[59] the relevant stipulations of the rule include the following:

- Covered employers must establish, implement, and enforce a mandatory coronavirus vaccination policy.
- Employees who are not fully vaccinated must undergo weekly testing and wear face coverings at the workplace or when occupying a vehicle with another person for work purpose.

- Exemptions are granted to those with religious or other legally recognized objections.

The rule applies to workers employed in workplaces that are under the authority and jurisdiction of OSHA, including industries as diverse as manufacturing, retail, health care, delivery services, warehouses, maritime, meatpacking, agriculture, construction, and logging, so long as the employer has a total of at least 100 employees.[60] Remarkably, and this is one of the most crucial aspects of the controversy surrounding forced coronavirus vaccination, the rule pre-empts and invalidates 'any State or local requirements that ban or limit an employer's authority to require vaccination, face covering, or testing' since OSHA considers contrary stipulations to be a barrier to its implementation of this rule and protection of workers in the US from COVID-19 infection.[61] In other words, compliance is mandatory for all employers of labour with the requisite number of workers, regardless of whether the law in the state or municipality where the industry or business is domiciled prescribes a contrary regime.

Relatedly, a subsequent executive order – this time requiring coronavirus vaccination for federal employees – was issued on 9 September 2021.[62] The executive order mandates the Safer Federal Workforce Task Force[63] to issue guidance within seven days of the date of the order on agency implementation of this requirement for all agencies covered by the order.[64] Consistent with this authority, the task force issued the guidance on 13 September 2021, which, aside from stipulating that all federal executive branch employees must be fully vaccinated, directs the relevant agencies to work expeditiously to ensure full compliance as quickly as possible, with 22 November 2021 specified as the deadline.[65]

Along similar trajectory, another executive order[66] mandates executive departments and agencies, including independent establishments dealing with the federal government, to comply with all guidance for contractor or subcontractor workplace locations published by the Safer Federal Workforce Task Force.[67] The mandate applies to any workplace locations in which an individual is working on or in connection with a federal government contract or contract-like instrument.[68] A subsequent guidance published by the task force was unequivocal as to the way it intends to fulfil this responsibility. It requires full vaccination of all covered contract employees and imposes upon covered contractors the responsibility for ensuring compliance.[69] Exemptions are restricted to employees claiming a medical or disability exemption or opposition to vaccination based on religious grounds.

Aside from federal civil servants and contractors, another demographic caught in the vaccine mandate imbroglio are health workers, including nursing home employees. On 5 November 2021, the Centers for Medicare & Medicaid Services (CMS) issued an interim final rule which revised the previous regulation that most Medicare- and Medicaid-certified providers and suppliers must comply with in order to remain eligible for funding under Medicare and Medicaid ~~Medicare~~ programmes.[70] This rule has octopus-like tentacles, encompassing hospitals, hospices, clinics, and nursing homes – all of whose staff are required to be vaccinated against coronavirus.[71] The rule, which was made under the authority granted to the secretary of Health and Human Services (HHS),[72] applies directly to providers regulated by CMS, whereas those not so regulated may be subject to OSHA regulations, such as the ones previously examined.[73] Exemptions are made, based on medical conditions or religious beliefs, observances, or practices.[74]

5.3.2 Vaccine mandate at the state level

Apparent from the introductory part of this section is that the approach regarding vaccine mandate and other coercive responses to the coronavirus pandemic in the US hinges greatly on the dominant political ideology in the jurisdiction in question. Accordingly, although mandatory vaccine programmes are favoured by the central government, permissive regimes are embraced by some, but not all, states. In some states – Montana and Tennessee, for instance – recently enacted legal and policy frameworks outrightly prohibit vaccine mandates.[75] As reported by the Associated Press, 'Republican-controlled Montana Legislature' has enacted a law[76] which prohibits 'requiring vaccines as a condition for employment', on the ground that to do otherwise would be discriminatory and a 'violation of the state's human rights laws'.[77] Tennessee, another Republican state, also passed legislation outlawing the vaccine mandate.[78] Tennessee law is noteworthy and illustrative of the ideological underpinning of vaccine mandate-nullifying statutes, such as this one and similar ones in other jurisdictions:[79]

i) The US Constitution does not prohibit the states from regulating health and medical practices, nor does it require any person to consent to any form of medical treatment, directly or indirectly, in relation to COVID-9.
ii) The right at common law to personal security and the liberty to be free from an unwanted touching of one's limbs and body was retained by the people of this state, and that right includes rights and duties with respect to medical treatment administered by other persons, such as through COVID-19 vaccinations.
iii) Informed consent between patients and healthcare practitioners protects the rights at common law of persons, and all such consent must be voluntary and not given under duress, coercion, misrepresentation, or fraud.
iv) Consistent with our constitutionally recognized and inalienable right of liberty, every person within this state is and must remain free to choose or to decline to be vaccinated against COVID-19 without penalty or threat of penalty.

These considerations are at the core of the opposition by Republican governors to the vaccine mandate of the Biden administration and are reflected in one form or the other in the legal regimes of affected states. Under the Tennessee statute, which was enacted on 12 November 2021,[80] governmental entity, school, or local education agency are forbidden from requiring proof of vaccination against coronavirus.[81] The same is true of private businesses.[82] Strikingly, the law exempts from being vaccinated or showing proof thereof any person that objects to being inoculated 'for any reason' whatsoever.[83]

The following week, the Republican governor of Florida signed a bill into law,[84] which bars all private employers, regardless of size, from compelling workers to be vaccinated.[85] The exemptions in the law, which departs significantly from the parochialism of the federal regulations examined previously, cover medical and religious reasons, employees who can demonstrate they have acquired natural immunity, those willing to undergo periodic testing, and so forth.[86]

Although the legislature in Texas is yet to act, the state's Republican governor issued an executive order on 11 October 2021, banning the vaccine mandate.[87] The sweeping order applies to any entity in the state, all of whom are barred from requiring vaccinations from employees or customers[88] who object 'for any reason of personal conscience, based on a religious belief, or for medical reasons, including prior recovery from COVID-19'.[89] Other states which have totally banned vaccine mandate or made exceptions regarding healthcare workers include Arizona, Arkansas,[90] Georgia, Indiana, New Hampshire, North Dakota, Oklahoma, and Utah.[91] Others include Alabama,[92] Iowa,[93] Kansas,[94] and West Virginia.[95]

What these states have in common is not geographical contiguity; they do not even have common boundaries. What unites them is a shared belief in limited government, in the republican ideals of freedom, explaining why all of them are conservative states, with Republican governors.[96] On 5 November 2021, more than half of the states in the country filed lawsuits challenging Biden administration's vaccine requirement for private businesses.[97] The lawsuits are seeking a determination by courts as to whether the Biden administration's COVID policy represents a proper exercise of legitimate authority or 'a federal power grab' that 'usurps the authority of states to set health policy'.[98]

Juxtaposing the foregoing with the situation in the rest of the country – Democratic states – reveals quite a completely different picture. On 26 July 2021, California Governor Gavin Newsom announced the imposition of the vaccine mandate on government employees, healthcare workers, and 'high-risk congregate' settings, all of whom must show proof of full vaccination or be tested at least once every week.[99] Two days later, New York Governor Andrew Cuomo followed suit.[100] Subsequent months witnessed the adoption of similar measures in other Democratic states, including Virginia, Washington, Hawaii, Oregon, and Maryland.[101]

5.3.3 Local authorities and compulsory vaccination

Multiple local authorities have enacted COVID regulations, affecting several aspects of normal life in the affected communities. In Washington, DC, individuals must present proof of vaccination before being allowed into certain establishments, namely, restaurants, nightclubs, taverns, coffee shops, movie theatres, live entertainment and sporting venues, gyms, and conference centres.[102] The rule applies to anyone 12 years and older and became operational on 15 February 2022.[103] The regulation in Chicago is even more draconian, requiring anyone five years and older to show proof of vaccination to dine indoors, visit gyms, or enter entertainment venues where food or drinks are served.[104] Boston's regulation took effect on 15 January 2022 and makes entry into certain indoor spaces contingent upon proof of vaccination.[105] People working in such establishments are also required to be vaccinated.[106] Similar mandates are also being implemented in Philadelphia, Los Angeles, Minneapolis, St. Paul, and New Orleans[107] as well as New York, San Francisco, and Seattle.[108]

Two commonalities among cities that have institutionalized vaccine mandates are that they are domiciled in Democratic states and led by Democrats. Conversely, cities in Republican states have refrained from imposing mandates on businesses and individuals. In fact, most of them have independently rolled back the impositions that heralded the onset of the pandemic in 2019 such as wearing of masks in public places, whereas others have acted in compliance with orders issued by their respective state governments. In May 2021, Republican states of Texas and Iowa enacted statutory frameworks precluding local government authorities from imposing their own mask mandates and schools from requiring students and teachers to wear face mask.[109] Other Republican states have passed a similar legislation.[110] Kansas Republican lawmakers went a step further by enacting a legislation permitting anyone aggrieved by coronavirus mandates to file a civil action against the state, local government, or school board, and the hearing of the suit must be expedited.[111]

5.3.4 Compulsory inoculation scheme and extant case law

Whereas the imposition of the COVID-19 vaccine mandate by the Biden administration was celebrated in some quarters, it was roundly rejected by others, especially in conservative circles.[112] Bemoans House Minority Leader Kevin McCarthy, a Republican, ~~stated~~ '[t]o Joe Biden, force is more important than freedom. Americans won't stand for it'.[113] Oklahoma Governor Kevin Stitt was even more resolute, '[a]s long as I am governor, there will be no government vaccine mandates in Oklahoma'.[114] Widespread condemnation of compulsory vaccination is to be understood in the context of a declaration by Biden the previous year, 'I don't think [vaccines] should be mandatory. I wouldn't demand it to be mandatory',[115] and a prior announcement by the White House that mandating vaccination is 'not the role of the federal government'.[116]

By the end of October 2021, four separate lawsuits had been filed challenging the administration's vaccine mandates.[117] Others are to follow, including from private businesses and non-profit organizations.[118] In one of the cases, *Missouri and other v. Biden and other*,[119] plaintiffs contended, *inter alia*, that the CMS vaccine mandate, which requires employees of health establishments receiving federal funding to be vaccinated, threatens the job of millions of healthcare workers who risked their lives in the early days of the pandemic to care for strangers and friends in their communities, and must be withdrawn.[120] The plaintiffs further argued that police power over compulsory vaccination has always been the province of – and still properly belongs to – the states and that federalism allows states to tailor such matters in the best interests of their communities, and, therefore, the court should set aside the CMS's nationwide mandate as an unlawful agency action under the Administrative Procedure Act.[121] Describing the vaccine mandate as 'arbitrary and capricious' and an exercise of power which the CMS does not have in the absence of congressional approval, US District Judge Matthew T. Schelp granted the prayer of the plaintiffs, enjoining the defendants from enforcing the vaccine mandate against the affected employees in the plaintiff states.[122] An appeal by the Biden administration for the injunction to be vacated was roundly rejected by the 8th Circuit Court of Appeals.[123]

In a different case, but on the same matter, which was brought by Louisiana and joined by 13 other states, a Louisiana US district judge issued a nationwide injunction against vaccine mandate for healthcare workers.[124] Still, in another case, the states of Missouri, Montana, Arizona, and Nebraska co-led an 11-state coalition, joined by five private employers, seeking an immediate halt to the implementation of the OSHA vaccine mandate on private employers with 100 or more employees pending judicial review.[125] That same month, the 5th US Circuit Court of Appeals in New Orleans issued an order blocking the OSHA mandate.[126] Several private entities have also filed lawsuits challenging the mandate, some against the federal government and others against local authorities. In one of such cases, firefighters, state troopers, and other state employees brought an action seeking nullification of a proclamation by Washington Governor Jay Inslee, a Democrat, that all healthcare, education, and state employees must be fully vaccinated by 18 October 2021 or face termination.[127] Rejecting the application for a temporary restraining order, the US District Court Judge Thomas Rice held that '[t]he Supreme Court has long endorsed state and local government authority to impose compulsory vaccines'.[128]

With all the lawsuits and conflicting decisions, what is the current situation regarding the two mandates, issued by OSHA and CMS respectively? As expected, the various lawsuits brought against the two mandates, including those not discussed in the preceding paragraphs, eventually wound up before the US Supreme Court. They were consolidated into two distinct cases.

In the first of the two cases, *National Federation of Independent Business v. Dep't of Labor*,[129] the US Supreme Court granted the application to stay the OSHA Rule which mandated businesses with 100 or more employees to require the workers to be vaccinated. One of the critical questions the court had to consider was whether the Occupational Safety and Health Act, which created the OSHA, plainly authorized the secretary's mandate. The court held that it does not, that the Act empowers the secretary to set workplace safety standards, not broad public health measures.[130] The court ruled that although Congress has indisputably given OSHA the power to regulate occupational dangers, it has not given that agency the power to regulate public health more broadly.[131]

Biden v. Missouri[132] was the second of the two consolidated cases. There, the US Supreme Court lifted the two injunctions restraining the Secretary of Health and Human Services (through the CMS) from enforcing the rule requiring facilities that participate in Medicare and Medicaid programmes to ensure that their workers are vaccinated against coronavirus. In a 5–4 decision, the court held that the secretary did not exceed his statutory authority in requiring that, in order to remain eligible for Medicare and Medicaid dollars, the facilities covered by the interim rule must ensure that their employees are vaccinated against COVID-19.[133] It held that the secretary has authority granted by Congress to require, as a condition for participation in the programmes, such conditions as he 'finds necessary in the interest of the health and safety of individuals who are furnished services'.[134] The court acknowledged that the vaccine mandate exceeded what the secretary has done in the past to control infection in the nation's health facilities but held the exercise justified because he has never had to address an infection of similar scale and scope as that brought about by COVID-19.[135]

5.4 Legal, ethical, and pragmatic considerations regarding the vaccine mandate

The aftermath of the rulings in *National Federation of Independent Business v. Dep't of Labor*[136] and *Biden v. Missouri*[137] is that pending judicial review of the substantive suits before the US Court of Appeals for the Fifth and Sixth Circuits, the OSHA mandate requiring businesses with 100 or more employees to ensure that the workers are vaccinated can no longer be implemented, whereas enforcement of the CMS rule requiring compulsory vaccination of workers in facilities receiving federal funding has been reinstated. Remarkably, the holdings by the US Supreme Court did not address the broader legal and ethical implications of compulsory vaccine mandate. Therefore, even if it is conceded, as the plaintiffs contended in *Missouri v. Biden*,[138] that police powers over compulsory vaccination fall within the powers of states and not the federal government, this does not address the question whether a competent adult may be compulsorily vaccinated against his will. Is compulsory vaccination consistent with protection of individual liberty? Is there a right of refusal?

To respond to this question, we seek insight from a case decided more than a century ago by the US Supreme Court – *Jacobson v. Massachusetts*.[139] At issue was whether a Massachusetts law which empowers towns and cities to compulsorily vaccinate their citizens against smallpox was constitutional. Having experienced adverse reaction to vaccination as a child, Jacobson refused vaccination and was fined five dollars. His central argument was that subjecting him to a fine or imprisonment on account of his refusal to be vaccinated constitutes an invasion of his liberty, the right of individuals to determine for themselves how to treat their health and bodies. The court disagreed, holding that although the constitution guarantees individual liberty, the guarantee is not absolute.[140] The court held that the statute in question is a health law and a legitimate exercise of the police power of the state of Massachusetts to protect the health and safety of its citizens. 'The safety and the health of the people of Massachusetts are' primarily 'for that Commonwealth to guard and protect . . . [and] do not ordinarily concern the National Government'.[141] This was the point canvassed all along by Republican governors against the vaccine mandates of the Biden administration. Apart from affirming that regulating public health and public safety falls within the police power of states, the court made two observations that are relevant to the thrust of this chapter.

Firstly, where the police power of a state is exercised in an arbitrary or oppressive manner, the courts would intervene. Therefore, where as a result of the particular condition of the health or body of an individual, subjecting him to vaccination would be cruel and inhuman, the courts would 'be competent to interfere and protect the health and life of the individual concerned'.[142] Secondly, where it is 'apparent or can be shown with reasonable certainty' that an individual 'is not at the time a fit subject of vaccination or that vaccination, by reason of his then condition, would seriously impair his health or probably cause his death', the court would intervene.[143] Given that that the court felt that Jacobson did not situate himself within the exempted class, his conviction was sustained. The court concluded that since he appears to be 'in perfect health and a fit subject of vaccination' and remains in the community, he cannot be allowed to refuse to obey the legal framework designed 'for the protection of the public health and the public safety, confessedly endangered by the presence of a dangerous disease'.[144]

Remarkably, although the US Supreme Court did not define what the term 'a fit subject of vaccination' means or when vaccination law becomes wrongful or oppressive, it seems likely that laws which do not respect these boundaries would likely be struck down as unconstitutional. But exactly how far the courts would be prepared to go in such cases is not at all clear, especially considering the rejection of a childhood adverse reaction to vaccination as a basis for the refusal of Jacobson to be vaccinated. One would have deemed this experience to have qualified Jacobson as not being 'a fit subject of vaccination', but the court held otherwise, in deference to the common good of the community. The question then becomes, would the supreme court restate the ruling in *Jacobson v. Massachusetts*,[145] by upholding the vaccine mandate of the Biden Administration or chart a different course, as canvased by the states suing the administration?

The ethical principle of autonomy empowers individuals to do anything that appeals to them, but this entitlement is subject to a very important caveat, namely, so long as the action in question does not harm another person. The same principle is expressed in law as liberty of the person or right to self-determination, which encapsulates the right to privacy (right to be let alone)[146] and the right to bodily integrity. The right to bodily integrity, institutionalized in *Schloendorff v. Society of New York Hospitals*,[147] confers upon '[e]very human being of adult years and sound mind . . . a right to determine what shall be done with his own body' and punishes any interference without consent as 'an assault for which [the person will be] liable in damages'.[148] Cases on the right to informed consent are legion[149] and need not be rehearsed. Nonetheless, it is crucial to specifically identify the right among the constellation of rights whose invasion is being resisted by opponents of compulsory vaccination.

But does forced inoculation really amount to a breach of human rights? Bioethicist Mathew Liao disagrees, reasoning that 'when you don't get vaccinated, you're putting people in danger'.[150] It is this line of thought that incubates arguments such as this one – that private business owners have a right to control their environments. 'They want to be able to tell everyone, "when you come here, you're safe" '.[151] The idea is that workers also have a right to feel safe at their places of employment.[152]

Concern about these interests is quite legitimate. The difficulty is how to balance them. This is certainly not an easy task. To hold, as does health law and policy scholar Mark Hall, that '[b]ecause one person's choice affects the health of other people and the public at large, people do not have a fundamental right to refuse vaccination',[153] clearly misses the point. There are solid ethicolegal grounds for refusing to submit oneself to COVID-19 vaccine or any vaccine or medical treatment for that matter – for instance, those imbedded in health and religious reasons.[154] But unlike OSHA and CMS regulations, which accommodate only these two grounds, the relevant laws in several Republican states are more permissive. As previously indicated, the executive order issued by Governor Greg Abbot, for example, exempts from vaccination anyone who objects 'for any reason of personal conscience, based on a religious belief, or for medical reasons, including prior recovery from COVID-19'.[155]

Recognizing prior recovery from exposure to coronavirus as a ground for refusal to be vaccinated is controversial. As pointed out in the introductory section, although WHO is opposed to compulsory vaccination, it does not support attaining herd immunity through exposing people to the virus, the reason being that it would result in unnecessary infections, suffering, and death.[156] Still, although WHO holds that exposing people to a virus in an attempt to reach herd immunity is scientifically and ethically problematic,[157] this position is not shared by everyone, explaining why the number of jurisdictions in the US granting mandate waivers to those who had suffered coronavirus infection is rising.[158] Opposition to recognizing natural immunity centres on three points. Firstly, there is no certainty as to how long naturally acquired immunity lasts; but the same deficit of knowledge exists regarding vaccines, explaining the need for booster shots. Moreover, there is a study by the US National Institutes of Health (NIH) which concludes that immunity acquired after coronavirus infection can last up to eight months.[159] The second objection is that there is no simplified means of identifying those with natural immunity. Third is the claim that even if it is conceded that survivors of prior infections acquire natural protection against the virus, vaccination would give them extra-strong protection – called hybrid immunity.[160] If so, the argument goes, why not just get vaccinated? An interesting response is provided by a professor at George Mason University, 'vaccinating the naturally immune is medically unnecessary'.[161] Although this claim is disputed, supporting evidence abound.[162]

Researchers in Israel have discovered that natural immunity confers longer lasting and stronger protection against coronavirus than immunity acquired through vaccination.[163] Dvir Aran, a biomedical data scientist involved in analysing Israeli data on vaccine effectiveness, affirms that available data suggest that the 'recovered have better protection than people who were vaccinated'.[164] This study has been corroborated.[165] Following the assessment of a database of the entire population for the purpose of comparing the efficacy of vaccination with previous infection, another set of Israeli researchers found nearly identical numbers.[166] Their conclusion is striking, '[o]ur results question the need to vaccinate previously infected individuals'.[167] There is another study from Malawi, a country where just 5% of the population has been fully vaccinated, which attributes very low cases of COVID-19 in that country to the high number of individuals who have been previously infected (as many as 80%) and thereby acquired immunity.[168] Similar studies have been carried out in other African countries including Kenya, Madagascar, and South Africa, with similar results.[169]

In light of the cacophony of opinions and positions, what is the correct approach to adopt? A helpful response is the principle enshrined in *Tarasoff v. Regents of the University of California*,[170] namely, '[t]he protective privilege ends where the public peril begins'.[171] But while this principle offers some guidance, its utility in resolving the controversy is quite limited. It is a general principle of law that does not easily lend itself to a precise definition. One might ask, for instance, at what point does the exercise of individual liberty cross into the domain of communal interest? Who determines this point?

Regarding public health challenges such as coronavirus, if it is affirmed, in line with case law, that the duty belongs to the states, it behoves these federating units to draw the appropriate boundary, where individual liberty must yield to communal interest. The fact that the vast majority of jurisdictions in the US (27 states)[172] are decidedly opposed to compulsory vaccination suggests that a different approach, one that respects individual choices, especially one that was the product of an informed medical opinion, is warranted. It is about respect for medical freedom. The claim by the George Mason University professor that subjecting him to vaccination was 'medically unnecessary' was based on the advice of an immunologist, on account of having tested positive for COVID-19 antibodies on five different occasions.[173] Moreover, medicine has advanced tremendously since 1905, when *Jacobson v. Massachusetts*[174] was decided, and this should be taken into consideration in fashioning the right approach to the pandemic.

Furthermore, coronavirus infection is treatable and does not represent the death sentence once attributed to it. Aside from controversial drugs such as ivermectin, lopinavir/ritonavir and hydroxychloroquine, there are proven therapies that have either received full approval by the US Food and Drug Administration (FDA) or been authorized for emergency use. Among these are antiviral therapies such as molnupiravir, Paxlovid, and remdesivir; monoclonal antibodies including REGN-COV2 (casirivimab and imdevimab), bamlanivimab, etesevimab, and sotrovimab; and immunomodulatory agents such as corticosteroids, tocilizumab, sarilumab, and siltuximab.[175] Moreover, in late 2021, it was announced that two companies have developed pills specifically for treating COVID-19. The pill produced by Merck is called molnupiravir, and the other one, known as Paxlovid, was manufactured by Pfizer.[176] In light of these developments, it is difficult to resist a departure from the stringency of the vaccine mandate of the Biden administration or similar measures elsewhere.

To wrap up this section, we consider this explication of the rights to privacy and bodily integrity, *to wit*, '[h]uman rights protect our bodies and our ability to be the masters of our bodies', and the 'consequence of this is our ability to determine our medical treatments'.[177] In substituting private discussions and agreements between patients and their doctors with government interposition, forced inoculation directly offends this very important principle of human rights and ethics. Nonetheless, as emphasized previously, human rights are not absolute, and this has two significant implications. Firstly, as human rights scholar Kanstantsin Dzehtsiarou explains, 'governments can interfere with [human rights] if they can justify such interference as necessary for and proportionate to the achievement of another valuable goal'.[178] This is indeed true and must be analysed in terms that if we accept, as we should, that the word 'necessary' means 'needed', the question then becomes, is the vaccine mandate needed for treatment of coronavirus infection? The response must be affirmative since the vaccines have proven useful, but the same is true of the other alternative methods of treatment previously enumerated.

The next question centres on whether forced vaccination is proportionate to the goal sought to be achieved, namely, eliminating coronavirus infection as a threat to public health? Since the word 'proportionate' connotes 'commensurability', one wonders how forceful invasion of the constellation of human rights indicated previously is proportionate to attaining a goal that could be achieved through other less coercive means. This concern leads directly to the second implication. Both human rights and constitutional law require that in limiting the rights of individuals for the purposes of attaining a higher goal, as in the vaccine mandate, the least restrictive means must be employed.[179] In this context, it must be noted that the availability of drugs for the virus provides an 'equally effective alternative to protect public health'.[180] Moreover, aside from the availability of drugs, there are other means of controlling the spread of the infection which respects medical freedom, for instance, by encouraging individuals to take up the vaccine through incentive schemes such as free or subsidized food, money awards, and gifts. These are clearly less restrictive means of fighting coronavirus and are consistent with human rights, particularly the right to health, as the next section demonstrates.

5.5 The right to health and the COVID-19 vaccine mandate

Though the arguments of the previous section that vaccine mandates amount to a breach of numerous rights, including privacy, informed consent, bodily integrity, and so forth, have obvious bearing upon the right to health, re-exploring them is not necessary. Instead, a more useful approach would be to focus on two questions which are critical to understanding the thrust of this work. What does the right to health mean in the context of a vaccine mandate? In electing to respond to COVID-19 challenges through forced inoculation, are governments acting in compliance with the obligations imposed by international human rights law?

The term 'right to health' refers to the entitlement of everyone to the enjoyment of a 'variety of facilities, goods, services, and conditions' that are necessary for maintaining or restoring health.[181] That an individual has a right to health does not mean that he has a right to be healthy,[182] since no person or institution can guarantee health. This is because even in abundance of healthcare facilities and complementary goods and services, other factors, such as genetics or pure carelessness, could and often play a significant role in one's health.[183] It was this understanding that prompted the rejection by the Third Committee of the UN General Assembly (Third Committee) of the definition of health contained in the preamble to the Constitution of WHO, as 'a state of complete physical, mental and social well-being and not merely the absence of disease or infirmity'.[184] Instead, the Third Committee considered, as more acceptable, the definition enshrined in the UDHR[185] in 1948 – as the entitlement of everyone 'to a standard of living adequate for the health of himself and of his family, including food, clothing, housing and medical care and necessary social services'.[186]

Consistent with the UDHR definition, the Third Committee developed the position that is now incorporated in Article 12 of the International Covenant on Economic, Social, and Cultural Rights (ICESCR), depicting the right to health as 'the right of everyone to the enjoyment of the highest attainable standard of physical and mental health' and specifying a number of 'steps to be taken by the States Parties . . . to achieve the full realization of this right'.[187] As to its contours, the Third Committee was unequivocal that the right to health should not be construed as a right to health care; instead, the right must be broadly interpreted to include of a gamut of socio-economic factors that promote conditions in which people can lead a healthy life, and extend to the underlying or social determinants of health, such as food and nutrition, housing, access to safe and potable water and adequate sanitation, safe and healthy working conditions, and a healthy environment.[188] This is very important, for often the conditions in which people live and work (social or underlying health determinants) are more important than access to health care.

Aside from the ICESCR, there are at least three major regional frameworks that are relevant to the right to health in Africa, namely, the African Charter on Human and Peoples' Rights (African Charter),[189] African Charter on the Rights and Welfare of the Child (ACRWC),[190] and the Protocol to the African Charter on Human and Peoples' Rights on the Rights of Women in Africa (Maputo Protocol).[191] Nevertheless, since the guarantees relating to health in these frameworks mirror the stipulations in ICESCR, discussing the provisions of the former is not necessary. More relevant to the goal of this chapter is elucidating how the right to health interfaces with the COVID-19 vaccine mandate – an interface that is intertwined with the obligations imposed by the right to health.

Like other human rights, a tripartite obligation, namely, the obligation to *respect, protect*, and *fulfil* (RESRPROFIL) the right to health, is imposed upon states parties to ICESCR and other related legal regimes.[192] To *respect* the right to health means that states are to refrain from denying or limiting equal access for all people, including the vulnerable population.[193] Included within this heading is the obligation to desist from 'applying coercive medical treatments, unless on an exceptional basis for the treatment of . . . or the prevention and control of communicable diseases'.[194] Whether this obligation is justificatory of coercive inoculation against coronavirus is subject to serious legal and ethical analysis, the kind that was pursued in the preceding section of this chapter. Particularly considering, as previously explained, that other less restrictive and equally effective responses to the infection are available, forcible administration of vaccines directly offends the obligation to respect the right to health. There is no 'exceptional basis' justifying a coercive response when non-coercive measures are available. The obligation to *protect*[195] foists a duty upon states to restrain third parties from interference with the enjoyment of the right to health.[196] Under this obligation, third parties, including private sector employers, are prohibited from obstructing the right to health, such as by requiring coronavirus inoculation as a condition of employment.

The third legal obligation, to *fulfil*, mandates states to adopt appropriate legislative, administrative, budgetary, judicial, promotional, and other measures towards the full realization of the right to health.[197] This obligation is perhaps the most important of the three in terms of its impact on the subject being discussed. It centres directly on the propriety or legitimacy of the means of responding to public health challenges such as the one presented by the pandemic. In this sense, a relevant question to ask regarding the duty to fulfil is whether regulations imposing vaccination on people are an appropriate means of discharging the obligation of states regarding the right to health in the context of coronavirus infection. The preceding section returned a negative response. States that choose to operationalize their response to the pandemic by adopting legal or policy frameworks that authorize forced inoculation (thereby deviating from the doctrine of informed consent) are flouting the obligation to fulfil the right to health. To be compliant, legislative or other measures must allow individuals to choose among the various options available to shield themselves from infections or attain recovery upon being infected.

Aside from the RESRPROFIL obligations, another means of assessing whether state parties to the ICESCR are compliant with the international human rights law is to gauge the compatibility of extant legal and policy frameworks in their jurisdictions with the essential elements of the right to health, namely, availability, accessibility, acceptability and quality (the AAAQ paradigm) of existing health services and delivery.[198] *Availability* means that for the right to health to be actualized, there must be available, in sufficient quantity within the territory of the state party, functioning public health and healthcare facilities, goods, and services, as well as complementary programmes.[199] A*ccessibility* implies that health facilities, goods, and services must not only be available in sufficient quantity, but they must also be accessible to everyone within the jurisdiction of the state party without discrimination.[200] *Acceptability*, the third element, requires all health facilities, goods, and services to be respectful of medical ethics and culturally appropriate, that is, respectful of the culture of the people, sensitive to gender and life-cycle requirements, and designed to respect confidentiality and improve the health status of the people.[201] *Quality* means that in addition to being culturally acceptable, health facilities, goods, and services must also be scientifically and medically appropriate and of good quality. Attaining quality requires having an adequate number of skilled medical personnel, scientifically approved and unexpired drugs and hospital equipment, safe and potable water, and adequate sanitation.[202]

Although the four elements – the AAAQ paradigm – are important for actualizing the right to health, the most relevant to the topic at hand are *Acceptability* and *Quality*. Regarding the former, which requires therapies to be respectful of medical ethics, the discussion in the previous section (on autonomy, privacy, and informed consent) has shown the shortcomings of forced inoculation when effective alternatives are available. Therefore, the vaccine mandate fails the test of acceptability of health services. The latter, which requires therapy to 'be scientifically and medically appropriate and of good quality',[203] is to be examined in the context of the question of whether the COVID-19 vaccines are safe. Two points must be made. Firstly, there is no consensus regarding the quality of available vaccines. Proof is the recently recommended booster shots, which were not envisaged at the time the drugs became available on the market and which has led to the question: How many booster shots are enough? Secondly, despite claims by the US and WHO regarding the safety of the vaccines, the reality is that there is no credible data on the long-term effects of the drug. This uncertainty, which is a major factor driving reluctance to submit to vaccination, casts doubt as to whether the vaccines meet the threshold of quality as an essential element of the right to health.

5.6 Conclusion

The polemic regarding the vaccine mandate can be summed up as a conflict between paternalistic inclinations of the government or government overreach, on one hand, and individual autonomy and yearning for human freedom, on the other. It is a dichotomy between an unrelentingly burdensome notion of protecting public health versus the protection of the right to health. The right to health encapsulates the doctrine of informed consent and medical freedom, the autonomous decision of competent individuals and their doctors regarding health care, free of intrusion by third parties, including the government. This is not to suggest that government intervention in healthcare is a violation of human rights. To the contrary, and as evident in the

RESPROFIL obligations and the AAAQ paradigm, government involvement in the delivery of health services is a necessity.

To set the record straight, the COVID-19 mandate is generally defended on the basis that the vaccine is safe and represents the most effective means of combating the virus, and there is no equally effective alternative therapy. But against this position are several counter-arguments, among which are the following:

(a) In contrast to the claim of mandate apologetics that vaccination is the most effective means of controlling coronavirus and that no equally effective alternatives exist, drugs are currently available to treat COVID-19 infection, as pointed out in Section 5.4 of this chapter. Moreover, naturally acquired immunity provides an equally (if not more) effective protection, explaining why, apart from several jurisdictions in the US, countries such as Italy[204] and Germany[205] are increasingly recognizing proof of natural immunity from a recent infection as sufficient to exempt individuals from forced inoculation.

(b) Data on the long-term effects of the vaccines are non-existent, and, therefore, it is reasonable to be concerned about possible adverse consequences or harm that may arise in the future.

(c) Compulsory vaccination is unethical in that, firstly, by discounting alternatives such as drugs and natural immunity, it fails the proportionality test; secondly, it is not unavoidably necessary or needed in light of alternatives and reasonable concerns about the long-term effect of the vaccines; thirdly, on account of its coercive nature versus other alternatives, it fails the least restrictive test; fourthly, it is unfair because it treats those with natural immunity as equally vulnerable to infection and equally threatening to others; and fifthly, it substitutes autonomously made individual preferences with paternalism, by permitting the intrusion of a third party (government/its agents) on physician–patient relationships.

(d) Multiple human rights are endangered when people are ordered to be vaccinated against their will, including the right to life, the right to health, right to personal liberty and self-determination, right to privacy and bodily integrity, and so forth.

(e) The *Tarasoff* principle, *to wit*, '[t]he protective privilege ends where the public peril begins',[206] which is often cited in defence of the position that the human rights said to have been compromised by the vaccine mandate are not absolute, is not tenable given the availability of drugs for the treatment of the infection and the efficacy of naturally acquired immunity.

(f) Vaccination, properly defined, is designed to inoculate recipients against infection from the targeted organism or illness. None of the coronavirus vaccines offers full immunity against infection; otherwise, there would be no need for booster shots, which are currently being encouraged (and likely to be mandated shortly) in several countries.

On the strength of the foregoing, a reasonable conclusion would be that individual preferences must be respected – in other words, a paradigm shift from the paternalism of compulsory vaccination to medical freedom. This is the path recommended to countries in Africa. In a BBC exclusive interview, following his refusal to be vaccinated and subsequent ban from competing in the Australian Open, Novak Djokovic, the top tennis player in the world, was asked whether he is 'prepared to forgo the chance to be the greatest player that ever picked up the racket, statistically', and he responded in the affirmative, '[y]es . . . I do' and that is '[b]ecause the principles of decision-making on my body are more important than any title or anything else'.[207] Deducible from this response is that individual preference or medical freedom, the right of individuals to decide for themselves in the realm of medicine, which is encapsulated within the ethicolegal regimes and pragmatic considerations explored in Sections 5.4 and 5.5 of this chapter, is of greater importance than any perceived benefit, whatsoever it is, to be derived from compulsory COVID-19 vaccination.

5.7 Acknowledgment

For their insightful questions and comments, which significantly improved the quality of this work, I thank my health law and human rights students and, of course, KasiemObi Nnamuchi, my able assistant. The usual caveats apply.

Notes

1 WebMD 'Coronavirus History' available at www.webmd.com/lung/coronavirus-history#:~:text=But%20how%20did%20SARS%2DCoV,set%20off%20a%20global%20pandemic (accessed 15 October 2023). www.chr.up.ac.za
2 See Biology/LibreTexts '9.3A: The international committee on taxonomy of viruses' available at https://bio.libretexts.org/Bookshelves/Microbiology/Book%3A_Microbiology_(Boundless)/9%3A_Viruses/9.3%3A_Classifying_Viruses/9.3A%3A_The_International_Committee_on_Taxonomy_of_Viruses (accessed 15 October 2023).
3 WHO 'Naming the coronavirus disease (COVID-19) and the virus that causes it' available at www.who.int/emergencies/diseases/novel-coronavirus-2019/technical-guidance/naming-the-coronavirus-disease-(covid-2019)-and-the-virus-that-causes-it (accessed 15 October 2023).
4 As above.
5 As above.
6 WHO 'Coronavirus Disease (COVID–19)' available at www.who.int/health-topics/coronavirus#tab=tab_1 (accessed 15 October 2023).
7 WHO 'Coronavirus Disease (COVID–19)' available at www.who.int/health-topics/coronavirus#tab=tab_3 (accessed 15 October 2023).
8 As above.
9 CDC 'People with certain medical conditions' 25 February 2022 available at www.cdc.gov/coronavirus/2019-ncov/need-extra-precautions/people-with-medical-conditions.html (accessed 15 October 2023).

10 As above.
11 Center for Disaster Philanthropy 'COVID-19 coronavirus' 23 December 2021 available at https://disasterphilanthropy.org/disaster/2019-ncov-coronavirus/?gclid=Cj0KCQiAw9qOBhC-ARIsAG-rdn4FFhXSN2PypJNEPMURVg0h-XJ7SsOv_OJ5Hc0atzRYGFZ5KquqMH4aAqZ0EALw_wcB (accessed 15 October 2023).
12 WHO 'WHO coronavirus (COVID-19) dashboard' available at https://covid19.who.int/ (accessed 15 October 2023).
13 CDC 'History of 1918 flu pandemic' available at www.cdc.gov/flu/pandemic-resources/1918-commemoration/1918-pandemic-history.htm (accessed 15 October 2023).
14 WHO 'Coronavirus disease (COVID-19): Herd immunity, lockdowns and COVID-19' 31 December 2020 available at www.who.int/news-room/questions-and-answers/item/herd-immunity-lockdowns-and-covid-19 (accessed 15 October 2023).
15 As above.
16 Jacobson v. Massachusetts 197 U.S. 11 (1905).
17 KFF 'Global COVID-19 Tracker – Updated as of February 12 2022' available at www.kff.org/coronavirus-covid-19/issue-brief/global-covid-19-tracker/ (accessed 15 October 2023).
18 As above.
19 As above.
20 As above.
21 As above.
22 WHO 'Advice for the public: Coronavirus disease (COVID-19)' Updated 1 October 2021 available at www.who.int/emergencies/diseases/novel-coronavirus-2019/advice-for-public#:~:text=Clean%20your%20hands%20frequently%20with,self%2Disolate%20until%20you%20recover (accessed 15 October 2023).
23 Reuters 'Egypt introduces ban on unvaccinated public sector employees' 15 November 2021 available at www.reuters.com/world/middle-east/egypt-introduces-ban-unvaccinated-public-sector-employees-2021-11-15/ (accessed 15 October 2023).
24 As above.
25 As above.
26 Egypt Today Staff 'Egypt: COVID-19 vaccination mandatory for those above 18 yrs' *Egypt Today* 26 December 2021 available at www.egypttoday.com/Article/1/111235/Egypt-COVID-19-vaccination-mandatory-for-those-above-18-yrs (accessed 15 October 2023).
27 Crisis24 'Morocco: Authorities introduce vaccine pass to access public buildings and businesses as of Oct. 26/update 75' 26 October 2021 available at https://crisis24.garda.com/alerts/2021/10/morocco-authorities-introduce-vaccine-pass-to-access-public-buildings-and-businesses-as-of-oct-26-update-75(accessed 15 October 2023).
28 As above.
29 As above.
30 Reuters 'Ghana to make COVID-19 vaccine mandatory for targeted groups from January' 28 November 2021 available at www.reuters.com/world/africa/ghana-make-covid-19-vaccine-mandatory-targeted-groups-january-2021-11–28/ (accessed 15 October 2023).
31 GhanaToday 'COVID-19 jabs won't be compulsory but will be required to access government facilities – Health Minister' 26 December 2021 available at https://allafrica.com/stories/202112260078.html (accessed 15 October 2023).
32 As above.

33 Reuters (n 30 above).
34 AL Dahir 'Kenya will impose widespread restrictions on the unvaccinated starting next month' *New York Times* 22 November 2021 available at www.nytimes.com/2021/11/22/world/africa/kenya-covid-vaccination-mandate.html (accessed 15 October 2023).
35 A Slimi 'Kenyan High Court temporarily suspends controversial vaccine mandate' *Foreign Brief* available at www.foreignbrief.com/daily-news/kenyan-high-court-temporarily-suspends-controversial-vaccine-mandate/ (accessed 15 October 2023).
36 The Conversation 'Vaccine mandates in South Africa: Where are they most needed?' 7 December 2021 available at https://theconversation.com/vaccine-mandates-in-south-africa-where-are-they-most-needed-173253 (accessed 15 October 2023).
37 X Mtembu 'Here are some of the country's companies who have announced mandatory COVID-19 vaccine policies for their employees' *IOL News* 6 December 2021 available at www.iol.co.za/business-report/companies/here-are-some-of-the-countrys-companies-who-have-announced-mandatory-covid-19-vaccine-policies-for-their-employees-24942608-3b6f-48269fe8-3b99123f8450 (accessed 15 October 2023).
38 I Lawrence & EM Okojie 'Mandatory vaccinations in the workplace: SA's CCMA hands down an important decision' *ENSafrica* 26 January 2021 available at www.ensafrica.com/news/detail/5173/mandatory-vaccinations-in-the-workplace-sas-c (accessed 15 October 2023).
39 G Makhafola 'UFS joins Wits and UWC in implementing vaccine mandate for staff, students on campus' *News24* 27 November 2021 available at www.news24.com/news24/southafrica/news/ufs-joins-wits-and-uwc-in-implementing-vaccine-mandate-for-staff-students-on-campus-20211127(accessed 15 October 2023).
40 As above.
41 J Erunke 'COVID-19: FG approves vaccine mandate policy for all staff' *Vanguard* 27 November 2021 available at www.vanguardngr.com/2021/11/covid-19-fg-approves-vaccine-mandate-policy-for-all-staff/ (accessed 15 October 2023).
42 A Odusote 'Compulsory COVID-19 vaccination in Nigeria? Why it's illegal, and a bad idea' *The Conversation* 8 September 2021 available at https://theconversation.com/compulsory-covid-19-vaccination-in-nigeria-why-its-illegal-and-a-bad-idea-167396 (accessed 15 October 2023).
43 D Ojerinde et al 'Compulsory vaccination: NMA, JOHESU kick as FG threatens sanction' *Punch* 1 September 2021 available at https://punchng.com/compul sory-vaccination-nma-johesu-kick-as-fg-threatens-sanction/ (accessed 15 October 2023).
44 As above.
45 As above.
46 As above.
47 As above.
48 As above.
49 Africanews 'Kenyan court suspends government's COVID vaccine certificate plan' 14 December 2021 available at www.africanews.com/2021/12/14/kenyan-court-suspends-government-s-covid-vaccine-certificate-plan// (accessed 15 October 2023).
50 As above.
51 J Savulescu 'Good reasons to vaccinate: Mandatory or payment for risk?' (2021) 47 *Journal of Medical Ethics* 78–85.
52 Z Rasheed 'Should COVID-19 vaccines be mandatory?' *Al Jazeera* 18 October 2021 available at www.aljazeera.com/news/2021/10/18/should-covid-19-vaccines-be-mandatory (accessed 15 October 2023).

53 A Kirzinger et al 'KFF COVID-19 vaccine monitor: The increasing importance of partisanship in predicting COVID-19 vaccination status' 16 November 2021 available at www.kff.org/coronavirus-covid-19/poll-finding/importance-of-partisanship-predicting-vaccination-status/ (accessed 15 October 2023).
54 TL Beauchamp & JF Childress *Principles of biomedical ethics* (Fifth Edition) (2001) 57–58.
55 T Gibson 'Gov. Kemp: Federal vaccine mandates "unlawful, dangerous overreach"' *News4JAX* 3 November 2021 available at www.news4jax.com/news/local/2021/11/03/gov-kemp-federal-vaccine-mandates-unlawful-dangerous-overreach/ (accessed 15 October 2023).
56 Executive Order 13999 of 21 January 2021 'Protecting worker health and safety' Federal Register Vol. 86, No. 15 Tuesday, 26 January 2021 sec 2(a), 7211.
57 As above sec 2(b).
58 COVID-19 Vaccination and Testing; Emergency Temporary Standard, Federal Register/Vol. 86, No. 212/Friday, 5 November 2021/Rules and Regulations, 61402
59 OSHA 'Emergency temporary standard, summary: COVID-19 vaccination and testing ETS' available at www.osha.gov/sites/default/files/publications/OSHA4162.pdf (accessed 15 October 2023).
60 As above.
61 United States Department of Labor 'Occupational safety and health administration, emergency temporary standard' available at www.osha.gov/coronavirus/ets2/faqs (accessed 15 October 2023).
62 'Executive order 14043 of 9 September 2021, requiring coronavirus disease 2019 vaccination for federal employees' Federal Register/Vol. 86, No. 175/Tuesday, 14 September 2021, sec 2, Presidential Documents, 50989.
63 Executive Order 13991 of 20 January 2021, Protecting the federal workforce and requiring mask-wearing, Federal Register/Vol. 86, No. 14/Monday, 25 January 2021/Presidential Documents, 7045. This executive order established the Task Force. See sec 4.
64 Executive Order 14043 (n 62 above) sec 2.
65 Safer Federal Workforce Task Force 'COVID-19 workplace safety: Agency model safety principles' 13 September 2021 available at https://www.saferfederalworkforce.gov/downloads/SFWTF_model%20agency%20safety%20principles_20220915.pdf.
66 Executive Order 14042 of 9 September 2021 'Ensuring adequate COVID safety protocols for federal contractors' Federal Register/Vol. 86, No. 175/Tuesday, 14 September 2021/Presidential Documents 50985.
67 As above sec 2.
68 As above.
69 Safer Federal Workforce Task Force 'COVID-19 workplace safety: Guidance for federal contractors and subcontractors' 10 November 2021.
70 Federal Register/Vol. 86, No. 212/Friday, 5 November 2021/Rules and Regulations, 61555.
71 As above, 61560.
72 As above.
73 As above, 61556.
74 As above, 61572.
75 L Mendelson 'Mandatory employee vaccines – coming to a state near you?' 27 January 2022 available at www.littler.com/publication-press/publication/mandatory-employee-vaccines-coming-state-near-you (accessed 15 October 2023).
76 Montana 'An Act prohibiting discrimination based on a person's vaccination status or possession of an immunity passport; Providing an exception and an exemption; Providing an appropriation, and providing effective dates' H.B.702 sec 1.

77 Associated Press 'Montana alone in banning vaccine requirements for employees' 20 August 2021 available at www.usnews.com/news/best-states/montana/articles/2021-08-20/montana-alone-in-banning-vaccine-requirements-for-employees (accessed 15 October 2023).
78 Tennessee Code sec 14–1–103.
79 Tennessee Code sec 14–1–102.
80 M Brown, DW Gang & YS Yu 'Tennessee Gov. Bill Lee signs sweeping COVID-19 legislation into law' *Nashville Tennessean* 12 November 2021 available at www.tennessean.com/story/news/politics/2021/11/12/tennessee-gov-bill-lee-covid-19-legislation-general-assembly-legislature-businesses-masks/6264103001/ (accessed 15 October 2023).
81 Tennessee Code sec 14–2–101, sec 14–2–102.
82 Tennessee Code sec 14–2–102.
83 Tennessee Code sec 14–2–102(a).
84 Florida H B 1B (2021).
85 A Castro & M L Janes 'What employers need to know about Florida's ban on vaccine mandates' 29 November 2021 available at www.shrm.org/resourcesandtools/legal-and-compliance/state-and-local-updates/pages/florida-ban-on-vaccine-mandates.aspx#:~:text=During%20a%20special%20legislative%20session,by%20the%20governor%20on%20Nov (accessed 15 October 2023).
86 As above.
87 R Allen 'Texas Gov. Greg Abbott bans any COVID-19 vaccine mandates – including for private employers' *Texas Tribune* 11 October 2021 availableatwww.texastribune.org/2021/10/11/texas-greg-abbott-covid-19-vaccine-mandate/ (accessed 15 October 2023).
88 As above.
89 Executive Order GA-40 relating to prohibiting vaccine mandates, subject to legislative action, sec 1, 11 October 2021.
90 Arkansas, H B 1977 'An Act concerning issues related to coronavirus (COVID-19); To provide employee exemption from federal mandates and employer mandates related to coronavirus 2019 (COVID-19); To declare an emergency; And for other purposes (2021)'.
91 H Mitchell '12 states banning COVID-19 vaccine mandates & how they affect healthcare workers' *Becker's Hospital Review* 12 October 2021 available at www.beckershospitalreview.com/workforce/11-states-banning-covid-19-vaccine-mandates-how-it-affects-healthcare-workers.html (accessed 15 October 2023).
92 Alabama, Act 2021–561.
93 Iowa, House File 902 'An Act relating to COVID-19 vaccination requirements by employers and unemployment insurance and including effective date provisions' (2021).
94 Kansas, H B 2001 (2021).
95 West Virginia, H B 335 (2021).
96 Mitchell (n 91 above).
97 DA Lieb, G Mulvihill & A Demillo 'At least 27 states file lawsuits over Biden's vaccine mandate for businesses' *Associated Press* 5 November 2021 available at www.10tv.com/article/news/nation-world/biden-vaccine-mandate-for-businesses-lawsuit/507-a15c24eb-a0eb-4f96-bed3-9823c79d1aa0 (accessed 15 October 2023).
98 As above.
99 E Davis Jr 'Governors start mandating the COVID-19 vaccine for state employees' *U.S. News* 29 July 2021 available at www.usnews.com/news/best-states/articles/2021-07-29/these-governors-are-mandating-the-covid-19-vaccine-for-government-employees (accessed 15 October 2023).
100 As above.

101 As above.
102 K Smith 'List: COVID-19 vaccine measures across U.S. cities, states' *News Nation* 3 January 2022 available at www.newsnationnow.com/health/coronavirus/covid-vaccine-requirements/ (accessed 15 October 2023).
103 As above.
104 As above.
105 As above.
106 As above.
107 F Brown 'Unlocking the world: Twin cities join other US tourist spots turning to indoor vaccine or testing mandates' *CNN* 13 January 2022 available at www.cnn.com/travel/article/major-us-cities-vaccine-test-mandates-covid-19/index.html (accessed 15 October 2023).
108 As above.
109 A Durkee 'Mask mandates now banned for local governments and schools in growing number of GOP states' *Forbes* 20 May 2021 available at www.forbes.com/sites/alisondurkee/2021/05/20/mask-mandates-now-banned-for-local-governments-and-schools-in-growing-number-of-gop-states/?sh=7157853266bf (accessed 15 October 2023).
110 As above.
111 T Wu 'New law limiting local COVID-19 orders accelerates rollback of restrictions across Kansas' *Topeka Capital-Journal* 10 April 2021 available at www.cjonline.com/story/news/coronavirus/2021/04/10/new-law-limiting-local-covid-19-orders-accelerates-restrictions-rollback-kansas-politics-county-city/7153366002/ (accessed 15 October 2023).
112 A Wise &T Keith 'Biden lays out plan to mandate vaccines or testing for millions of workers' *National Public Radio* 9 September 2021 available at www.npr.org/2021/09/09/1035149651/biden-will-require-vaccines-for-federal-workers-as-part-of-a-new-covid-strategy (accessed 15 October 2023).
113 As above.
114 As above.
115 M Braun & S M Capito 'Biden promised no vaccine mandates; the Senate will vote to overturn his private employee mandate' *Washington Examiner* 8 December 2021 available at www.washingtonexaminer.com/opinion/op-eds/joe-biden-promised-no-vaccine-mandates-the-senate-will-vote-to-overturn-his-private-employee-mandate (accessed 15 October 2023).
116 The White House 'Press briefing by press secretary Jen Psaki' 23 July 2021 available at www.whitehouse. gov/briefing-room/press-briefings/2021/07/23/press-briefing-by-press-secretary-jen-psaki-july-23-2021/ (accessed 15 October 2023).
117 The Associated Press '19 states sue Biden administration over COVID vaccine rule' 30 October 2021 available at https://federalnewsnetwork.com/management/2021/10/10-states-sue-biden-administration-over-covid-vaccine-rule/ (accessed 15 October 2023).
118 See for instance In re MCP No. 165, 20 F. 4th 264 (2021).
119 Missouri & Ors v. Biden & Ors, No. 4:21 CV 1300 DDN (E.D. Mo. 20 December 2021).
120 Plaintiffs' Brief, Missouri & Ors v. Biden & Ors, No. 4:21-cv-01329 (E.D. Mo. 10 November 2021) para 1–2.
121 As above para 4.
122 A Durkee 'Appeals court refuses to put Biden's vaccine mandate for healthcare workers back into effect' *Forbes* 13 December 2021 available at www.forbes.com/sites/alisondurkee/2021/12/13/appeals-court-refuses-to-put-bidens-vaccine-mandate-for-healthcare-workers-back-into-effect/?sh=5d78ff5f60bd (accessed 15 October 2023).
123 As above.

124 G Hilburn 'Louisiana judge blocks nationwide COVID-19 vaccine mandate for health care workers' *Lafayette Daily Advertiser* 30 November 2021 available at www.theadvertiser.com/story/news/2021/11/30/louisiana-federal-judge-blocks-biden-national-covid-vaccine-mandate-healthcare-workers/8806478002/ (accessed 15 October 2023).
125 J Lagasse 'Eleven states file lawsuit over vaccine mandate for private businesses' *Healthcare Finance* 8 November 2021 available at www.healthcarefinancenews.com/news/eleven-states-file-lawsuit-over-vaccine-mandate-private-businesses (accessed 15 October 2023).
126 Hilburn (n 124 above).
127 M Hunt 'Federal judge denies lawsuit brought by state employees to stop Washington vaccine mandate' *KREM Television* 25 October 2021 available at www.krem.com/article/news/health/coronavirus/vaccine/federal-judge-spokane-denies-motion-washington-vaccine-mandate/293-97f611bc-64fb-4187-9788-1e4d0e747f7f (accessed 15 October 2023).
128 As above.
129 National Federation of Independent Business v. Dep't of Labor (consolidated with Ohio, et al, v. Dep't of Labor) 595 U. S. ____ (2022)
130 As above, 6.
131 As above, 9.
132 Biden v. Missouri (consolidated with Becerra v. Louisiana), 595 U. S. ____ (2022)
133 As above, 8.
134 As above, 5, citing 42 U. S. C. sec1395x(e)(9).
135 As above, 7.
136 National Federation of Independent Business v. Dep't of Labor (consolidated with Ohio, et al, v. Dep't of Labor) 595 U. S. ____ (2022)
137 Biden v. Missouri (consolidated with Becerra v. Louisiana), 595 U. S. ____ (2022)
138 Plaintiffs' Brief (n 120 above) para 4.
139 Jacobson v. Massachusetts (n 16 above).
140 As above, 27, citing Crowley v. Christensen, 137 U.S. 86, 89 (1890).
141 As above, 38.
142 As above, 38–39.
143 As above, 39.
144 As above.
145 As above.
146 SD Warren & LD Brandeis 'The right to Privacy' (1890) 4(5) *Harvard Law Review* 195. See also Olmstead v. U.S., 277 U.S. 438, 478 (1928) (Justice Brandeis, dissenting).
147 Schloendorff v. Society of New York Hospital, 211 N.Y. 125 (N.Y. Ct. App. 1914).
148 As above, 129–130.
149 See for instance Canterbury v. Spence, 464 F.2d 772 at 282–283 (1972).
150 S Todd 'Do mandatory vaccines violate human rights?' *Quartz* 2 August 2021 available at https://qz.com/2042743/do-mandatory-vaccines-violate-human-rights/ (accessed 15 October 2023).
151 As above.
152 As above.
153 As above.
154 As above.
155 Executive Order GA-40, sec 1, Relating to prohibiting vaccine mandates, subject to legislative action, 11 October 2021.
156 WHO (n 14 above).
157 As above.

158 A Izaguirre 'GOP embraces disputed argument for natural immunity as substitute for vaccines' *AP/Los Angeles Times* 21 November 2021 available at www.latimes.com/world-nation/story/2021-11-21/gop-embraces-natural-immunity-as-substitute-for-vaccines/ (accessed 15 October 2023).
159 S Reynolds 'Lasting immunity found after recovery from COVID-19' *NIH* 26 January 2021 available at www.nih.gov/news-events/nih-research-matters/lasting-immunity-found-after-recovery-covid-19#main-content/ (accessed 15 October 2023).
160 Izaguirre (n 158 above)
161 K Clarey 'George Mason University grants vaccine exemption following prof's lawsuit' *Dive* 26 August 2021 available at www.hrdive.com/news/george-mason-university-grants-vaccine-exemption-following-profs-lawsuit/605382/ (accessed 15 October 2023).
162 See JM Dan 'Immunological memory to SARS-CoV-2 assessed for up to 8 months after infection' *Science* 6 January 2021 available at www.ncbi.nlm.nih.gov/pmc/articles/PMC7919858// (accessed 15 October 2023).
163 S Gazit et al 'Comparing SARS-CoV-2 natural immunity to vaccine-induced immunity: Reinfections versus breakthrough infections' *MedRxiv Preprint* available at https://doi.org/10.1101/2021.08.24.21262415 (accessed 25 August 2021).
164 J Block 'Vaccinating people who have had COVID-19: Why doesn't natural immunity count in the US?' (2021) 374 *British Medical Journal* 2272 available at www.bmj.com/content/374/bmj.n2101.full (accessed 15 October 2023).
165 Y Goldberg et al 'Protection of previous SARS-CoV-2 infection is similar to that of BNT162b2 vaccine protection: A three-month nationwide experience from Israel' *medRxiv* 2021.04.20.21255670 available at https://doi.org/10.1101/2021.04.20.21255670 (accessed 4 April 2021).
166 As above.
167 As above.
168 N Aizenman 'Africa may have reached the pandemic's holy grail' *National Public Radio* 28 January 2022 available at www.npr.org/sections/goatsandsoda/2022/01/28/1072591923/africa-may-have-reached-the-pandemics-holy-grail (accessed 15 October 2023).
169 As above.
170 Tarasoff v. Regents of the University of California, 551 P. 2d 334 (Cal. 1976).
171 As above, 347.
172 Lieb et al (n 97 above).
173 Clarey (n 161 above).
174 Jacobson v. Massachusetts (n 16 above).
175 M Cascella et al 'Features, evaluation, and treatment of coronavirus (COVID-19)' *StatPearls [Internet]* 5 January 2022 available at www.ncbi.nlm.nih.gov/books/NBK554776/ (accessed 15 October 2023).
176 P Autwaerter & A Casadevall 'Is COVID-19 treatable?' *John Hopkins Medicine* 23 November 2021 available at www.hopkinsmedicine.org/health/conditions-and-diseases/coronavirus/coronavirus-treatment-whats-in-development (accessed 15 October 2023).
177 Z Rasheed 'Should COVID-19 vaccines be mandatory?' *Al Jazeera* 18 October 2021 available at www.aljazeera.com/news/2021/10/18/should-covid-19-vaccines-be-mandatory (accessed 15 October 2023).
178 As above.
179 See for instance Huffman v. State, 204 P. 3d 339, 347 (Alaska 2009).
180 Rasheed (n 177 above).
181 UN Committee on Economic, Social and Cultural Rights, General Comment 14, The Right to the Highest Attainable Standard of Health (Twenty-second

session, 2000), para 9, UN Doc. E/C.12/2000/4 (2000), reprinted in Compilation of General Comments and General Recommendations Adopted by Human Rights Treaty Bodies, U.N. Doc. HRI/GEN/1/Rev.6 at 85 (2003) (General Comment No 14).

182 As above, para 8.

183 As above, para 9.

184 As above, para 4.

185 Universal Declaration of Human Rights, G.A. res. 217A (III), U.N. Doc A/810, 71 (1948).

186 As above, art 25.

187 International Covenant on Economic, Social and Cultural Rights, Art. 12, G.A. res. 2200A (XXI), 21 UN GAOR Supp. (No. 16) at 49, U.N. Doc. A/6316 (1966), 993 UNTS 3, *entered into force* 3 January 1976.

188 General Comment No 14 (n 181 above) para 4.

189 African [Banjul] Charter on Human and Peoples' Rights, adopted 27 June 1981, OAU Doc. CAB/LEG/67/3 rev. 5, 21 *International Legal Materials* 58 (1982), *entered into force* 12 October 1986. See art 16.

190 African Charter on the Rights and Welfare of the Child, Art. 14, OAU Doc. CAB/LEG/24.9/49 (1990), *entered into force* 29 November 1999.

191 Protocol to the African Charter on Human and Peoples' Rights on the Rights of Women in Africa, Art. 14, Adopted by the 2nd Ordinary Session of the Assembly of the Union, Maputo, CAB/LEG/66.6 (13 September 2000), *entered into force* 25 November 2005.

192 General Comment No 14 (n 181 above) para 33.

193 As above, para 34.

194 As above.

195 As above, para 35.

196 As above, para 33.

197 As above, para 34.

198 As above, para 12.

199 As above, para 12(a).

200 As above, para 12(b).

201 As above, para 12(c).

202 As above, para 12(d).

203 As above.

204 L Lonas 'Italy requires all workers to present COVID-19 health passes' *The Hill* 16 September 2021 available at https://thehill.com/policy/healthcare/572646-italy-requires-all-workers-to-present-covid-19-health-passes (accessed 15 October 2023)

205 BBC 'COVID-19: Germany puts strict curbs on unvaccinated and families criticise 'sickening' No 10 party' 2 December 2021 available at www.bbc.com/news/uk-59498880 (accessed 15 October 2023).

206 Tarasoff v. Regents (n 170 above).

207 A Rajan 'Novak Djokovic willing to miss tournaments over vaccine' *BBC* 16 February 2022 available at www.bbc.com/news/world-60354068 (accessed 15 October 2023).

6

AN INTERSECTIONAL PERSPECTIVE ON INEQUALITIES IN ACCESS TO COVID-19 VACCINES IN AFRICA

The case of migrants

Aisosa Jennifer Omoruyi

6.1 Introduction

While the world is no longer in crisis mode due to COVID-19,[1] the WHO Director-General also warned that given the risk of new variants emerging and causing new surges, countries must not let their guard down but sustain and strengthen the health system capacity gains in response to the pandemic for the future. The Director-General also highlighted the need to build stronger and more resilient people, communities, and health systems from now on.[2] The impact of COVID-19, especially on vulnerable and marginalized individuals and groups, cannot be ignored, especially as they demonstrated distinct and intensified dimensions of vulnerability. States must also learn from the human rights and service delivery failures during the pandemic and design measures to build back better.

The COVID-19 pandemic exacerbated existing vulnerabilities relating to income, gender, education, and disability, among others, leaving already marginalized or disadvantaged groups in a dire position. This manifested in loss of livelihood, the disproportionate impact of lockdowns, limited access to online education, inability to maintain necessary hygiene and social distance or isolation due to poor housing conditions, food insecurity, and limited access to healthcare services and vaccines. The experiences, failures, good practices, and lessons are essential for the design of measures to protect these groups from mutually reinforcing shocks, especially in the case of possible future public health crises.

Vaccination was a significant pillar of the global recovery from the COVID-19 pandemic, and this required access and uptake to be substantial to achieve herd immunity. However, inequality was very glaring in access to

DOI: 10.4324/9781032671437-8

vaccines between countries globally, demonstrated in vaccine nationalism by high-income countries (HICs). The situation of Africa in the race for access to vaccines was not unexpected, given that the continent had usually lagged in the queue for new health technologies, including vaccines. The capacity to produce medicines and vaccines is low in Africa, as less than 2% of drugs consumed in Africa are made on the continent.[3] As of April 2022, more than a year after many HICs already began vaccine administration, many African countries were yet to meet the 70% population target, placing the continent at the bottom of the global vaccine coverage.[4] Beyond the vaccine inequality at the global level, a critical issue was how countries implemented vaccination plans. Within countries, inequalities existed in rollout plans that excluded certain disadvantaged groups. The allocation and access to vaccines should be based on the right to enjoy the highest attainable standard of health without distinction based on race, religion, political belief, economic, or any other social condition.

Despite equality and non-discrimination being critical components in the realization of the right to health, there were real concerns about COVID-19 vaccines reaching historically vulnerable and marginalized communities in Africa who had also been largely neglected or underrepresented in the COVID-19 response in terms of both safeguarding their health and cushioning the socio-economic impact. Vulnerable and marginalized persons in this circumstance would include racial/ethnic minorities, people living with disabilities, the elderly, groups affected by humanitarian emergencies, migrants, refugees, asylum seekers, indigenous communities, and nomadic pastoralists, among others.[5] Several conditions characterize these groups, including being poor; dire living conditions; having a high disease burden; having disadvantage in accessing social services, including health care; and sometimes hard to reach due to geographical location[6] or transient movements.[7] The disadvantages experienced by various groups were often the result of an intersection of multiple factors such as gender, socio-economic status, race, age, migration status, and disability. It is also important to note that the pandemic had somewhat redefined vulnerability as persons or groups could become vulnerable or face marginalization due to the effects of the pandemic.[8] Vaccine rollout plans in Africa demonstrated government blind spots, and where some marginalized groups were included on paper, little was done to ensure they got vaccinated.[9] Given that vaccination is part of healthcare delivery, it was unsurprising that these groups encountered challenges in accessing COVID-19 vaccination. However, their exclusion made COVID-19 a disease of poverty, further exacerbating existing inequalities.

Among the obligations of states in realizing the right to health is to ensure universal immunization against major infectious diseases and take measures to prevent, treat, and control epidemic and endemic diseases.[10] The African Commission has also emphasized the need to ensure access to essential medicines to all without discrimination.[11] Based on these obligations, this chapter adapts the theory of intersectionality as a framework to assess the marginalization of certain groups of people in accessing COVID-19 vaccines in Africa. It draws insights from the challenges faced by migrants in the vaccine rollout process. While migration occurs within countries, the analysis here refers to foreign nationals with various temporary or permanent residence permits, such as migrant workers, asylum seekers, refugees, and undocumented migrants.[12] It emphasizes the need to contextualize the impact of a public health emergency on various groups and design responses accordingly. While the discussions here relate to the COVID-19 pandemic and access to vaccines for vulnerable groups, the lessons can be applied in future public health crises to ensure everyone can access needed health services rather than just vaccines.

6.2 Contextualizing the problem

Amid global health inequalities, access to COVID-19 vaccines in adequate quantities in Africa was a significant challenge.[13] This was, however, not surprising given that the continent has always fallen behind in the queue for new technologies and medicines, including vaccines.[14] While the rates of infection and death from COVID-19 may not have been as severe in Africa as in the US and Europe, the threat posed by the emergence of new variants and the pandemic's health, economic, and social effects could not be ignored.[15] Access to the COVID-19 vaccine, in addition to adequate testing and necessary hygiene and social distancing measures, was critical to bringing the infection rates under control.[16] However, the absence of equity in distribution and access posed a significant challenge, intensifying the need to level uneven power dynamics and ensure equitable access.[17] The issue of equitable access to COVID-19 vaccines is related to equity between countries in the global supply of vaccines and within countries in ensuring no population group was unfairly marginalized in the rollout process.[18] The focus of this chapter is on the latter.

Several HICs were criticized for hoarding vaccines and practicing vaccine nationalism at a time when most low- and middle-income countries (LMICs) had received nothing.[19] Another important issue was for governments to ensure that similar unequal access is not the case at the country level through rollout plans that exclude certain vulnerable groups,[20] hence the calls for effective and fair prioritization of groups for vaccination.[21] With a boost in supply worldwide, COVID-19 vaccines became increasingly available to all (except young children), unlike during the early rollout phase where certain groups such as health and essential workers, older persons, and people with co-morbidities were prioritized. With booster doses recommended and what seemed like a periodic vaccination in the future, countries had to grapple with ensuring that vaccines reached all groups on an equal basis and in a sustainable and timely manner. The exclusion of certain groups in the vaccination programme because of little to no consideration of their plight or structural barriers to access remained a concern.

The COVID-19 pandemic had the effect of deepening inequality and exacerbating vulnerabilities of ordinarily marginalized people in various ways, and a response that factors in these differential impacts and varied limitations is essential. The theory of intersectionality prompts such contextual understanding. The idea finds application where there is a need to contextualize or understand the differential experience of a phenomenon to respond to it adequately. Taking the COVID-19 pandemic as an example, while everyone is at risk of contracting the disease and has been impacted in some way, the experience varied across groups, even those historically vulnerable and marginalized. Existing gender and social inequalities were exacerbated by the pandemic and affected various groups in different ways.[22] In managing the pandemic and its effects, there were tendencies for governments to be race-blind, class-blind, and even gender-blind, including being blind to its impact on other identities such as persons with disabilities and ethnic minorities, among others, as well as persons in difficult situations such as armed conflict, humanitarian emergency, and people experiencing homelessness.[23] The absence of viewing how the COVID-19 pandemic overlaps with pre-existing disadvantages rather than a blanket attribution of the nature of vulnerability or marginalization often led to a failure in the response, especially in access to vaccines.

6.3 Adapting the theory of intersectionality to understand the impact of the COVID-19 pandemic on vulnerable and marginalized groups

Rooted in Black feminism[24] and critical race theory,[25] the feminist theory of intersectionality originates in the work of Kimberly Crenshaw.[26] Crenshaw drew attention to the intersectionality of race and gender in defining the experience of black women in the US as opposed to white women and black men whose experiences were used to inform the law and discourses against race and sex discrimination. Intersectional discrimination had mainly remained hidden due to the essentialist understanding of identity, which reduced people to a few traits constituting the identity, thus excluding features not associated with the group.[27] This gave rise to the exclusionary tendencies inherent in forming groups and their interests.

The theory of intersectionality stems from the premise that people have layered identities derived from social relations and the operations of power structures. The approach provides a framework or methodology for understanding how intersecting power systems influence the experience of groups of people bound by similar identities in society. Power in this regard is the process of privileging, normalizing, and placing a more excellent value on specific identities over others. Power in most societies is organized along the axes of identities such as gender, race, and class, as well as sexuality, ability, age, nationality, and religion, among others.[28] In this structure, some identities are more valued or normalized than others because they are differentiated from those considered less valued or less normal, creating privileges and disadvantages. These hierarchies are socially constructed rather than reflecting traits, capacities, or experiences.[29] These power structures go beyond distinguishing individuals but determine to a large extent access to resources and various social institutions such as government, work, education, family, law, media, and medicine, among others. This structure creates the existence of privileged identities alongside marginalised intersecting identities.[30] An intersectional perspective aids the analysis of how systems of privilege and disadvantage interact in people's lives based on their peculiar identities and how these structures of power inseparably link with and shape each other to create unique and qualitatively different experiences of oppression.[31]

From its initial conceptions, intersectionality has evolved into an understanding that all grounds of discrimination could interact with each other and produce unique experiences of discrimination. The definition of intersectionality offered by Carbado *et al.* as a method and a disposition, a heuristic and analytic tool'[32] captures how the theory has evolved as an analysis in progress.[33] The idea is among few that have applied widely beyond its initial conception to various social identities and issues across disciplines and geographical boundaries.[34] The way the intersectionality theory has evolved has been considered as creating a lively and provocative travelogue reflecting its adaptation, redirection, and contestation.[35] Although criticized as ambiguous and open-ended, this attribute has been considered the secret of its success and an essential contribution to feminist scholarship.[36] Given that the theory is not an effort to identify an exhaustive list of intersectional social categories, it is not confined to any subjects or identities.[37] This travelogue has also shown that the theory was not completed by its initial comprehension, articulation, or movement; instead, it has been an ongoing analysis. Scholars and activists have broadened intersectionality to various issues, social identities, power dynamics, and political and legal systems in multiple jurisdictions beyond the US.[38] Beyond black women, the theory has also been used to understand how intersecting identities affect the experience of discrimination or marginalization of other groups such as men,[39] children,[40] and older people.[41] The engagement with intersectionality has also been employed across disciplines, creating interdisciplinary links and pushing theoretical and normative debates.[42]

It has been suggested that African experiences need to be considered in theory building,[43] and the theory of intersectionality has found expression in understanding the concerns of women in Africa despite its origin in Western feminist thought and experience. Intersectionality presents an interesting paradox because it facilitates a contextual understanding of experiences rather than a blanket attribution of the source of their marginalization.

It has been applied widely in Africa to understand the influence of multiple forms of discrimination that shape the lived experiences of several groups of women, men, and children in various African contexts. A special issue in the 2017 edition of *Agenda* journal[44] was dedicated to exploring the meaning and application of intersectionality in different African contexts, primarily focused on South Africa. It reflected issues, including how intersectionality is lived and subjectively experienced in various contexts.[45] Scholars in Africa have applied the theory to different identities, including men,[46] children,[47] and multiple groups of women, including older people,[48] refugees, and migrants.[49] Several contexts have also been explored, such as education,[50] marriage,[51] disability,[52] employment and earning inequality,[53] and access to water.[54] These identity groups and contexts studied in Africa draw attention to unique challenges faced by different groups of persons on the continent.[55] The literature demonstrates how context, including place and history, social status, marital status, profession or occupation, and nationality, might be essential identity categories in African contexts. Applying the theory in Africa resonates with the earlier travelogue described as one of adaptation and redirection.[56] It demonstrates both the durability of the concept and the possibilities and richness that African perspectives can offer scholarship on intersectionality.[57]

This chapter adapts the theory to the COVID-19 pandemic as a tool to assess the unique challenges of migrants in accessing COVID-19 vaccines and the failure of states to recognize group disadvantages in the vaccine rollout process. The travelogue, to a large extent, demonstrates that the theory finds application where there is a need to contextualize or understand the differential experience of a phenomenon to respond to it adequately. Some people were disadvantaged in accessing COVID-19 vaccines for various reasons, and understanding these peculiarities helps develop a holistic response plan or strategy that ensures no one is left behind. This would require designing approaches to address the fundamental limitations of specific groups where necessary rather than a one-size-fits-all or essentialist approach.

Despite the familiar reassurance that everyone is 'in this together' or that COVID-19 'is the great equalizer',[58] one clear impact of the COVID-19 pandemic has been the deepening of inequality and vulnerabilities for people marginalized by the intersection of various factors such as race, ethnicity, national origin, immigration status, disability, gender, age, and income, among others.[59] Structural inequalities befall several marginalized groups who bear the hardest and disproportionate effect of shocks, including climate change, drought, and COVID-19. In several ways, the results of the pandemic and restrictions aimed at curbing the spread exacerbated the suffering of already marginalized and vulnerable populations such as the poor, indigenous communities, rural dwellers, people with disabilities, people affected by armed conflict or other humanitarian emergencies, asylum seekers and refugees, and migrants, among others. In the same vein, the lack of attention to their specific needs in the pandemic response plans also further marginalized and heightened the sufferings of these groups, especially in the absence of adequate social safety protections. Before the pandemic, they were already experiencing unequal access to social services, including health care, precarious housing conditions, food insecurity, tenuous living and working conditions, and a higher risk of exploitation and abuse due to their peculiar circumstances. The impact on the labour market was also dire for these groups due to job losses, given that working remotely, which became very popular, is highly correlated with education and formal employment, under which they are not significantly represented.

Studies have demonstrated the disadvantage suffered by various groups, including people with disabilities,[60] indigenous groups,[61] refugees, migrants, and rural dwellers, among others, in access to COVID-19 vaccines.[62] How each person or group experiences the effect of the COVID-19 pandemic is seen as a manifestation of the intersection of structures of inequality.[63] The following section highlights how the pandemic impacted migrants and how their peculiar circumstances defined exclusion from the response plan including in accessing vaccines.

6.4 Inequalities in accessing COVID-19 vaccines in Africa – migrants

This section highlights the experience of migrants in accessing COVID-19 vaccines in Africa, specifically the barriers they encountered. Migrants have no internationally accepted definition but generally comprise persons living outside their countries, usually to seek greener pastures, seek education, or be with family.[64] Although there are legal differences between migrants such as refugees and asylum seekers,[65] for this chapter, migrants mean foreign nationals comprising those with various temporary or permanent residence permits such as migrant workers, asylum seekers, refugees, and undocumented migrants.

Many migrants live in situations of vulnerability from having to contend with poverty, xenophobia, racism and discrimination, trafficking, inadequate housing conditions, lack of or inadequate support networks, insecure and challenging conditions of employment, risk of detention, language barriers, and challenges in access to health-care and other social services compared to citizens.[66] Besides the pandemic, many members of this group are often vulnerable to poor health because of their low socio-economic status, immigration status, and non-national status,[67] indicating multiple intersecting points of vulnerability. Undocumented migrants[68] face significant challenges in accessing social services, including health care and an enduring threat of arrest and deportation.[69]

The African Commission has noted the severe and disproportionate impact of the COVID-19 pandemic on migrants.[70] Refugees, asylum seekers, and undocumented migrants especially were at risk of contracting COVID-19 in camps and reception centres with tenuous living conditions with little to no means of socially distancing or maintaining proper hygiene or self-isolating in the event of an illness.[71] These groups face challenges accessing healthcare services for several reasons, including language barriers, lack of identity documents and their legal status. They are often excluded from national health promotion and disease prevention programmes, even during the COVID-19 pandemic.[72] In a study exploring the exclusion of migrants in health care in Gauteng Province, South Africa, 19.2% of health workers reported discrimination against migrants, while 20% reported differential treatment of migrants.[73] In Libya, a survey of migrants and refugees in Tripoli found that 45% of respondents were unsure how to seek care if they experienced symptoms of COVID-19 in addition to reduced access to work and lack of basic needs.[74] Sadly, such exclusions have public health implications that transcend this group, impacting citizens alike, especially in COVID-19, which requires very cautious infection control measures that must include everyone.

As of March 2022, the United Nations High Commissioner for Refugees (UNHCR) noted that while over 160 countries included refugees in vaccination plans on paper, the reality was far from inclusive due to administrative barriers, capacity, and logistics issues that hindered refugees from accessing vaccines.[75] The International Organization for Migration (IOM) further confirmed this, highlighting the discrepancy between migration inclusion plans and practice linked to several factors, including administrative/policy barriers, financial, technical, vaccine availability, information barrier/mistrust, xenophobia, and discrimination.[76] This was amplified by the fact that 80% of refugees are hosted in LMICs that faced critical vaccine inequity and implementation challenges.[77] The UNHCR reports showed that total vaccination rates of refugees in countries such as Ethiopia, Sudan, and Uganda were as low as 0.05%.[78] Only a few vaccination plans in Africa fit migrants into the rollout process, and even where they were, in reality, access remained a challenge.[79] Restricting their access to vaccination in the face of vulnerability was another form of discrimination against these groups. As such, there were calls for including migrants in the COVID-19 response, particularly regarding vaccine access, considering their often-precarious legal status and increased vulnerabilities to COVID-19 and associated health risks.[80] This required countries to adopt a 'migration aware' approach to COVID-19 vaccination plans in which population movement is considered in designing and implementing policies and other interventions.[81]

In South Africa, the High Court in Pretoria in *Scalabrini Center of Cape Town and Another v. Minister of Social Development and Others*[82] declared as unconstitutional the directives issued by the Minister of Social Development, given that it excluded asylum seekers and special permit holders from accessing the COVID-19 social relief of distress grant. This case is significant in highlighting the social exclusions migrants face, and it was also a wake-up call to the government to avoid excluding vulnerable groups in response plans, including COVID-19 vaccination. It was suggested that in creating criteria for vaccine prioritization, attention must be given to those migrants who are most exposed and vulnerable to infection for several reasons, including being in irregular situations; having low-income; living in camps or unsafe conditions, in immigration detention; and those in transit.[83]

The absence of documentation, identification, or irregular status was another hurdle to accessing COVID-19 vaccines. Given the need to track who was vaccinated, record the vaccine received, and follow up where necessary, a person receiving the COVID-19 vaccine must be registered on the Electronic Vaccination Data System, which requires a valid identification number such as passport number and refugee or asylum seeker permit number. Many undocumented migrants could not receive vaccines because of the absence of identity documents. The COVID-19 pandemic affected the timing of permit renewal or decisions on migration status.[84] Many also avoided vaccination centres due to the fear of arrest, detention, and possible deportation, especially when there have been prior xenophobic experiences with healthcare staff due to a lack of documentation.[85] This prompted calls for states to ensure that legal status is not a hindrance in accessing COVID-19 vaccines.[86] Ensuring this required guaranteeing the safety of everyone seeking vaccination services.[87] This limited access was a clear example of discrimination, necessitating the need to remove barriers, including the compulsory identification requirement for this group. Failure by governments, as with other instances of exclusion, demonstrated a disregard for how the virus spread, the threat of mutations, and a lack of clarity about government obligations in this regard.[88]

6.5 The right to health and equitable access to COVID-19 vaccines

States have an obligation in Article 12 of the ICESCR in realizing the right to health to, among others, take steps to ensure the prevention, treatment, and control of epidemic and endemic diseases. The Committee on Economic, Social, and Cultural Rights (CESCR), in its General Comment No. 14, explained that control of epidemic and endemic diseases requires States' individual and joint efforts to, among others, 'ensure the implementation or enhancement of immunisation programmes and other infectious disease control strategies'.[89] In the context of pandemics, a reasonable global, continental, and national vaccine governance programme is critical to fulfilling this obligation. The African Charter requires states to take measures to protect the health of their people.[90] In expounding on states' obligations in this regard, the African Commission, in its guidelines, has highlighted as a minimum core obligation of states in realizing the right to health to, among others, ensure universal immunization against major infectious diseases and take measures to prevent, treat, and control epidemic and endemic diseases.[91] With COVID-19 being a highly contagious disease, appropriate attention from states in protecting their people and maintaining the infection rates was essential.

Despite their legal status, migrants must be protected from discrimination regarding health services.[92] The Sustainable Development Goal (SDG) 3.8 targets Universal Health Coverage (UHC). This approach requires states to provide access to quality essential healthcare services, medicines, and vaccines for all without discrimination. The United Nations Political Declaration of the High-Level Meeting on UHC also emphasized eliminating the root causes of discrimination in access to health services and for countries to strive towards UHC.[93] These are reflected in various international human rights instruments and soft laws that outline the obligations of states to realize the right to health. The CESCR and the African Commission have emphasized that states must ensure non-discrimination in access to health care as central elements to realizing the right to health.[94] According to the Committee on Migrant Workers, states must provide equitable access to healthcare services irrespective of nationality or migration status, in line with the obligation concerning the right to health and non-discrimination.[95]

This principle of non-discrimination is also reflected in the United Nations Global Compact for Safe, Orderly and Regular Migration which is grounded in human rights and reaffirms commitments of states to uphold the principle of non-discrimination and eliminate xenophobia, racism, and intolerance against migrants and ensure access to essential services including health.[96] The World Health Assembly (WHA), in its Resolution 61.17 of 2008 on the Health of Migrants, noting the healthcare challenges of migrants, called upon states to promote migrant-sensitive health policies and equitable access to health promotion and disease prevention and care for migrants without discrimination. In health emergencies like the COVID-19 pandemic, disease containment plans and healthcare services must be migrant-sensitive and ensure they are not excluded.[97] In Resolution 70.15 on Promoting the Health of Refugees and Migrants, the WHA emphasized the importance of international collaboration in addressing migrant health challenges.[98] These culminated in the WHO Draft Global Action Plan 2019–2023 on promoting the health of refugees and migrants.[99]

In the context of the pandemic, the African Commission emphasized the centrality of rights guaranteed in the charter for a successful response to and recovery from the impacts of the pandemic. It highlighted the importance of attention being paid to the right to health and life under Articles 16 and 4 of the charter in the context of the COVID-19 pandemic.[100] In its Resolution 449,[101] the Commission emphasized that these rights should guide public health measures, the protection of the most vulnerable from severe complications, and the safety of health workers, and ensure safe access to health care for COVID-19-related issues as well as other health challenges and adequate access to water, soap, and other preventive cleaning products. Although vaccines were not yet available when this resolution was issued, the principles of human rights upon which the resolution was founded apply in this context. In its Resolution 470 on the Protection of Refugees, Asylum Seekers, and Migrants in the fight against the COVID-19 pandemic in Africa,[102] the African Commission condemned all violations of rights to which migrants have been directly or indirectly subjected in the context of management of the COVID-19 pandemic in Africa. It, therefore, noted that state parties to the African Charter must ensure that these vulnerable categories benefit from all preventive measures, including COVID-19 vaccines.

6.6 Responding to the COVID-19 vaccine inequality through an intersectional lens

Health equity is attained when every person can achieve optimum health, and no one is disadvantaged due to social position or other socially determined circumstances.[103] Ensuring equal opportunity for all persons to enjoy the highest attainable state of physical and mental health is at the core of the right to health for preserving lives and ensuring the dignity of all persons. Public health emergency response strategies should aim to reduce existing healthcare disparities rather than create new ones by giving all persons equal opportunity to be vaccinated. More so, lessons learnt from the pandemic have shown that excluding some persons from public health protection measures, such as limiting vaccinations based on several factors such as legal status or omitting to ensure access to ordinarily marginalized or vulnerable groups, is counterproductive. This is particularly so as continued spread provided avenues for viral mutations that could withstand existing treatment methods and vaccines.[104] The obligation to protect public health requires government commitment to removing unfair disabling criteria that affect certain groups and surmounting existing challenges that affect vulnerable and marginalized groups in accessing healthcare services.

This chapter provided the perspective of the peculiar challenges facing migrants. The aim was to highlight the need for efforts to identify and remove obstacles and barriers to receiving the COVID-19 vaccine, including limited access to health care. A first step in addressing the discrimination in access to vaccines is developing policies and plans that consider their realities or a 'migration aware' response. The legal status of refugees, asylum seekers, and migrants, worse still, where undocumented, should not be a barrier to accessing vaccines and delaying the protection of these groups. Increasing coverage among this group should include strengthening vaccination and surveillance activities at border crossings, transit sites, and camps; identifying groups in remote areas; tracking migration patterns; and integrating vaccine provision with humanitarian assistance. Engaging with groups is critical to determining their challenges, and they can equally proffer solutions and build trust. Appropriate responses can also be developed in consultation with civil society – international organisations working with these vulnerable groups.

Some good examples exist of addressing barriers to vaccine access for some vulnerable groups. The IOM highlighted some efforts that targeted the hindrances that some migrants encountered. They include removing the requirement of identification for COVID-19 vaccination; creating of a firewall between health and immigration officials as a guarantee that they will not be arrested when seeking vaccination; making vaccine accessible to all at all clinics; categorizing migrants as a priority group; reaching out to migrant and refugee communities in the appropriate language and through trusted communication channels; and mobile vaccination to reach communities where primary health services remain scarce.[105]

The identification requirement was a significant challenge for people without identity documents, especially undocumented migrants and those who, due to COVID-19 interruptions, could not renew their permits. Their exclusion undermined the efforts of various African governments to curb the spread of the virus. The South African government made efforts to ensure undocumented migrants received the vaccine by waiving the need for identity documents. Rather, the government set up vaccination centres on various sites, allowing an undocumented person to be given a unique identifier to be vaccinated and tracked for health purposes only.[106] In bypassing the need for a second dose and uncertainty about their return for it, the Western Cape Department of Health chose to prioritize the Johnson & Johnson single dose for undocumented persons.[107] This demonstrated recognition of and responses suited to peculiar challenges faced by this group. This is an important intervention that targets specific challenges rather than a one-size-fits-all approach. The efforts highlighted demonstrate an understanding of unique patterns of discrimination or disadvantage in access to COVID-19 vaccines to respond to it adequately.

The COVID-19 pandemic widened existing inequalities and created new challenges for migrant inclusion within host societies.[108] The IOM noted that during a crisis like the COVID-19 pandemic, in which the global community struggled to come to terms with the pandemic and the uncertainties regarding the future, it was easy for minority groups, including migrants, to become marginalized and to be the targets of discrimination or to experience a high degree of vulnerability. More so, the economic fallout caused heightened tensions about scarce jobs and services. However, the integration process that is key to developing a harmonious relationship between a host county and migrants should not fall away in emergency periods. This integration covers essential aspects, including the rights and obligations of migrants and host societies, including access to health and social services. Countries need to put in place appropriate measures to address xenophobic attacks and discrimination against migrants and ensure migrants have unhindered access to public services and support; migrant communities have adequate access to information; public health response measures are respectful of the human rights of migrants; and awareness campaigns to address misinformation and counter prejudices against migrant groups.

6.7 Conclusion and future perspectives

While the WHO has lifted the 'public health emergency of international concern' status of COVID-19, it insists the disease continues to pose a global threat. States have thus been urged to sustain health gains and strengthen the health system to respond to future emergencies while boosting the resilience of communities. The COVID-19 pandemic is an example of a disaster that occurs when a hazard (natural or man-made) meets vulnerability. Important considerations would revolve around how countries address these vulnerabilities. There is a need to boost individual, community, national, regional, and global resilience to possible future epidemics, pandemics, or other infectious disease outbreaks within countries.

The lessons learned from the COVID-19 pandemic underscore the need for global cooperation as health is a shared responsibility.[109] It also demonstrates the need for countries to implement effective policies to improve the health and well-being of all,[110] strengthen health systems, address inequalities, boost economic resilience, and design comprehensive risk management strategies. Given that the health crisis was by far the most challenging element of the pandemic to manage, it is also a wake-up call to countries to improve capacity, human and financial resources, and emergency preparedness within the health system as responses to public health emergencies are centred on a well-functioning health system.[111] During the outbreak of COVID-19, even HICs were overwhelmed and had to initiate strategies like lockdowns mainly to gain time to build capacity for response. COVID-19 was sudden; its magnitude was the first of its kind. However, it also served as a warning for all countries to boost health system resilience to combat future health shocks.

The pandemic has shown that to be effective, human rights considerations must be a significant part of the response to public health emergencies. Importantly, states must pay more attention to ensuring access to health care for all, especially groups from lower socio-economic backgrounds who were worst hit by the impact of the pandemic. The experience of COVID-19 has shown that exclusionary response strategies for health emergencies are counterproductive. While the pandemic again showed that vaccines are powerful tools to combat diseases, groups that found it difficult to access COVID-19 vaccines remained unprotected. This was not only at variance with the elements of universal health coverage[112] but also meant keeping them as a reservoir of the virus with a risk of contracting and transmitting and the greater risk of emerging variants that may evade immunity provided by existing vaccines. It also showed that efforts to ensure fair distribution of vaccines/medical technologies globally would be futile if rollout strategies were not inclusive at the country level. As such, while global health inequality is a significant concern, local disparities in access to healthcare services are an even more substantial challenge.

Importantly, states must adopt a migration-sensitive or migration-aware health system in which population movement is embedded in intervention, policy, and research design.[113] Vearey defines migration-aware responses as 'the rights of migrants to access public healthcare services' and 'the broader social and structural determinants of the health of migrants', which 'change over time and place'.[114] The WHA has called on states to raise health service providers' and professionals' cultural and gender sensitivity to migrants' health issues and identify and fill gaps in health service delivery.[115] The importance of international cooperation in this regard has been emphasized.[116] This is especially important given that migrants are not a static population requiring cross-border, multi-country strategies to address their health challenges. There should be strengthened collaboration in promoting the exchange of information on migrant health, cooperation on strengthening health systems, and helping countries that host many migrants.

The lessons from the COVID-19 pandemic are not only relevant for future pandemics or health emergencies. Instead, the pandemic was another wake-up call for countries to rethink health policies, health financing, human resource strengthening, and its human rights approach to issues relating to public health and access to health services. This is even important to deal with compounding risks associated with climate change and other natural hazards. The SDGs 2030 aim to ensure no one is left behind. The pandemic has affected the attainment of the SDGs by many countries, notably the SDGs relating to ending poverty (SGD 1), health and well-being (SDG 3), quality education (SDG 4), and decent work and economic growth. Building back better thus requires that no group is marginalized, especially those most impacted by the pandemic. It also necessitates rethinking how health service platforms are sensitive to the needs of various groups, such as migrants, and the barriers they face in accessing healthcare services.

Notes

1 The WHO officially, in May 2023, ceased categorizing the COVID-19 pandemic as a public health emergency of international concern ending its status as a global health emergency. This came after marked improvement with less mortality and increased immunity against the virus. For the entire declaration, see WHO 'Statement on the fifteenth meeting of the IHR (2005) emergency committee on the COVID-19 pandemic' 5 May 2023 available at www.who.int/

news/item/05-05-2023-statement-on-the-fifteenth-meeting-of-the-international-health-regulations-(2005)-emergency-committee-regarding-the-coronavirus-disease-(covid-19)-pandemic

2 As above.

3 T Pheage 'Dying from lack of medicines' *African Renewal* 2017 available at www.un.org/africarenewal/magazine/december-2016-march-2017/dying-lack-medicines (accessed 17 November 2020).

4 Africa Centre for Disease Control and Prevention 'COVID-19 vaccine dashboard' 21 April 2022 available at https://africacdc.org/covid-19-vaccination/

5 S Kuy et al 'Focusing on vulnerable populations during COVID-19' (2020) 95(11) *Academic Medicine* 2–3.

6 J Barjis, G Kolfschoten & J Maritz 'A sustainable and affordable support system for rural healthcare delivery' (2013) 56 *Decision Support Systems* 223–233.

7 Nomadic pastoralists are good examples of movement barriers. A Sheik Mohamed & JP Velema 'Where health care has no access: The nomadic populations of sub-Saharan Africa' (1999) 4(10) *Tropical Medicine and International Health* 695.

8 T Lancet 'Redefining vulnerability in the era of COVID-19' (2020) 397(10230) *Lancet* 1089.

9 R Walker, N Maple & J Vearey 'Migrants and the COVID-19 vaccine roll out in Africa: Hesitancy and exclusion' Migration and Coronavirus in Southern Africa Coordination Group (MiCoSA) Occasional Paper June 2021 available at www.mahpsa.org/wp-content/uploads/2021/06/MiCoSA-Migrants-the-Covid-19-vaccine-OccasionalPaper-June2021.pdf 7.

10 Article 12 of the International Covenant on Economic, Social and Cultural Rights.

11 African Commission 141 Resolution on Access to Health and Needed Medicines in Africa ACHPR/RES.141(XXXXIV)08 issued at its 44th Ordinary Session held in Abuja, Nigeria from the 10–24th of November 2008.

12 See J Vearey 'Migrants' right to health: A legislative and policy review from Southern Africa' International Organisation for Migration, report (2022).

13 A Aborode et al 'Equal access of COVID-19 vaccine distribution in Africa: Challenges and way forward' (2021) 93(9) *Journal of Medical Virology* 5212–5215.

14 M Senthilingam 'COVID-19: Why Africa's pandemic is different' (2021) *BMJ* 375; MM Kavanagh et al 'Access to life-saving medical resources for African countries: COVID-19 testing and response, ethics, and politics' (2020) 395 *The Lancet* 1735.

15 A Fontanet et al 'SARS-CoV-2 variants and ending the COVID-19 pandemic' (2021) 397(10278) *The Lancet* 952–954; SSA Karim & QA Karim 'Omicron SARS-CoV-2 variant: A new chapter in the COVID-19 pandemic' (2021) 398(10317) *The Lancet* 2126–2128.

16 C van Oosterhout et al 'COVID-19 evolution during the pandemic – Implications of new SARS-CoV-2 variants on disease control and public health policies' (2021) 12(1) *Virulence* 507–508.

17 AJ Alaran 'Uneven power dynamics must be levelled in COVID-19 vaccine access and distribution' (2021) 2 *Public Health in Practice*.

18 Walker et al (n 10 above).

19 A Otu et al 'Beyond vaccine hesitancy: Time for Africa to expand vaccine manufacturing capacity amidst growing COVID-19 vaccine nationalism' (2021) 2(8) *The Lancet Microbe* 347–348; G Nhamo et al 'COVID-19 vaccines and treatments nationalism: Challenges for low-income countries and the attainment of the SDGs' (2021) 16(3) *Global Public Health* 319–339; JDN Lagman 'Vaccine nationalism: A predicament in ending the COVID-19 pandemic' (2021) 43(2) *Journal of Public Health* 375–376.

20 EG Martin, GS Birkhead & DR Holtgrave 'Maintaining a focus on health equity during the COVID-19 vaccine rollout' (2021) 27(3) *Journal of Public Health Management and Practice* 226–228.
21 S Sekalala et al 'An intersectional human rights approach to prioritising access to COVID-19 vaccines' (2021) 6(2) *BMJ Global Health* 1–8; G Persad, ME Peek & EJ Emanuel 'Fairly prioritising groups for access to COVID-19 vaccines' (2020) 324(16) *JAMA* 1601.
22 See WHO *Addressing human rights as key to the COVID-19 response* (2020) 1.
23 It has been emphasized that it is crucial to consider the population-level impacts of COVID-19 and give special attention to disproportionate risks faced by marginalized and disadvantaged populations. D Puras et al 'The right to health must guide responses to COVID-19' (2020) 395 *Lancet* 1888–1890.
24 Black feminism examines the interlocking relationship between gender, race, and class which was largely ignored by white feminists. It was borne out of the fact that black women's experience of gender discrimination was shaped by race and class inequality which was different from the experience of white middle-class women. See EM Simien 'Black feminist theory: Charting a course for Black women's studies in political science' (2004) 26(2) *Women & Politics* 83–85.
25 See DW Carbado 'Colorblind intersectionality' (2013) 38(4) *Signs: Journal of Women in Culture and Society* 815. The critical race theory is a framework that questions the ways that race and racial power are constructed by law and culture engendering white supremacy and privilege. See R Delgado & J Stefancic *Critical race theory: An introduction* (Third Edition) (2017) 3–4.
26 K Crenshaw 'Demarginalizing the intersection of race and sex: A black feminist critique of antidiscrimination doctrine, feminist theory and antiracist politics' (1989) 1 *University of Chicago Legal Forum* 139; K Crenshaw 'Mapping the margins: Intersectionality, Identity politics, and violence against women of color' (1991) 43(6) *Stanford Law Review* 1241.
27 T Makkonen 'Multiple, compound and intersectional discrimination: Bringing the experiences of the most marginalized to the fore' Unpublished LLM thesis, Institute for Human Rights, Abo Akademi University, 2002, 18.
28 G Barak, P Leighton & J Flavin *Class, race, gender, and crime: The social realities of justice in America* (2010) 69–133. Despite the fight for increased equality and changes to the structures of society initiated by social movements mobilized based on several marginalized identity categories, these structures are still very evident in most societies and still affect how persons of certain identity categories are valued and can access social institutions and services.
29 GJS Dei, LL Karumanchery & N Karumanchery-Luik *Playing the race card: Exposing white power and privilege* (2004) 5; CE James 'The paradox of power and privilege: Race, gender and occupational position' (1994) 14(2) *Canadian Woman Studies* 50.
30 WM Liu 'White male power and privilege: The relationship between white supremacy and social class' (2017) 64(4) *Journal of Counselling Psychology* 349.
31 D Roberts & S Jesudason 'Movement intersectionality: The case of race, gender, disability, and genetic technologies' (2013) 10(2) *Du Bois Review: Social Science Research on Race* 314.
32 DW Carbado et al 'Intersectionality: Mapping the movements of a theory' (2013) 10(2) *Du Bois Review: Social Science Research on Race* 303.
33 S Cho 'Post-intersectionality: The curious reception of intersectionality in legal scholarship' (2013) 10(2) *Du Bois Review: Social Science Research on Race* 386.
34 Carbado et al (n 33 above) 303.
35 As above, 304.

36 K Davis 'Intersectionality as buzzword: A sociology of science perspective on what makes a feminist theory successful' (2008) 9(1) *Feminist theory* (67–85) 68–69; L McCall 'The complexity of intersectionality' (2005) 30(3) *Signs: Journal of Women in Culture and Society* 1771.

37 Carbado et al (n 26 above) 815. Given that there exists a range of intersecting power structures in society that the theory cannot address all at once, it has been rightly suggested that any analysis must restrict itself to specific structures of power. See Carbado et al (n 26 above) 304.

38 Carbado et al (n 26 above) 304. For a discourse around intersectionality that has emerged in Europe, see S Bilge 'Intersectionality undone: Saving intersectionality from feminist intersectionality studies' (2013) 10(2) *Du Bois Review: Social Science Research on Race* 405.

39 P Butler 'Black male exceptionalism? The problems and potential of black male-focused interventions' (2013) 10 *Du Bois Review: Social Science Research on Race* 485; Makkonen (n 28 above) 34; B Moolman 'Rethinking "masculinities in transition" in South Africa considering the "intersectionality" of race, class, and sexuality with gender' (2013) 11(1) *African Identities* 93.

40 CI Ravnbol 'Intersectional discrimination against children: Discrimination against Romani children and anti-discrimination measures to address child trafficking' (2009) United Nations Children's Fund 3.

41 M Makiwane, C Ndinda & H Botsis 'Gender, race and ageing in South Africa' (2012) 26(4) *Agenda* 15.

42 AY Clarke & L McCall 'Intersectionality and social explanation in social science research' (2013) 10(2) *Du Bois Review* 349; PA Goff & KB Kahn 'How psychological science impedes intersectional thinking' (2013) 10(2) *Du Bois Review* 365; R Chadwick 'Thinking intersectionally with/through narrative methodologies' (2017) 31(1) *Agenda* 5.

43 O Oyewumi 'Conceptualising gender: Eurocentric foundations of feminist concepts and the challenge of African epistemologies' in *African gender scholarship: Concepts, methodologies and paradigms* (2004) 3.

44 This journal is focused on gender and feminism in its broad and complex diversity.

45 A Gouws 'Feminist intersectionality and the matrix of domination in South Africa' (2017) 31(1) *Agenda* 19. Gouws engaged in a critical analysis of the concept of intersectionality to provide more clarity on its genealogy and to contextualize its use in the South African context. A Mahali 'Without community, there is no liberation': On #BlackGirlMagic and the rise of Black woman-centred collectives in South Africa' (2017) 31(1) *Agenda* 28. Mahali explored the coming together of Black women collectives with shared experiences of what it means to be a Black woman in contemporary South Africa. The author argued that the deliberate act of adopting 'a politics of recognition' – where race, class, and gender intersect – is a necessary step towards justice. His focus on the #BlackGirlMagic as a politics of recognition is a claim for social justice.

46 B Dworzanowski-Venter 'An intersectional analysis of male caregiving in South African palliative care' (2017) 31(1) *Agenda* 78. This paper explores the intersection of gender and class in understanding the experience of male care givers in a profession that is often feminized and invisible.

47 I Tshabangu 'The intersectionality of educational inequalities and child poverty in Africa: A deconstruction' (2018) 17 *Education Research Policy Practice* 69. See also F Reygan & M Steyn 'Diversity in basic education in South Africa: Intersectionality and critical diversity literacy' (2017) 14(2) *Africa Education Review* 68.

48 Makiwane et al (n 42 above).

49 J Moodley & L Graham 'The importance of intersectionality in disability and gender studies' (2015) 29(2) *Agenda* 24–33.
50 W Domingo '"We're watching you with interest": Reflections of a black law professor' (2017) 31(1) *Agenda* 64. Domingo, in determining how institutions of higher education in South Africa can be transformed, particularly for black women, considered the intersectionality of gender, race, culture, and religion as an innate and organic feature of her experiences as a black associate professor of law at a historically white institution of higher learning. E Prah 'Stratifications of blackness: Meditations on the intersect of gender, race and age' (2017) 31(1) *Agenda* 71. Prah, in this paper, explored the unique challenges of a young black female academic based on the influence of her age, gender, and race, in an academic field where performance is measured by identities inherited from centuries of interlocked suppressive systems which perceive her as subordinate.
51 E Moore & C Himonga 'Centring the intersection of race, class, and gender when a customary marriage ends' (2017) 31(1) *Agenda* 104–115. E Stern & J Mirembe 'Intersectionalities of formality of marital status and women's risk and protective factors for intimate partner violence in Rwanda' (2017) 31(1) *Agenda* 116.
52 Moodley & Graham (n 50 above) 24–33; M Humphrey 'The intersectionality of poverty, disability, and gender as a framework to understand violence against women with disabilities: A case study of South Africa' Unpublished LLM Research, Clark University, Worcester, MA, 2016.
53 E Amber & W Warnat 'Intersectionality and Employment Equity in South Africa' Unpublished LLM thesis Faculty of Humanities, University of Cape Town, 2012.
54 JA Thompson, SJ Gaskin & M Agbor 'Embodied intersections: Gender, water and sanitation in Cameroon' (2017) 31(1) *Agenda* 140.
55 These identities and contexts mentioned are not necessarily exhaustive of all the applications of the theory in Africa, rather it reflects the literature that has been engaged in this discussion.
56 Carbado et al (n 33 above) 304.
57 T Meer & A Müller 'Considering intersectionality in Africa' (2017) 31(1) *Agenda* 3–4.
58 SG Berkhout & L Richardson 'Identity, politics, and the pandemic: Why is COVID-19 a disaster for feminism(s)?' (2020) 42(4) *History and Philosophy of the Life Sciences* 49.
59 L Bowleg 'We're not all in this together: On COVID-19, intersectionality, and structural inequality' (2020) 110(7) *American Journal of public health* 917–917.
60 T Shakespeare, F Ndagire & QE Sekete 'Triple jeopardy: Disabled people and the COVID-19 pandemic' (2021) 397 *Lancet* 1331–1333.
61 Z Aranda et al 'A call for COVID-19 immunization campaigns that address the specific circumstances of indigenous peoples of Latin America and the Caribbean' (2021) 3 *The Lancet Regional Health – Americas* 1–2.
62 BB Braganza et al 'Prioritizing the marginalized in the COVID-19 vaccine rollout' (2021) 43(2) *Journal of Public Health* 368–369.
63 L Maestripieri 'The COVID-19 pandemics: Why intersectionality matters' (2021) 6 *Frontiers in Sociology* 52.
64 Habitat for Humanity 'Refugees, asylum seekers and migrants: A crucial difference' available at www.habitatforhumanity.org.uk/blog/2016/09/refugees-asylum-seekers-migrants-crucial-difference/
65 Refugees, asylum seekers, and migrants are generally referred to as people on the move, although they have legal differences. See Convention Relating to the Status of Refugees adopted 28 July 1951. Refugees are persons who flee their country due to conflict, risk, persecution, or human rights violations. Asylum seekers are persons who for the same reasons as a refugee flee their country but are yet to be legally recognized as refugees. See Convention Relating to the Status of Refugees adopted 28 July 1951.

66 This does not downplay the similar challenges that citizens also have to contend with. However, foreign nationals could sometimes experience these challenges in varied and more intense dimensions.
67 Report Special Rapporteur on the human rights of migrants, A/HRC/14/30, 16 April 2010, para 23
68 These are persons who lack valid documents required to be in a country legally.
69 FC Mukumbang, NA Anthony & BO Adebiyi 'Unspoken inequality: How COVID-19 has exacerbated existing vulnerabilities of asylum-seekers, refugees, and undocumented migrants in South Africa' (2020) 19(1) *International Journal for Equity in Health* 141.
70 African Commission on Human and Peoples' Rights 470 Resolution on the Protection of Refugees, Asylum Seekers and Migrants in the fight against the COVID-19 pandemic in Africa. ACHPR/Res.470 (LXVII) 2020 adopted at its 67th Ordinary Session held virtually, from 13 November to 3 December 2020.
71 C Greenaway et al 'COVID-19: Exposing and addressing health disparities among ethnic minorities and migrants' (2020) 27(7) Journal *of Travel Medicine* 113.
72 OHCHR A pandemic of exclusion: The impact of the COVID-19 pandemic on the human rights of migrants in Libya (2021) available at www.ohchr.org/sites/default/files/Documents/Issues/Migration/A_pandemic_of_exclusion.pdf; WHO 'Refugee and migrant health' 2 May 2022 available at www.who.int/news-room/fact-sheets/detail/refugee-and-migrant-health
73 JA White, D Blaau & LC Rispel 'Social exclusion and the perspectives of health care providers on migrants in Gauteng public health facilities, South Africa' (2020) 15(12) *PLoS ONE*.
74 Mixed Migration Centre 'MMC North Africa 4Mi Snapshot: Understanding the Impacts of COVID-19 on Refugees and Migrants in Tripoli' April 2020 available at https://mixedmigration.org/wp-content/uploads/2020/04/096_covid_snapshot_NA.pdf.
75 UNHCR Africa 'UNHCR highlights great progress on refugee vaccine inclusion but inequities hamper rollout' available at www.unhcr.org/news/press/2022/3/621e499f4/unhcr-highlights-great-progress-refugee-vaccine-inclusion-inequities-hamper.html
76 IOM 'Migrant inclusion in COVID-19 vaccination deployment' March 2022 available at www.iom.int/sites/g/files/tmzbdl486/files/documents/iom-vaccine-inclusion-mapping-global-march-2022-external-final.pdf
77 UNHCR Africa (n 76 above).
78 UNHCR Africa 'COVID-19 pandemic' available at www.unhcr.org/afr/corona virus-covid-19.html
79 T Lekubu 'Vaccinating migrants is the constitutional thing to do' *The Dialogue Online* The Southern African Liaison Office available at www.salo.org.za/wp-content/uploads/2021/03/DO-Vaccines-and-Migrants-.pdf
80 FC Mukumbang 'Are asylum seekers, refugees and foreign migrants considered in the COVID-19 vaccine discourse?' (2020) 5(11) *BMJ Global Health*; A Amani et al 'Migrant health is public health: A call for equitable access to COVID-19 vaccines' (2021) 6(3) *The Lancet Public Health* 144; IOM 'Striving for equitable access to COVID-19 vaccines to leave no migrant behind' 3 March 2021 available at www.iom.int/news/striving-equitable-access-covid-19-vaccines-leave-no-migrantbehind
81 J Vearey, M Modisenyane & J Hunter-Adams 'Towards a migration-aware health system in South Africa: A strategic opportunity to address health inequity' (2017) *South African Health Review* 1.
82 2021 (1) SA 553 (GP) (18 June 2020).
83 UN Committee on Migrant Workers, UN Special Rapporteur on the Human Rights of Migrants, United Nations High Commissioner for Human Rights and the Inter-American Commission on Human Rights 'Joint guidance note on

equitable access to COVID-19 vaccines for all migrants' 2021 available at https://reliefweb.int/sites/reliefweb.int/files/resources/JointGuidanceNoteCOVID-19-Vaccines-for-Migrants.pdf.

84 WHO 'Refugee and migrant health' 2 May 2022 available at www.who.int/news-room/fact-sheets/detail/refugee-and-migrant-health; Southern African Liaison Office 'Access to COVID-19 vaccines for migrants in South Africa' *Policy Dialogue Report* 25 March 2021 available at www.salo.org.za/wp-content/uploads/2021/04/25-03-2021-PD-Report-Vaccines-and-Migrants-Illustrated_final.pdf

85 VOA 'South Africa rolls out COVID-19 vaccines for undocumented immigrants' December 22 2021 available at www.voanews.com/a/south-africa-rolls-out-covid-vaccines-for-undocumented-immigrants/6365760.html

86 M Zard et al 'Leave no one behind: Ensuring access to COVID-19 vaccines for refugees and displaced populations' (2021) 27 *Nature Medicine* 747.

87 Walker et al (n 10 above) 7.

88 LM Lee, AE Lowe & MK Wynia 'COVID-19 vaccine exclusion based on legal residence is unwise and unethical' (2021) 42 *Journal of Public Health Policy* 346–349.

89 CESCR General Comment 14, para 16.

90 Article 16 African Charter on Human and Peoples' Rights.

91 African Commission 'Principles and guidelines on the implementation of economic, social and cultural rights in the African Charter on human and peoples' rights' (2011) 24 available at https://www.escr-net.org/resources/principles-and-guidelines-implementation-economic-social-cultural-rights-african-charter.

92 See United Nations Convention Relating to the Status of Refugees 1951; International Convention on the Protection of All Migrant Workers and Members of their Families 1990.

93 United Nations 'Political declaration of the high-level meeting on universal health coverage "Universal health coverage: Moving together to build a healthier world"' United Nations (2019).

94 CESCR General Comment No. 14 para 12(b); African Commission Principles and Guidelines on Implementation of Economic Social and Cultural Rights para 67.

95 Committee on Migrant Workers General Comment No. 2 on the rights of migrant workers in an irregular situation and members of their families, CMW/C/GC/2, 28 August 2013, para 18.

96 United Nations Global Compact for Safe, Orderly and Regular Migration, 2018 A/RES/73/195

97 World Health Assembly Resolution 61.17: Health of Migrants, WHA (2008).

98 As above; W. H. Assembly 'WHA resolution 70.15 promoting the health of refugees and migrants' WHA (2017).

99 WHO Promoting the Health of Refugees and Migrants. Draft Global Action Plan, 2019–2023. A72/25 Rev. 1, World Health Organization (2019).

100 449 Resolution on human and peoples' rights as central to successful response to COVID-19 and recovery from its socio-political impacts – ACHPR/Res. 449(LXVI) 2020.

101 As above.

102 African Commission 470 Resolution on the Protection of Refugees, Asylum Seekers and Migrants in the fight against the COVID-19 pandemic in Africa adopted at its 67th Ordinary Session held virtually from 13 to 30 December 2020.

103 N McClung et al 'The advisory committee on immunization practices' ethical principles for allocating initial supplies of COVID-19 vaccine – United States, 2020' (2020) 69(47) *Morbidity and Mortality Weekly Report* 1783.

104 SP Otto 'The origins and potential future of SARS-CoV-2 variants of concern in the evolving COVID-19 pandemic' (2021) 31(14) *Current Biology* 918–929.
105 IOM 'Migrant inclusion in COVID-19 vaccination deployment' March 2022 available at www.iom.int/sites/g/files/tmzbdl486/files/documents/iom-vaccine-inclusion-mapping-global-march-2022-external-final.pdf
106 VOA (n 86 above).
107 J Bornman 'Undocumented people neglected in plans to vaccinate' *Mail and Guardian* 3 September 2021 available at https://mg.co.za/coronavirus-essentials/2021-09-03-undocumented-people-neglected-in-plans-to-vaccinate/
108 L Patuzzi *Driving migrant inclusion through social innovation: Lessons for cities in a pandemic* (2020).
109 World Economic Forum '7 lessons leaders should take from the COVID-19 crisis' 5 January 2021 available at www.weforum.org/agenda/2021/01/7-things-leaders-can-learn-from-the-covid-19-crisis/
110 WHO 'Lessons learned from COVID-19: How did the pandemic affect children's health and habits?' 22 May 2023 available at https://who.int/europe/news/item/22-05-2023-lessons-learned-from-covid-19–how-did-the-pandemic-affect-children-s-health-and-habits#:~:text=%E2%80%9CThe%20lessons%20we%20have%20learned,and%20well-being%20of%20families.
111 European Centre for Disease Prevention and Control 'Lessons from the COVID-19 pandemic' Stockholm: ECDC; 2023 available at www.ecdc.europa.eu/en/publications-data/lessons-covid-19-pandemic-may-2023
112 DT Mosca et al 'Universal health coverage: Ensuring migrants and migration are included' (2020) 20(2) *Global Social Policy* 247–253.
113 J Veary, M Modisenyane & J Hunter-Adams 'Towards a migration-aware health system in South Africa: A strategic opportunity to address health inequity' (2017) 1 *SAHR* 89–98.
114 Vearey (n 1 above).
115 WHA Resolution 61.17 (2008).
116 WHA Resolution 70.15 (2017).

7

A HUMAN RIGHTS APPROACH TO BUDGETARY ALLOCATION AND THE RIGHT TO HEALTH

COVID-19 and health systems in Africa

Ashwanee Budoo-Scholtz

7.1 Background

COVID-19 is a health crisis that has led to an economic crisis[1] in many countries. It has brought out the weakness of the health systems in Africa, which have struggled to combat the pandemic.[2] It was exacerbated by the usual inadequate allocation of resources to health and has put into distress health systems, which were already struggling.[3] As Paintsil puts it, the preparedness of health systems in sub-Saharan Africa was only 'the eye of the crocodile' in a lake full of crocodiles, implying that the health systems were not ready to tackle the issue.[4] Indeed, health systems across Africa were considered as fragile due to inadequate allocation of financial resources.[5] However, health spending is one of the most important aspect for a country's health system to function properly. Even before COVID-19, there were struggles across the world, especially in developing countries,[6] to make sure that sufficient resources were allocated towards health.[7] According to Frenk, there is the 'black hole' misconception that no amount of resources will ever be enough to reach the goals of functional health systems since the latter is like a sponge that just absorbs resources.[8] Nevertheless, there is evidence that 'limited resources' allow systems to spend more judiciously and be more 'efficient'.[9] Nevertheless, many African states have failed to efficiently allocate sufficient resources towards strengthening the health systems, which threw them into a pit with COVID-19.

In 2001, African Heads of States adopted the Abuja Declaration on HIV/AIDS, Tuberculosis and Other Related Infectious Diseases (Abuja Declaration) where they pledged to allocate 15% of their national budgets to the health sector. Moreover, as is discussed later in the chapter, African states

DOI: 10.4324/9781032671437-9

have also ratified and agreed to be bound by global and regional laws that require them to allocate sufficient budgetary resources to realize the right to health. However, despite these treaties and soft laws, and the Abuja Declaration, African states are still lagging behind in allocating sufficient resources to realize the right to health, with some of them even reducing their budget towards health.[10] As African countries were hit by the COVID-19 pandemic, they immediately realized that there was a need to increase their budgetary allocations towards strengthening the health systems. However, in some instances, even these allocations did not prevent health systems of countries such as South Africa,[11] Mauritius,[12] and Nigeria[13] from facing failures.

A human rights approach to budgetary allocation has been considered as an important aspect for the realization of rights such as the right to health.[14] This chapter analyses whether allocation of extra resources during the COVID-19 pandemic had adopted a human rights approach or whether most of the budget was for personnel and overheads, which is the case for many African budgets. To do so, the chapter firstly explains what a health system is. Secondly, it elaborates on the motivations for a human rights approach to budgetary allocation to ensure the realization of rights. While so doing, it does not provide the challenges of adopting a human rights approach to budgetary allocations since a previous publication does so already.[15] Thirdly, it assesses the extent to which COVID-19 has had an impact on health systems in Africa, and fourthly, it expands on the violations of the right to health due to the impact of COVID-19 on health systems. Fifthly, the research analyses the obligations of states to allocate budgetary resources to realize the right to health and examine whether budgetary allocations during COVID-19 adopted a human rights approach. Sixthly, it explains how a human rights approach to budgetary allocation will ensure better preparedness for future pandemics, and seventhly, there is a conclusion section.

The research is mainly a desktop review of primary sources and secondary sources in the form of academic publications and reports on the impact of COVID-19 on health systems in Africa and on human rights approaches to resource allocations. It is to be noted that the chapter does not perceive a human rights approach to allocation of resources as a solution to the impact of COVID-19 on health systems in Africa but rather as contributing towards a holistic approach to the pandemic. Moreover, while the pandemic had an impact on almost every aspect of one's life, this chapter studies only its impact on health systems.

7.2 What is a health system?

Health systems exist because human beings need to ensure that they are in good health, free of any illness.[16] While health systems exist since time immemorial, they were formalized just over a century ago.[17] The World Health

Organization (WHO) defines a health system 'as comprising all the organizations, institutions and resources that are devoted to producing health actions'.[18] It consists of 'all the people and actions whose primary purpose is to improve health'.[19] It therefore comprises both the private and public sectors, who work together to ensure that the system is functional.[20] The above definitions have been considered as a 'laundry list, where there is only a list of those working towards providing health without really understanding the way they interact with each other towards a final product.[21] According to them, there is a need to broaden one's view of a health system to include the following: the 'interrelations' between the different components and the 'population' as a core component; in addition to improving health, the objectives should also be to meet the 'legitimate expectations of the population' and to provide sufficient finance for the same. Also, in line with the provision of health services, they should perform other 'enabling functions such as stewardship, financing, and resource generation'.[22]

7.3 A human rights approach to budgetary allocation[23]

A human rights approach to budgetary allocation finds its origin in the human rights approach to the theory of fiscal sociology. According to the theory of fiscal sociology, taxes collected by the government are collective properties that need to be distributed among the citizens.[24] The idea of taxes being collective properties stemmed from the theory of fiscal sociology.[25] Towards the end of World War I, Goldscheid defined fiscal sociology as 'the functional interdependence between state finances and social development, as well as the nature of the state in any particular historical setting'.[26] Schumpeter elaborated on the issue of fiscal sociology and analysed Goldscheid's approach. He stated that a state's 'fate' depends heavily on 'the economic bleeding which the needs of the state necessitates' and on 'the use to which its results are put to use'.[27] He further noted that the 'fiscal history' of a country determines the 'spirit of a people, its cultural level, its social structure, the deeds its policy may prepare', among others.[28] Both of them examined the taxation system and how it should be used to redistribute the income to the citizens.

Fiscal sociology's scope includes 'constitutional, legal and institutional influences on the budget', among others.[29] It has been considered as the effective provision of 'the synthetic unification of economic, sociological, political and legal approaches to public policy issues'.[30] It therefore provides for the framework for public budgeting.

Despite the fact that the theory of fiscal sociology was developed in the field of economics and to determine the manner in which a state should repay its debts, the theory is relevant for this chapter since both Goldscheid and Schumpeter have acknowledged that the state's intervention is important for the economy to function properly.[31] Both of them recognized that '[t]he character of the state depends upon the character of public finances'.[32] As such, a state that wants to be compliant with its human rights obligations has to manifest this in its public finance system.

Recognizing the link between human rights and public finance, Waris extrapolated human rights from fiscal sociology 'as a measure of the complex social interactions through their participation of society and citizens in the institutional processes of the fiscal state'.[33] She stated that the allocation of resources 'is decided upon by the "rulers" often with no requirement that reference be made to the people/citizens who contributed to the funds now at the state's disposal'.[34] She further noted that 'the use of limited resources and its prioritisation has been left traditionally to the state'.[35] Waris has explained the relationship between the revenue of the state and realization of rights in international conventions by stating that the state has the responsibility to make provision for the realization of the rights, and this requires resources.[36]

Waris' extrapolation of human rights from fiscal sociology can be interpreted to mean that the theory of fiscal sociology lays the basis to make governments accountable for the distribution of their resources. Waris' inclusion of human rights in the theory of fiscal sociology indicates that the public finance system of a country has to take human rights into consideration. Despite the fact that her work focuses on taxation and human rights, she has clearly established that the state has to use the taxes collected to realize human rights. Thus, the resource allocation process has to take into account human rights.

Hence, resource allocation must take into account the way in which all rights, including the right to health, are affected. A human rights approach to budgetary allocation ensures that sufficient resources are allocated to realize human rights, the right to health in this instance. This was emphasized by the Committee on Economic, Social and Cultural Rights (CESCR) in their General Comment No. 14.[37]

7.4 Impact of COVID-19 on health systems in Africa

The WHO has defined 'building blocks and priorities' for a framework that ensures an efficient health system.[38] They are service delivery, health workforce, information, medical product, vaccines and technologies, financing, and leadership and governance.[39] This section analyses the extent of the impact of COVID-19 on each of the building blocks and priorities to assess whether the pandemic has had a negative effect on health systems.

7.4.1 Service delivery

The service delivery aspect of health systems is the provision of 'effective, safe, good quality' care to those in need, with utmost efficiency.[40] It includes 'trained staff working with the right medicines and equipment, and with adequate financing'.[41] During the COVID-19 pandemic, many health systems across Africa struggled to ensure the provision of health services,[42] be it related to COVID-19 or others. Many people either were scared to go to the hospital during the COVID-19 pandemic or could not access the same due to transportation issues.[43] Even if they did manage to reach the hospital, many health providers were focused on COVID-19 issues and other health services being limited or stopped for that period.[44] For instance, according to the WHO, there was a decline in health services such as 'outpatient consultation, inpatient admission, skilled birth attendance, treatment of confirmed malaria cases and provision of the combination pentavalent vaccine in 14 countries' across Africa during the peak of the COVID-19 pandemic.[45] Such decline led to non-provision of essential healthcare services in many African countries. Across Nigeria, for example, during the COVID-19 pandemic, there was a decline in 'the provision of essential reproductive, maternal, child and adolescent health . . . services in primary health care facilities'.[46] In Egypt, the hospitals neither were properly equipped (be it in terms of quantity or quality) nor had the manpower to deal with the pandemic, especially with the virus affecting medical personnel.[47] In the initial stages of the pandemic, Uganda's essential healthcare services deteriorated with 'reduced case finding for HIV/AIDS and malaria', unavailability of refills for those with chronic conditions, and lack of treatment for cancer patients, among others.[48] Hence, one can deduce that the COVID-19 pandemic had a negative impact on health service delivery in the continent, with some countries, such as South Africa, facing a collapse of the health system.[49]

7.4.2 Health workforce

The health workforce comprises 'health service providers and health management and support workers'.[50] A functional health workforce is one that is 'available, competent, responsive and productive'.[51] However, during the COVID-19 pandemic, many healthcare workers in African countries did not have the required knowledge to deal with this infectious disease. In Kenya, many of them were scared to work in the healthcare environment, given the lack of information and lack of appropriate personal protective equipment.[52] Moreover, these countries were also facing shortages of the health workforce.[53] While the initial vaccine rollout in Africa targeted frontline workers, including those working in the healthcare sector, such action came too late. By that time, many health workers had lost their lives to the virus,[54] thereby leading to a reduction in the health workforce to assist in combatting the virus. To date, many African frontliners are not yet vaccinated against the virus, with only 11% of the population being vaccinated.[55] This is despite healthcare workers in countries such as Morocco showing interest in getting vaccinated.[56] Therefore, even the health workforce aspect of the public health system has been negatively affected by the COVID-19 pandemic.

7.4.3 Information

Health systems must be able to generate and use health information.[57] Such information should be disseminated and be used frequently and in situations of emergencies.[58] This information dissemination is two-fold: firstly, among the different stakeholders of the health systems providing health services and secondly, to the public. Many countries in Africa failed to provide both information during the COVID-19 pandemic.[59] On the one hand, once COVID-19 was declared a 'global public health emergency of international concern',[60] the WHO has been requesting data from countries around the world. However, many African countries, especially in the beginning of the pandemic, were not in a position to do so due to insufficient data gathering techniques or lack of testing. Tanzania did not even try to collect data on COVID-19 in the first year until there was a change in presidency.[61]

On the other hand, even though countries were popularizing measures to combat COVID-19, many African countries were not providing transparent information to the public on the situation of COVID-19 in the country, either because they did not want to instil fear or because there is/was a challenge to register such information.[62] According to the WHO, in 2021, six in seven COVID-19 cases went undetected in Africa.[63] Countries such as 'Burundi, Cote d'Ivoire, Democratic Republic of the Congo, Guinea-Bissau, Mozambique, Republic of the Congo, Senegal, and Zambia' had to wait for financial support of the WHO to start tracking the virus. Additionally, many people in Africa are hesitant to get the vaccine due to many reasons, such as being generally against vaccine, the speed with which the vaccine was created, non-belief in the seriousness of COVID-19, fake news, and religion.[64] Many governments have indeed targeted these reasons for vaccine hesitancy.[65] However, such campaigns did not reach far and wide in many countries. As such, information was not optimally generated and used during the pandemic.

7.4.4 Medical product, vaccines, and technologies

A health system must be able to provide 'equitable access to essential medical products, vaccines and technologies of assured quality, safety, efficacy and cost-effectiveness, and their scientifically sound and cost-effective use'.[66] In the context of the COVID-19 pandemic, this would refer to treatment and vaccines for COVID-19. Yet, one major challenge in combatting COVID-19 was the lack of testing kits and vaccines in African countries, with few of them producing and having access to the same.[67] Furthermore, oxygen supply and ventilators, which were essential in severe cases of COVID-19, were not readily available in many hospitals across the continent.[68] In some African countries, the number of functional ventilators was appalling, with, for instance, South Sudan having only four ventilators, the Central African Republic having three, and Liberia having six.[69]

7.4.5 Financing

Sustainable financing is key to a health system so that it can provide the population with the required services.[70] This might be the most important aspect of a health system since without financing, the other aspects of a health system will not function. Indeed, the already inadequate healthcare financing has been identified as the crux of the failure of health systems in Africa during the pandemic. In 2019, sub-Saharan Africa spent only an average of 4.95% of its budget on health, which demonstrates the unpreparedness of the continent to tackle the pandemic from a health system perspective.

Human Rights Watch, through interviews, established the following:[71]

> [A] chronic lack of investment in healthcare infrastructure and equipment has made it harder for African nations to retain skilled healthcare workers, provide essential medicines, and reduce the mortality rates of perennial diseases like malaria.

This inadequate financing of the healthcare system was reflected by, among others, the shortages in COVID-19 testing kits,[72] ventilators,[73] and protective equipment, and the lack of space for isolation.[74] Despite this, countries such as South Africa have cut down their budget in real terms when it comes to health despite the wake-up call by the COVID-19 pandemic.[75]

7.4.6 Leadership and governance

Health systems' leadership and governance range from a myriad of stakeholders, but it basically relates to the branch of government working in the area of health.[76] It incorporates the political and the technical aspects of providing health services. Such leadership and governance need to make decisions about priorities concerning the health system. Hence, there was a need for leadership and governance to have an immediate and effective response to the virus to ensure that there is 'good coordination' among the different stakeholders.[77] Some African countries did show leadership and governance in combatting COVID-19. For instance, South Africa actively ensured that it has testing capacity and proactively started contact tracing,[78] and Morocco created an application to monitor the virus.[79] However, in countries like Tanzania,[80] the former president had declared the country coronavirus-free, and hence no steps were taken to combat the virus.

As a conclusion to the impact of COVID-19 on health systems in Africa, this section has demonstrated that the pandemic has had a negative impact on most aspects of the health system. These impacts have resulted in violations of the right to health as discussed in the section below.

7.5 The violations of the right to health due to the impact of COVID-19 on health systems

The right to health is protected at both the global level and the regional level through Article 12 of the International Covenant on Economic, Social, and Cultural Rights (ICESCR), Articles 12 and 14 of the Convention on the Elimination of All Forms of Discrimination Against Women (CEDAW), Article 24 of the Convention on the Rights of the Child, Article 25 of the Convention on the Rights of Persons with Disabilities, Article 16 of the African Charter on Human and Peoples' Rights (African Charter), and Article 14 of the Protocol to the African Charter on the Rights of Women in Africa. There are general comments that lay emphasis on the sexual and reproductive health rights at the African level.[81] The Committee on Economic, Social and Cultural Rights (ESCR Committee) has elaborated that the right to health includes the 'right to the enjoyment of a variety of facilities, goods, services and conditions necessary for the realization of the highest attainable standard of health'.[82] It assesses the realization of the right to health in terms of its availability, accessibility, acceptability, and quality.[83] This right is also applicable in the context of COVID-19 as demonstrated by the ESCR Committee's statement on COVID-19 and economic, social, and cultural rights adopted in 2020.[84] At the African Commission level, similar to the ESCR Committee, there was a press release on the impact of the COVID-19 pandemic on economic, social, and cultural rights in Africa, where African states were called upon to strengthen their healthcare systems.[85]

Despite the above treaty provisions and soft laws, the impact of COVID-19 on health systems led to a deterioration in all four components of realizing the right to health. Concerning availability, many health services were unavailable due to, firstly, the focus being on combatting the virus and, secondly, the lack of capacity in terms of personnel and equipment to deal with the virus.[86] As noted in Section 7.4 of this chapter, many public transport systems were shut down, and hence hospitals were not accessible. Moreover, in many African countries, some health facilities such as community health centres were shut down,[87] and patients had to travel longer distances to access health services. As for acceptable health care, patients were, in many instances, left unattended due to the high rate of transmission, with many of them losing their lives due to non-acceptable healthcare standards. These include overcrowding in hospitals or unwillingness to accept those who are positive with the virus. Concerning the quality of health services, since the health systems were at the verge of collapsing in many African countries, services were restricted to a bare minimum, with countries failing to provide quality healthcare services.

7.6 Budgetary allocation to realize the right to health

As can be deduced from Section 7.4 of this chapter, COVID-19 has had a negative impact on health systems due to mostly lack of financial resources, which has affected the different components. In the current section, the research argues that had African countries adopted a human rights approach to COVID-19 budgetary allocations, these impacts could have been mitigated. As indicated in the introductory part, the chapter does not presume that a human rights approach would have eliminated the impact of COVID-19 on health systems but rather argue that it could have reduced the same. To do so, the chapter firstly elaborates on African countries' obligations to allocate budgetary resources to realize the right to health. Secondly, it analyses the different budgetary steps adopted to respond to the COVID-19 pandemic in the context of health systems in African countries to assess whether they adopted a human rights approach.

7.6.1 Obligations to allocate budget for the realization of economic, social, and cultural rights88

This section focuses on the global and regional instruments that impose an obligation on states to allocate budgetary resources to realize economic, social, and cultural rights such as the right to health. It firstly elaborates on the treaties and soft laws at the United Nations (UN) level and, secondly, discusses the treaties and soft laws at the African Union level.

7.6.1.1 UN level

At the UN level, the primary document regulating economic, social, and cultural rights is the ICESCR, as discussed earlier. Concerning resource allocation, Article 2(1) of the ICESCR provides the following:

> Each State Party to the present Covenant undertakes to take steps, individually and through international assistance and co-operation, especially economic and technical, to the maximum of its available resources, with a view to achieving progressively the full realization of the rights recognized in the present Covenant by all appropriate means, including particularly the adoption of legislative measures.

Article 2(1) of the ICESCR makes reference to appropriate measures that include financial measures.[89] Non-realization of the rights protected by the ICESCR has to be justified by demonstrating that 'every effort has been made to use all resources that are at its disposition in an effort to satisfy' the obligation imposed by the covenant.[90]

In the concluding observations concerning Philippines,[91] the ESCR Committee uses a 'comparative analysis'[92] to demonstrate that the state had not respected its obligations under Article 2(1) of the ICESCR. It was noted that the proportion of the national budget spent on military was far higher than the allocation to housing, agriculture, and health combined.[93] The same observation was made in relation to the Republic of Korea's state report, where the ESCR Committee expressed concern about 'the high level of defence expenditure' that was 'in contrast with the shrinking budget for key areas of economic, social and cultural rights'.[94] These concluding observations are relevant in the context of the COVID-19 pandemic to assess whether the state has allocated sufficient resources to realizing the right to health.

The fact that countries have not spent the resources allocated to a specific item due to 'inefficient administration or corruption' is also an indicator that they are not respecting their obligations under Article 2(1) of the ICESCR.[95] This was highlighted in the concluding observations for Colombia where the ESCR Committee stated that the Colombian government must utilize 'budget items earmarked for social expenditure in the State's overall budget and ensure that such appropriations are used for the purposes for which they were budgeted'.[96] Such an observation was also made for Kenya, where the ESCR Committee recommended that the state improves 'its budget execution process with a view to spending all the allocated funding in a timely, effective and transparent manner'.[97] Therefore, 'maximum available resources' encompass the appropriations in the budget that have still not been spent.

The concluding observations on Uganda's initial report[98] highlighted the importance of national budget allocation for the realization of the rights provided by the ICESCR. It specifically recommended the following:[99]

> . . . the State party reprioritize its allocation of resources and steadily increase the share of the public budget available to these sectors with a view to ensuring the progressive realization of the rights contained in the Covenant.

States are therefore recommended to allocate budgetary resources to realize the rights in the ICESCR. The ESCR Committee also made reference to budgetary allocation for specific rights protected by the ICESCR.[100]

Moreover, the ESCR Committee has recommended states to ensure that there is no decrease in resources that are allocated to the realization of economic, social, and cultural rights.[101] It has further stated that even when the government is trying to stabilize the economic situation, it must always ensure 'the core content of the rights'.[102] In the event a state does not have the necessary resources, the ESCR Committee has recommended states to consider economic, social, and cultural rights in their negotiations with international financial institutions.[103] This is applicable to the COVID-19 context where African states have to ensure that they are not regressive in their resource allocation for the realization of the right to health.

More specific to the right to health, in 2020, the ESCR Committee adopted a general comment on the right to highest attainable standard of health.[104] This general comment clearly includes budgetary steps as part of the obligation to fulfil the right to health.[105] States have to further demonstrate that they have used the maximum available resources to realize the right to health.[106] Many African countries were given loans and aids from financial institutions and donors to combat the COVID-19 pandemic.[107] Hence they have the duty to ensure that these financial resources were directed towards strengthening public health systems to realize the right to health.

In addition to the concluding observations and general comments above, in 2007 the ESCR Committee made a statement concerning the obligation of states to take steps to make use of the maximum of available resources (2007 ESCR Committee statement).[108] Paragraph 7 of the 2007 ESCR Committee statement provides that to combat discrimination, states should take 'budgetary measures in order to prevent third parties from interfering with the rights' protected by the ICESCR 'or to facilitate, provide and promote the enjoyment of these rights'. This statement further states that 'the obligation to protect and, to a greater extent, the obligation to fulfil, on the other hand, often require positive budgetary measures'.[109] Thus, the realization of the rights protected by a treaty necessitates budgetary allocations on behalf of the government.

As can be derived from the interpretation of Article 2(1) of the ICESCR by the ESCR Committee, realization of the rights provided by the ICESCR requires not only legislative measures but also financial resources. In addition to Article 2(1) of the ICESCR, the general comments and concluding observations of the ICESCR Committee have been more comprehensive about the steps, including budgetary steps, that states must take so that rights such as the right to health are realized.

More specific to COVID-19, the ESCR Committee in 2020 issued a statement on COVID-19 and economic, social, and cultural rights (ESCR Committee statement).[110] The very first paragraph of the statement mentions how COVID-19 is 'threatening to overwhelm public healthcare systems' across the world. It emphasized on how the right to health of the most marginalized in societies have been impacted due to failures or shortcomings of health systems.[111] Paragraph 14 of the ESCR Committee statement requires states to allocate sufficient resources to realize economic, social, and cultural rights and emphasizes on the right to health due to the disproportionate impact of COVID-19 on the same.

7.6.1.2 African Union level

The primary document protecting the right to health is the African Charter. In relation to allocation of budgetary resources to realize human rights,

Article 1 of the African Charter provides that states 'shall undertake to adopt legislative or other measures' to give effect to the rights protected by the African Charter. Furthermore, under Article 16 of the African Charter concerning the right to health, states have the obligation to take 'necessary measures to protect the health of their people and to ensure that they receive medical attention when they are sick'.

These articles do not expressly mention the allocation of budgetary resources to realize the rights in the African Charter. The African Commission on Human and Peoples' Rights (African Commission) has interpreted the obligations under the African Charter to include budgetary allocation of resources. One of the functions of the African Commission is to 'formulate and lay down, principles and rules aimed at solving legal problems relating to human and peoples' rights and fundamental freedoms upon which African Governments may base their legislations'.[112] Such documents can be in the form of resolutions, general comments, declarations, and guidelines. Some of them are the Pretoria Declaration on Economic, Social, and Cultural Rights in Africa and the Guidelines and Principles on Economic, Social, and Cultural Rights in the African Charter. In the context of the COVID-19 pandemic, Resolution 449 adopted in 2020 puts human and peoples' rights at the centre of COVID-19 responses.[113]

Moreover, another avenue for the African Commission to expand on the normative standards is through the state reporting procedure under Article 62 of the African Charter. According to this article, each state party needs to present a report to the African Commission containing the legislative and other steps taken to implement the obligations under the African Charter every two years. Once the African Commission has reviewed the report, it can issue concluding observations and recommendations to the state party concerned.[114] The African Commission has mentioned budgetary allocation to realize the right to health in the concluding observations of many countries such as Angola,[115] Burkina Faso,[116] Eritrea,[117] and the Gambia.[118] This means that even if there is no express mention of budgetary resources for the realization of the right to health, states are expected to adopt such steps for the realization of this right.

Additionally, on 24 March 2020, the African Commission's chairperson released a press statement on a human rights approach to respond to the COVID-19 pandemic.[119] One of the areas of concern was the right to health where states were reminded of their obligation to realize the same and to ensure that everyone has access to health services, irrespective of whether they have insurance or not. Furthermore, states were required to strategize to ensure that enough financial resources are being directed to the different aspects of the health systems.

Moreover, on 4 June 2020, the Working Group on Economic, Social, and Cultural Rights of the African Commission released another press statement[120] that emphasized on the impact of COVID-19 on health systems. The press statement called on states to take steps to make sure that economic, social, and cultural rights are realized and to[121]

> Strengthen health care systems including increased budgetary allocation, provision of ventilators, test kits, personal protective equipment, medical supplies and consumables required for the prevention and treatment of COVID-19, address maternal and infant health as well as other diseases.

This statement is crucial to this research because it shows that the African Commission recognizes that there is a need for budgetary allocation of resources for there to be a functional health system during the COVID-19 pandemic. These two statements imply that states have to ensure that they adopt a human rights approach to budgeting to strengthen health systems, which will lead to a better realization of the right to health in Africa.

In addition to these documents, at the African Union level, even before the COVID-19 pandemic, African states had recognized the importance of budgetary allocation of resources towards the right to health and had adopted the Abuja Declaration on HIV/AIDS, Tuberculosis and Other Related Infectious Diseases of 2001 (Abuja Declaration 2001). To combat HIV/AIDS, tuberculosis, and other infectious diseases, the states committed to 'take all necessary measures to ensure that the needed resources are made available from all sources and that they are efficiently and effectively utilized'.[122] Going a step further, the states also pledged to allocate 'at least 15%' of their annual budget to 'the improvement of the health sector'.[123] In addition to the above, the states also undertook to mobilize all resources, including financial resources, for the provision of 'care and support and quality treatment' to that section of the population that is affected with HIV/AIDS, tuberculosis, and other related infections.[124] However, before the COVID-19 pandemic, in 2014, only four countries, namely Malawi, Ethiopia, the Gambia, and Eswatini, were above the 15% threshold, with the African average being around 10%.[125]

Thus, many African countries were lagging behind in implementing their obligations to realize the right to health through the allocation of sufficient budgetary resources.

7.6.2 Analysing the budgetary steps to respond to the COVID-19 pandemic in the context of health systems in Africa

Many countries around the world, including Africa, restructured their budget to combat the COVID-19 pandemic.[126] Most of them created funds related to COVID-19 to allocate resources to combat the pandemic.[127] The funds covered a wide range of expenditure such as social programmes and unemployment support, and debt, unemployment, and tax reliefs, and varied in amounts.[128] Most of the interventions had a component related to strengthening or building resilience of the health systems. This section only focuses on the expenditures relating to health systems since this is the focus of the chapter.

As soon as the pandemic hit the world, many African countries responded by adopting legal, policy, and budgetary measures. Many of the budgetary measures included increases in spending in the health sector.[129] For instance, the 2020 amended Nigerian budget aimed to, among others, upgrade 'healthcare facilities'[130] through 'building health infrastructure and strengthening capacity within the healthcare system'.[131] In South Africa, a National Treasury Fund was created to, among others, capacitate the health systems to test and to send community health workers across the country.[132] Egypt adopted stimulus packages to ensure that its health systems have medical supplies and for 'bonuses to medical staff'.[133] In Ghana, most of the strategy pillars to combat COVID-19 concerned contact tracing, isolation to stop the spread of the virus, and treatment.[134] Many countries also invested in telemedicine technologies to make sure that patients still have access to treatment even if they cannot access hospitals.[135] Many countries also earmarked percentages of the budget to buy vaccines, even if many African countries received vaccines as donations.

A human rights approach to these allocations towards health systems would have taken into account whether the allocations would make health services more available, accessible, and adaptable, and increase the quality of health. However, most of the allocations were done hastily and did not really do this test.

Furthermore, the already existing weak health systems in Africa contributed to a slow response to the budgetary measures to combat COVID-19. In Ghana, even though the COVID-19 response focused on budgetary allocations for health, it has been argued that such a step was too late given that the health sector has been long deprived of funding. Hence, even the extra allocations during the COVID-19 pandemic did not assist Ghana to effectively combat the virus since only one main centre was responsible for testing.[136] Moreover, there was a shortage in protective gear.[137] Hence, countries' noncompliance with the Abuja Declaration and their obligations under global and regional laws to allocate sufficient budgetary resources to realize the right to health led to weak systems that could not bear the weight of COVID-19. Had they, before the pandemic, strengthened and built resilience of the health systems through allocation of sufficient budgetary resources, the extra COVID-19 funds could have efficiently assisted in combatting the virus and ensured that health services were of good quality and were available, accessible, and acceptable during the pandemic.

7.7 Future pandemics and a human rights approach to budgetary allocation to realize the right to health

Most of the budgetary measures for COVID-19 in relation to health concerned increasing the budget for health to ensure that there is enough contact tracing, testing, isolation, and availability of equipment and vaccines. However, while the whole COVID-19 budget was consequential in many countries, most of them allocated only a small proportion to health systems. For instance, in South Africa, the COVID-19 Fiscal Response Package allocated only 4% of the budget to health systems to combat COVID-19,[138] and while Egypt did allocate extra funds to the health sector, almost half of its stimulus package went to the tourism sector.[139] These minimal proportions of the budget demonstrate that COVID-19 budgetary allocations gave less weight to strengthening health systems and hence were not made from a human rights perspective to realize the right to health. As indicated in the introductory sentence of this chapter, COVID-19 is firstly a health crisis, and hence, most efforts should have logically been geared towards health systems to be able to provide health services for the same. Nevertheless, this was not done, and hence, even with increased budgetary allocations, the four components of the realization of the right to health were not optimally met. Countries need to adopt a human rights approach to budgetary allocation to realize the right to health because this ensures an adequately funded health system that is strong enough to deal with pandemics.

One advantage of the human rights approach to budgetary allocation is that it ensures transparency in the resource allocation process. Many African budgets are presented in a broad manner, and it is difficult to assess the amount that is actually being directed to a particular line item unless it is clear in the policies of the government. In many instances, such allocations are done on a departmental/ministerial basis, with the majority of the budget being for overheads and personnel. With COVID-19 also, the budget was broad with no specifics as to how much is exactly being allocated to ensure that health services are available, accessible, acceptable, and of a good quality. Many government officials have used the opportunity that COVID-19 presented and misappropriated COVID-19 funds.[140] In Nigeria, while some of the budget was earmarked for health, such budget was an opportunity to make the rich richer through corruption, with many even believing that the COVID-19 pandemic was an opportunity for 'political leaders to make good money' instead of improving the health sector.[141] This was also the case in South Africa where there was corruption concerning procurement of COVID-19-related equipment and supplies.[142] A human rights approach to budgetary allocation would create more accountability and ensure that resources earmarked for a particular right is correctly spent on the same. As a result, there will be maximal scrutiny on how the funds are being spent, with little leeway for corruption. This will lead to a stronger health system, which can better bear the weight of future pandemics.

Countries must already adopt a human rights approach to budgetary allocation to realize the right to health to ensure that they are better prepared for future pandemics. They should not wait for another pandemic to start allocating more resources in an erratic manner to health care. Such a step will also ensure that they are implementing their obligations under global and regional laws.

7.8 Conclusion

COVID-19 has generally had a negative impact on health systems in Africa since it adversely affected the components of the same. These impacts led to violations of the right to health since health services were not of a good quality and were unavailable, inaccessible, and unacceptable during the pandemic with many African countries facing a collapse of their health systems when they were hit by the COVID-19 pandemic. This chapter argues that states have an obligation to allocate sufficient budgetary resources to realize the right to health, and hence, African states must ensure that their budgets reflect that they are working towards the realization of the right to health. One way of doing this is through a human rights approach to public budgeting.

If African countries had adopted a human rights approach to budgeting, the impacts of COVID-19 on health systems could have been mitigated. This is so because, firstly, they would have ensured that sufficient resources are allocated towards the realization of the right to health and as a consequence to health systems. Secondly, if such an approach was adopted before the pandemic, health systems across the continent would not be so fragile and would have been able to bear the brunt of the COVID-19 pandemic. Thirdly, a human rights approach to budgetary allocation ensures that there is transparency and accountability in resource allocation. Such transparency and accountability would have led to less corruption both before and during the COVID-19 pandemic and led to more resources being directed towards strengthening health systems.

Notes

1 National Treasury 'Briefing by National Treasury on financial implications of COVID-19 on both the economy and the budget' (30 April 2020) 26 available at www.treasury.gov.za/comm_media/press/2020/JT%20SCoF%20and%20SCoA%20briefing%20COV19.pdf (accessed 22 February 2022).

2 SA Lone & A Ahmad 'COVID-19 pandemic – an African perspective' (2020) 9(1) *Emerging Microbes and Infections* 1302.

3 CA Nnaji & J Moodley 'Impact of the COVID-19 pandemic on cancer diagnosis, treatment and research in African health systems: A review of current evidence and contextual perspectives' (2021) 15(1170) *Ecancermedicalscience* 1.

4 E Paintsil 'COVID-19 threatens health systems in sub-Saharan Africa: The eye of the crocodile' (2020) 130(6) *Journal of Clinical Investigation* 2741.

5 EE Elebesunu et al 'COVID-19 calls for health systems strengthening in Africa: A case of Nigeria' (2021) 36(6) *The International Journal of Health Planning and Management* 2036.

6 OB Da'ar et al 'Coronavirus disease 2019 (COVID-19): Potential implications for weak health systems and conflict zones in Middle East and North Africa' (2020) 35(5) *The International Journal of Health Planning and Management* 1242.
7 JE Ataguba & D McIntyre 'Paying for and receiving benefits from health services in South Africa: Is the health system equitable?' (2012) 27(1) *Health Policy and Planning* 36.
8 J Frenk 'The global health system: Strengthening national health systems as the next step for global progress' (2010) 7(1) *PLoS Medicine*.
9 As above.
10 FR Zimano 'The catch-22 in pre-set budgetary allocations: The case of 2001 Abuja Declaration' (2020) 7(2) *International Journal of Human Rights and Constitutional Studies* 149–157.
11 C Staunton, C Swanepoel & M Labuschaigne 'Between a rock and a hard place: COVID-19 and South Africa's response' (2020) 7(1) *Journal of Law and Biosciences* 1–12.
12 A Budoo-Scholtz 'Is COVID-19 bringing out the inequalities in the delivery of health services in Mauritius?' *AfricLaw* 11 October 2021 available at https://africlaw.com/2021/10/11/is-covid-19-bringing-out-the-inequalities-in-the-delivery-of-health-services-in-mauritius/ (accessed 11 April 2022).
13 D Odubanjo 'Where COVID-19 has left Nigeria's health system' *The Conversation* 13 December 2020 available at https://theconversation.com/where-covid-19-has-left-nigerias-health-system-151346 (accessed 11 April 2022).
14 Committee on Economic, Social and Cultural Rights 'General Comment No. 14: The right to highest attainable standard of health' adopted on 11 August 2000 E/C.12/2000/4 para 33.
15 See Section 4.3 of A Budoo 'Adoption of a human rights approach to budgeting as a step to realise the right to education in African countries' in AC Onuora-Oguno, WO Egbewole & TE Kleven (eds) *Education law, strategic policy and sustainable development in Africa: Agenda 2063* (2018) 38–43.
16 WHO 'Strengthening health systems to improve health outcomes: WHO's framework for action' (2007) 9 available at https://iris.who.int/handle/10665/43918.
17 As above.
18 World Health Organization 'The World Health Report 2000: Health systems: Improving performance' (2000) xi available at https://www.who.int/publications-detail-redirect/924156198X.
19 As above, 1.
20 WHO 2007 (n 16 above) 14.
21 Frenk (n 8 above) 1.
22 As above, 1–2.
23 This section is adapted from Chapter 3 of the author's unpublished doctoral thesis submitted to the University of Pretoria: A Budoo 'The role of gender budgeting in implementing the obligation to provide resources to realise women's human rights in Africa' (2016) under the supervision of Prof Magnus Killander (University of Pretoria) and Prof Attiya Waris (University of Nairobi).
24 RE Wagner *Fiscal sociology and the theory of public finance: An exploratory essay* (2007) 25.
25 JG Backhaus 'Fiscal sociology: What for?' (2001) 10 available at www.uni-erfurt.de/fileadmin/user-docs/Finanzwissenschaft/bibliothek/valedictory_lecture.pdf (accessed 20 February 2022).
26 R Goldscheid as quoted by RA Musgrave 'Schumpeter's crisis of the tax state: An essay in fiscal sociology' (1992) 2 *Journal of Evolutionary Economics* 99.
27 JA Schumpeter 'The crisis of the tax state' in R Swedberg (ed) *The economics and sociology of capitalism* (1991) 100.

28 As above, 101.
29 M McLure 'Fiscal sociology' Discussion paper available at https://ecompapers.biz.uwa.edu.au/paper/PDF%20of%20Discussion%20Papers/2003/03_16_McLure.pdf (accessed 20 February 2022) 2.
30 As above, 7–8.
31 Waris' argument below.
32 As above.
33 A Waris *Tax and development: Solving Kenya's financial crisis through human rights: A case study of Kenya's constituency development fund* (2013) 9–10.
34 As above, 4.
35 As above.
36 As above.
37 Committee on Economic, Social and Cultural Rights, General Comments No. 14 (n 14 above).
38 WHO 2007 (n 16 above) 14.
39 As above.
40 As above.
41 As above.
42 G Shapira et al 'Disruptions in maternal and child health service utilization during COVID-19: Analysis from eight sub-Saharan African countries' (2021) 36 *Health Policy and Planning* 1140.
43 L Holtz 'COVID-19's impact on overall health care services in Africa' *Brookings* 12 October 2021 available at www.brookings.edu/blog/africa-in-focus/2021/10/12/covid-19s-impact-on-overall-health-care-services-in-africa/ (accessed 16 February 2022).
44 As above.
45 Website of the World Health Organization available at www.afro.who.int/news/covid-19-hits-life-saving-health-services-africa (accessed 16 February 2022).
46 B Adelekan et al 'Effect of COVID-19 pandemic on provision of sexual and reproductive health services in primary health facilities in Nigeria: A cross-sectional study' (2021) 18 *Reproductive Health* 1.
47 MI Kamel 'A view of health services after COVID-19: An Egyptian perspective' (2020) 56(1) *Alexandria Journal of Medicine* 122.
48 NM Tumwesigye et al 'Effects of the COVID-19 pandemic on health services and mitigation measures in Uganda' Working Paper 571 for the Centre for Global Development (2021) 8.
49 See generally J Nyasulu & H Pandya 'The effects of coronavirus disease 2019 pandemic on the South African health system: A call to maintain essential health services' (2020) 12 *African Journal of Primary Health Care and Family Medicine* 1.
50 WHO 2007 (n 16 above) 16.
51 As above.
52 E Barasa et al 'Indirect health effects of the COVID-19 pandemic in Kenya: A mixed methods assessment' (2021) 21 *BMC Health Services Research* 12.
53 L Nepomnyashchiy et al 'COVID-19: Africa needs unprecedented attention to strengthen community health systems' (2020) 396(10245) *The Lancet* 150.
54 Website of WHO available at www.who.int/news/item/20-10-2021-health-and-care-worker-deaths-during-covid-19 (accessed 16 February 2022).
55 Website of the WHO available at www.afro.who.int/news/africa-needs-ramp-covid-19-vaccination-six-fold (accessed 16 February 2022).
56 M Khalis et al 'Acceptability of COVID-19 vaccination among health care workers: A cross-sectional survey in Morocco' 17 *Human Vaccines and Immunotherapeutics* 12 5076–5081.
57 WHO 2007 (n 16 above) 18.
58 As above.

59 Amnesty International 'East and Southern Africa: Media freedoms curtailed as COVID-19 regional crises expose urgent need or access to information' 3 May 2021 available at www.amnesty.org/en/latest/news/2021/05/east-and-southern-africa-media-freedoms-curtailed-as-covid19-regional-crises-expose-urgent-need-for-access-to-information/ (accessed 11 April 2022).
60 WHO 'Social and behavioural insights: COVID-19 data collection tool for Africa' (2021) available at https://www.who.int/news/item/25-08-2021-social-and-behavioural-insights-covid-19-data-collection-tool-for-africa.
61 K Houreld & D Lewis 'In Africa, lack of coronavirus data raises fear of 'silent epidemic' *Reuters* 8 July 2020 available at www.reuters.com/article/us-health-coronavirus-africa-data-insigh-idUSKBN24910L (accessed 11 April 2022).
62 E Yam 'Why we don't know the real number of COVID-19 deaths in Africa' *International Growth Centre* (26 October 2020) available at www.theigc.org/blog/why-we-dont-know-the-real-number-of-covid-19-deaths-in-africa/ (accessed 16 February 2022).
63 WHO Africa 'Six in seven COVID-19 infections go undetected in Africa' 14 October 2021 available at www.afro.who.int/news/six-seven-covid-19-infections-go-undetected-africa (accessed 11 April 2022).
64 See generally G Troiano 'Vaccine hesitancy in the era of COVID-19' 194 *Public Health* 245–251.
65 Website of WHO 'Key lessons from Africa's COVID-19 vaccine roll-out' (24 December 2021) available at www.afro.who.int/news/key-lessons-africas-covid-19-vaccine-rollout (accessed 16 February 2022).
66 WHO 2007 (n 16 above) 20.
67 B Bright et al 'COVID-19 preparedness: Capacity to manufacture vaccines, therapeutics and diagnostics in sub-Saharan Africa' (2021) 17 *Gobalization and Health* 2.
68 OO Ogunleye et al 'Response to the novel corona virus (COVID-19) pandemic across Africa: Successes, challenges, and implications for the future' 6 available on the website of Frontiers in Pharmacology available at www.frontiersin.org/articles/10.3389/fphar.2020.01205/full?&utm_source=Email_to_authors_&utm_medium=Email&utm_content=T1_11.5e1_author&utm_campaign=Email_publication&field=&journalName=Frontiers_in_Pharmacology&id=568873 (accessed 20 February 2022).
69 R Maclean & S Marks '10 African countries have no ventilators. That's only part of the problem' *The New York Times* 18 April 2020 available at www.nytimes.com/2020/04/18/world/africa/africa-coronavirus-ventilators.html (accessed 11 April 2022).
70 WHO 2007 (n 16 above) 21.
71 Website of Human Rights Watch available at www.hrw.org/news/2020/06/08/africa-covid-19-exposes-healthcare-shortfalls (accessed 16 February 2022).
72 Paintsil (n 4 above) 2742.
73 A Woodyatt 'The world is scrambling to buy ventilators in the COVID-19 pandemic. One country has only four of them – for 12 million people' *CNN* 18 April 2020 available at https://edition.cnn.com/2020/04/18/africa/covid-19-ventilator-shortage-intl-scli/index.html (accessed 16 February 2022).
74 Human Rights Watch (n 71 above).
75 T Lencoasa, K Mapipa & J Chaskalson 'Opinion: Health needed a recovery budget, we got the opposite' *Spotlight* 18 March 2022 available at www.spotlightnsp.co.za/2022/03/18/opinion-health-needed-a-recovery-budget-we-got-the-opposite/ (accessed 11 April 2022).
76 WHO 2007 (n 16 above) 23.
77 AMO Al Saidi et al 'Decisive leadership is a necessity in the COVID-19 response' (2020) 396(10247) *The Lancet* 295.

78 As above, 296.
79 As above, 297.
80 M Oduor 'President Magufuli warns Tanzanians against COVID-19 vaccines' *Africanews.com* 27 January 2021 available at www.africanews.com/2021/01/27/president-magufuli-warns-tanzanians-against-covid-19-vaccines// (accessed 17 February 2022).
81 General Comments No. 1 on Article 14 (1) (D) and (E) of the Protocol to the African Charter on Human and Peoples' Rights on the Rights of Women in Africa; and General Comment No. 2 on Article 14.1 (A), (B), (C) and (F) and Article 14. 2 (A) and (C) of the Protocol to the African Charter on Human and Peoples' Rights on the Rights of Women in Africa.
82 ESCR Committee General Comment No 14: The Right to the Highest Attainable Standard on Health (Article 12) adopted on 11 August 2020 E/C.12/2000/4 para 9.
83 ESCR Committee General Comment No. 14 para 12.
84 ESCR Committee 'Statement on the coronavirus disease (COVID-19) pandemic on economic, social and cultural rights' adopted on 11 April 2020.
85 African Commission 'Press release on the impact of the COVID-19 pandemic on economic, social and cultural rights in Africa' adopted on 4 June 2020.
86 G Tassema et al 'The COVID-19 pandemic and healthcare systems in Africa: A scoping review of preparedness, impact and response' (2021) 6 *BMJ Global Health* 1; and BM Biccard 'COVID-19: Why critically ill patients in Africa are taking a big hit' *The Conversation* 22 May 2021 available at https://theconversation.com/covid-19-why-critically-ill-patients-in-africa-are-taking-a-bigger-hit-161382 (accessed 20 February 2022).
87 For example in Mauritius: A Budoo 'Rescuing human rights in Mauritius during the COVID-19 Tsunami' *Verfassungsblog* 22 April 2020 available at https://verfassungsblog.de/rescuing-human-rights-in-mauritius-during-the-covid-19-tsunami/ (accessed 20 February 2022).
88 This section is adapted from Chapter 2 of the author's unpublished doctoral thesis submitted to the University of Pretoria: A Budoo 'The role of gender budgeting in implementing the obligation to provide resources to realise women's human rights in Africa' (2016) under the supervision of Prof Magnus Killander (University of Pretoria) and Prof Attiya Waris (University of Nairobi).
89 Committee on ESCR 'General Comment No 3: The nature of states parties' obligations' adopted on 14 December 1990 E/1991/23; and Committee on ESCR 'General Comment No 17: The right of everyone to benefit from the protection of the moral and material interests resulting from any scientific, literary, or artistic production of which he or she is the author' adopted on 12 January 2006 E/C.12/GC/17 para 34: States have the obligation to take 'financial and other positive measures which facilitate the formation of professional and other associations representing the moral and material interests of authors, including disadvantaged and marginalized authors'.
90 General Comment 3 of the ESCR Committee (n 89 above) para 10.
91 ESCR Committee's concluding observations of Philippines in 'Report on the twelfth and thirteenth sessions' (1996) E/1996/22.
92 M Sepulveda *The nature of the obligations under the International Covenant on Economic, Social and Cultural Rights* (2003) 316.
93 Concluding observations of Philippines (n 91 above) para 121.
94 ESCR Committee concluding observations of the Republic of Korea (2001) E/C.12/1/Add.59 para 9; See also ESCR Committee concluding observations of Senegal (2001) E/C.12/1/Add.62 para 23.
95 Sepulveda (n 92 above) 317.
96 ESCR Committee concluding observations of Colombia in its 'Report on the twelfth and thirteenth session' (1996) E/1996/22 para 200(b).

97 ESCR Committee concluding observations on the combined second to fifth report of Kenya adopted during its 57th session (4 March 2016) E/C.12/KEN/CO/2–5 para 18.
98 ESCR Committee concluding observations on the initial report of Uganda adopted during its 50th session (19 June 2015) E/C.12/UGA/CO/1.
99 As above, para 8.
100 ESCR Committee concluding observations of Kenya (n 97 above) paras 46, 50, 52 and 58; ESCR Committee concluding observations on the initial report of Namibia adopted during its 57th session (4 March 2016) E/C.12/NAM/CO/1 paras 18, 20, 37, 48, 62 and 72; and ESCR Committee concluding observations on the initial report of Gabon adopted during its 51st session (29 November 2013) E/C.12/GAB/CO/1 para 26.
101 ESCR Committee concluding observations on the fourth and fifth periodic report of Angola adopted during its 58th session (24 June 2016) E/C.12/AGO/CO/4–5 para 8.
102 As above.
103 ESCR Committee concluding observations on the second to fourth periodic report of Egypt adopted during its 51st session (29 November 2013) E/C.12/EGY/CO/2–4 para 6.
104 General Comment No 14 of the ESCR Committee.
105 As above, para 33.
106 As above, para 47.
107 'SA needs to know who it is paying and for what: An open letter to finance minister Enoch Godongwana about SA's international loans' 21 February 2022 available at www.chr.up.ac.za/latest-news/2949-sa-needs-to-know-who-it-is-paying-and-for-what-an-open-letter-to-finance-minister-enoch-godongwana-about-sa-s-international-loans (accessed 21 February 2022).
108 ESCR Committee statement 'An evaluation of the obligation to take steps to the "maximum of available resources" under an optional Protocol to the Covenant' adopted during the 38th Session in 2007 E/C.12/2007/1.
109 As above, para 7.
110 ESCR Committee 'Statement on the coronavirus disease (Covid-19) pandemic and economic, social and cultural rights' (6 April 2020) E/C.12/2020/1.
111 Para 2 of the ESCR Committee Statement.
112 Article 45(1)(b) of the African Charter.
113 African Commission 'Resolution 449 on Human and Peoples' Rights as central pillar of successful response to COVID-19 and recovery from its socio-political impacts' ACHPR/Res.449 (LXVI) 2020 available at www.achpr.org/sessions/resolutions?id=480 (accessed 21 February 2022).
114 African Commission 'Rules of Procedure of the African Commission on Human and Peoples' Rights' 2020 Rule 82.
115 African Commission 'Concluding observations on the cumulative periodic reports (2nd, 3rd, 4th and 5th) of the Republic of Angola' adopted at the 12th extraordinary session (30 July – 4 August 2012) Recommendation No. XIV.
116 African Commission 'Concluding observations and recommendations on the combined periodic report of Burkina Faso on the implementation of the African Charter on Human and Peoples' Rights 2011–2013' adopted during the 21st extraordinary session (23 February – 4 March 2017) para 31(vi).
117 African Commission 'Concluding observations and recommendations on the initial and combined periodic report of the State of Eritrea on the implementation of the African Charter on Human and Peoples' Rights' adopted during the 63rd ordinary session (24 October – 13 November 2018) para xlvi.
118 African Commission 'Concluding observations and recommendations on the combined periodic report of the Republic of the Gambia on the implementation

of the African Charter on Human and Peoples' Rights (1994–2018) and the initial report on the Protocol to the African Charter on Human and Peoples' Rights on the Rights of Women in Africa (the Maputo Protocol) (2005–2014)' adopted during the 31st extraordinary session held virtually (19–25 February 2021) para 56 (vi).

119 African Commission 'Press statement on human rights based effective response to the novel COVID-19 virus in Africa' 24 March 2020 available at www.achpr.org/pressrelease/detail?id=483 (accessed 21 February 2022).

120 As above.

121 As above.

122 Abuja Declaration 2001, para 26.

123 As above.

124 As above, para 30.

125 WHO 'Public financing for health in Africa: From Abuja to the SDGs' (2016) 14 available at https://www.afro.who.int/publications/public-financing-health-africa-abuja-sdgs.

126 F Rahim et al 'COVID-19 funds in response to the pandemic' (2020) 1 available at file:///C:/Users/a321/Downloads/en-special-series-on-covid-19-covid-19-funds-in-response-to-the-pandemic%20(3).pdf.

127 For a list of the different funds, see Rahim et al (n 126 above) 11–12, who summarized data from a 2020 WHO survey.

128 G Grossi et al 'Budgetary responses to a global pandemic: International experiences and lessons learnt for a sustainable future' (2020) 32(5) *Journal of Public Budgeting, Accounting and Financial Management* 738.

129 As above.

130 A Ejiogu et al 'Nigerian budgetary response to the COVID-19 pandemic and its shrinking fiscal space: Financial sustainability, employment, social inequality and business implications' (2020) 32(5) *Journal of Public Budgeting, Accounting and Financial Management* 921.

131 As above, 925.

132 C de Villers et al 'The South African government's response to COVID-19' (2020) 32(5) *Journal of Public Budgeting, Accounting and Financial Management* 802.

133 Em Elkhashen et al 'Egyptian budgetary responses to COVID-19 and their social and economic consequences' (2020) 33(1) *Journal of Public Budgeting, Accounting and Financial Management* 80.

134 LGA Amoah 'COVID-19 and the state in Africa: The state is dead, long live the state' (2021) 43(3) *Administrative Theory and Praxis* 355.

135 I Chitungo 'Towards virtual doctor consultations: A call for the scale up of telemedicine in sub-Saharan Africa during COVID-19 lockdowns and beyond' (2021) 21 *Smart Health* 4.

136 Amoah (n 134 above) 359.

137 As above.

138 National Treasury (n 1 above) 31.

139 Elkhashen et al (n 133 above) 80.

140 M Odour 'Africa's COVID-19 corruption that outweighs pandemic' 25 May 2021 available at www.africanews.com/2021/05/25/africa-s-covid-19-corruption-that-outweighs-pandemic// (accessed 22 February 2022).

141 OJ Eze et al 'Health sector corruption and COVID-19 outbreak: Evidence from Anambra and Enugu States, Nigeria' (2022) 40(1) *Journal of Contemporary African Studies* 43.

142 See generally G Mathiba 'Corruption, public sector procurement and COVID-19 in South Africa: Negotiating the new normal' (2020) 55(4) *Journal of Public Administration* 642–661.

PART III

Impact of COVID-19 on the right to health of disadvantaged and marginalized groups

8

TALE OF TWO PANDEMICS

Interrogating the impact of COVID-19 on access to maternal healthcare rights for rural women in Kenya and Uganda

Muwanguzi M. Robert, Ayeranga Godfrey, and Miyienda Pauline

8.1 Background

Not in recent memory can most people recall something that has been as devastating to the entire world as the COVID-19 pandemic, leaving in its wake the dramatic loss of human life, unprecedented disruptions to states' economies, public health, sources of livelihoods, and food chains. The COVID-19 pandemic is caused by a novel coronavirus called 'severe acute respiratory syndrome coronavirus 2' or SARS-CoV-2.[1] The origin of the virus is unknown with there being two schools of thoughts regarding the origin of the virus, with one being that a zoonotic spill over through which the virus transferred to humans caused the disease,[2] while the second school of thought being that the virus was likely a lab leak engineered by the Peoples' Liberation Army of China.[3] It was initially reported by the World Health Organization (WHO) on 31 December 2019.[4] On 30 January 2020, given the threats posed to the global community, COVID-19 was declared a global health emergency by WHO.[5]

Meanwhile, WHO declared COVID-19 a global pandemic on 11 March 2020, its first such designation since declaring H1N1 influenza a pandemic in 2009.[6] The virus has since spread, leaving the world at a standstill with little or no hope of a quick return to normal life, given its rapid mutational nature, with various variants, the latest one being omicron.[7]

Uganda reported her first confirmed COVID-19 case on 21 March 2020.[8] Similar to most African states, Uganda largely avoided the high infection rates and death toll(s) resulting from contraction of the COVID-19 virus during the first global wave,[9] with 84,116 confirmed cases and 1966 deaths reported as of 6 July 2021.[10]

DOI: 10.4324/9781032671437-11

Today the statistics stands at 170,000 confirmed cases and 3,632 deaths.[11] While this is likely under-representative of the true morbidity and mortality,[12] Uganda had successfully minimized the spread and direct impact of COVID-19 within its borders through its early, rapid, and severe response.[13] However, maternal health services were severely impacted by these measures during the height of the lockdown, which may have indirectly affected morbidity and mortality in this group.

Similarly, Kenya confirmed her first case of COVID-19 on 13 March 2020, through a traveller arriving from the UK. As of 27 April 2020, there were 363 confirmed cases, 114 recoveries, and 14 deaths (12 males and 2 females).[14] To date, the total number of confirmed cases in Kenya is 343,955.[15]

The global outbreak of COVID-19 and its subsequent declaration by WHO as a global pandemic led to the adoption of various restrictions/measures by states, including lockdowns and curfews, in a bid to contain the spread of the virus. Such measures however hindered access to various important services and rights, among which were those associated with maternal health care by women, especially those residing in rural areas of Africa, given the dynamics of geographical settings and access to essential services.

In this chapter, the authors shall interrogate the impact of these restrictions and measures on the realization/enjoyment of the right to health, but with an emphasis on maternal healthcare rights of women and child mothers in rural areas of Kenya and Uganda.

8.2 Unpacking the key dimensions of rural women living in Kenya and Uganda

To fully understand the kind of people that this study sought to investigate or study, it is prudent to start by unpacking very briefly who they actually are, the rural women. Attempting to define the term 'rural' will always present challenges, leading to unnecessary confusion and unwanted mismatches by both scholars and practitioners, since it is a term fraught with distinct meanings used in different contexts and also differing to different people, institutions, and states. Simply defined, the term 'rural area' refers to an open swath of land that has few homes or other buildings, and not very many people.[16] However, the definitions of 'rural' or 'rural areas' in both policy-oriented and scholarly literature are terms often taken for granted or left undefined, leading to difficulties or confusion in the process of ascertaining their actual meaning within the context of the instant research being conducted. In essence, from the above definition, it is apparent that rural areas include all geographical locations, segments of a country's population, infrastructure, and housing that are outside a designated urban area. It therefore goes without saying that the term 'rural' primarily encompasses a composition of populations or communities, properties or infrastructure, and environs that exclude the urban territory. It is a common characteristic among especially the rural communities in the developing countries that they primarily depend on informal agricultural and pastoral sources of livelihood, and they struggle to access state social services such as healthcare services and infrastructure.[17]

As of 21 January 2022, Africa's current population is 1,390,387,820; of this, approximately 43.8% of the population live in the urban areas.[18] Globally, rural women represent more than a quarter of the world's population (roughly 1.6 billion). According to UN Women, it is estimated that 'women make up more than 50% of Africa's population and 80% of them reside in rural areas'.[19] A rural woman is an active agent of economic and social change and environmental protection, who in many ways and to various degrees is constrained by her roles as a farmer, producer, investor, caregiver, and consumer.[20] Women form the backbone of rural and national economies, comprising 43% of the world's agricultural labour force and up to 70% in some countries.[21]

By 2019/2020, the population of Kenya and Uganda was estimated to be approximately 47.6 million and 41.22 million inhabitants, respectively. The percentage of rural population against total population in Kenya and Uganda was reported at 72% and 75.05% respectively in 2020.[22] Of the above, the percentage of rural women population in Kenya and Uganda was reported at 37.53% and 42% respectively in 2015.[23]

8.3 Deconstructing the basis and dynamics of maternal healthcare rights

8.3.1 Understanding the notion of maternal health (Care)

WHO generally defines health as the enjoyment of the highest attainable standard of health, and health is one of the fundamental rights of every human being.[24] It further defines maternal health as the health of women during pregnancy, childbirth, and the postpartum period. Maternal health therefore refers to women's health before and during pregnancy, in the course of delivery and post-delivery.[25] It also encompasses the absence of maternal morbidity and maternal mortality.[26] The Special Rapporteur on the right of everyone to the enjoyment of the highest attainable standard of physical and mental health maintains that women are entitled to reproductive healthcare services, goods, and facilities that are (a) available in adequate numbers, (b) accessible physically and economically, (c) accessible without discrimination, and (d) of good quality.[27]

On the other hand, maternal health care seeks to reduce complications that may affect the maternal health of a woman before and during pregnancy, delivery and post-delivery, and includes prenatal care, delivery, and perinatal care.[28] The determinants of the state of maternal health care in a country include maternal mortality and maternal morbidity,[29] under-five child mortality, access to antenatal care (ANC), availability of skilled attendants at birth, and access to family planning services, among others.[30] Therefore, the enjoyment of maternal health care is hinged upon the absence of maternal morbidity and maternal mortality.

Maternal morbidity denotes any condition attributed to or heightened by pregnancy and childbirth which has a negative impact on the woman's well-being and/or functioning.[31] It implies any condition or symptom arising from or made worse by pregnancy.[32] Maternal mortality refers to deaths caused by complications from pregnancy or childbirth.[33] The three key components and parameters of a good and properly functioning maternal healthcare delivery system are assessed based on accessibility of women to skilled birth attendants, an enabling environment, and a functional referral system.[34] Uganda's current maternal mortality rate stands at '189 deaths per 100,000 live births',[35] while the maternal morbidity rate is that 'for every woman who dies, six survive with chronic and debilitating ill health'.[36] The maternal mortality rate in Kenya stands at '355 deaths per 100,000 live births',[37] and the maternal morbidity ratio is that for every woman who dies, another 30 suffer long-term injuries and illness due to pregnancy- and childbirth-related complications.[38]

In Kenya, maternal mortality and morbidity arise from the interchange between social, cultural, economic, and logistical barriers, combined with a high fertility rate and inadequate and under-funded health services,[39] as well as limited use of skilled care, inadequate skills among healthcare providers, and low health facility coverage.[40] However, the leading causes of maternal deaths in Uganda include unsafe abortions, obstetric haemorrhage, sepsis, and obstructed labour.[41]

8.3.2 *Probing the inequities of African healthcare systems in comparison with other parts of the world*

According to WHO, a good healthcare system must meet the six pillars of healthcare delivery, which include service delivery, healthcare workforce, medicines and technologies, financing, healthcare information systems, and leadership/governance.[42] WHO defines health inequities as differences that exist in the health status or distribution of health resources between different population groups, arising from the social conditions in which people are born, grow, live, work, and age.[43] Western-centric authors tend to use 'inequalities' to denote differences between groups and 'inequities' to denote unjust differences between groups.

The underlying root drivers of health inequity are varied, intricate, ever-changing, and symbiotic by nature and can be categorized in two ways: the first is the intrapersonal, interpersonal, institutional, and systemic drivers that shape and drive power centres and resource bases across age, geographical location, race, gender, class, sexual orientation, gender expression, and other dimensions of individual and group identity, and second is the uneven distribution through the key social determinants of health, such as access to goods, services, and societal status that also tend to drive health inequities.[44] So unpalatable is the negative effect of health inequalities in Africa that it will follow the victims 'from womb to tomb'. Without a doubt, health inequities run contrary to the basic principles of human rights since they could have been avoided by victims, having not occurred accidentally but rather being socially determined by obtaining circumstances that population groups find themselves in, and over which they have no control over.

In Africa, healthcare systems face different challenges including under-funding and non-prioritization of healthcare activities, healthcare system corruption, and poor leadership and management,[45] thereby making it hard to attain the above six WHO pillars of healthcare delivery.[46] Furthermore, the WHO 2021 report on government health spending between 2000 and 2019[47] states that Africa and South-Asia had a lower healthcare spending rate, while Europe, East Asia, and North America had a higher healthcare spending rate. This is a clear indication of the existing inequity of health care in Africa compared to the other parts of the world.

Furthermore, healthcare systems in Africa suffer from problems of limited health infrastructure and workforce, including the lack of enough specialized hospitals that are well equipped with intensive care units and shortage of well-trained professionals.[48] For example, in urban areas of Africa, due to shortages in staff, health facilities end up being overcrowded with patients, while in rural areas, the poor road infrastructure and unreliable transport means make it hard for patients to access healthcare facilities.[49] It is also important to note that although Africa bears over 24% of the global disease burden, it only spends less than 1% of the world's financial resources on health, and only has 3% of the global health workforce, while the Americas which bear only 10% of the world's disease burden spend about 50% of the world's financial resources on health and have 37% of the global health workforce.[50]

To further elaborate this inequity, WHO estimates that Africa has around 1.3 million nurses and 300,000 doctors who must provide healthcare services to about 1.4 billion people, whereas Europe has around 7.4 million nurses and 3.4 doctors who must serve a population of 749 million people, which implies that there's an estimate of about 37 doctors per every 10,000 people in Europe as opposed to Africa which has three doctors, and Europe has about 83 midwives and nurses per 10,000 people, while Africa has 13 midwives and nurses who serve around 10,000 people.[51] Furthermore, according to WHO, Africa still has the lowest density of medical doctors, that is, around 2 doctors per 10,000 people, while Europe has the highest density of medical doctors, that is, around 43 serving a population of 10,000 people.[52]

Relatedly, many people in Africa, especially the poor, experience financial barriers in their quest to obtain healthcare service, and they, thus, end up facing huge out-of-pocket expenditures before they can obtain the required medical attention due to the ineffective health insurance systems,[53] which tend to leave out the poor,[54] thereby making the poor in many sub-Saharan African countries suffer from high crippling healthcare expenditures.[55]

According to WHO, in 2020, the out-of-pocket expenditure out of the current health expenditure for Africa was at 36.04%, the Americas spent 29.22%, Southeast Asia spent 37.94%, East Mediterranean spent 35.3%, Europe spent 26.87%, and the Western Pacific region spent 16.63%. This shows that during 2020, people in the African region had the second highest out-of-pocket spending in the world as opposed to Europe, the Americas, and the Western Pacific region,[56] which depicts the existing inequities between the African healthcare systems and the other parts of the world as elaborated earlier.

This study will show that the measures adopted by the governments of Kenya and Uganda in the quest to contain the spread of the COVID-19 pandemic further exacerbated the inequality gap between women living in rural and urban areas of both countries, since rural women could not easily access maternal healthcare services as compared to those living in urban areas.

8.3.3 Establishing the linkage between the right to health and maternal health care through international human rights instruments

The right to health is recognized under several international and regional human rights instruments in Africa including the Universal Declaration of Human Rights (UDHR); International Covenant on Economic, Social, and Cultural Rights (ICESCR); Convention on the Rights of the Child (CRC); Convention on the Elimination of All Forms of Discrimination against Women (CEDAW); International Convention on the Elimination of All Forms of Racial Discrimination (CERD); African Charter on the Rights and Welfare of the Child (African Children's Charter); Convention on the Rights of Persons with Disabilities (CRPD); African Charter on Human and Peoples' Rights; and Protocol to the African Charter on Human and Peoples' Rights on the Rights of Women in Africa (Maputo Protocol). These instruments create the basis for the worldwide recognition of the right to health which includes maternal health care (rights) as will be elaborated later.

The idea that every human being is entitled to have the physical needs of their body satisfied is central to the enjoyment of many other human rights, including the right to survive and live free of suffering. Article 25 of the UDHR recognizes the right of all persons to enjoy an adequate standard of living, which encompasses their health and well-being as well as that of their family, which includes access to maternal healthcare services.

Article 12 of the ICESCR stipulates that every person has the right to enjoy the highest attainable standard of physical and mental health. The ICESCR further obliges state parties to undertake steps aimed at reducing infant mortality and ensuring the provision of medical services to the sick.[57] The above duty requires states to take measures directed towards the promotion of maternal health.[58] This provision applies to all women, including all Kenyan and Ugandan women living in rural areas. The Committee on Economic, Social and Cultural Rights (CESCR) has construed the right to health to encompass sexual and reproductive health,[59] which includes maternal health care.

Article 24 of the CRC recognizes the right of every child to enjoy the highest attainable standard of health, which includes the right to access facilities required for the treatment of illness and rehabilitation of health. The CRC also obliges states to undertake various steps to ensure the realization of the right to health of the child.[60] This provision is key in advancing maternal health care, which includes child health care.

Relatedly, the CEDAW requires states to ensure that all persons have access to healthcare services, without discrimination.[61] It further recognizes other rights related to pregnancy, including maternity, education,[62] and maternity leave,[63] thereby guaranteeing all women living in the rural areas of Kenya and Uganda the right of access to maternal healthcare services. Furthermore, reproductive health is a key component of health care, which is a basic human right.[64]

Similarly, the CRPD stipulates that persons with disabilities have the right to enjoy the highest attainable standard of health without discrimination.[65] This includes the right to access maternal healthcare services by all Kenyan and Ugandan rural women living with disabilities. Article 5 (e) (iv) of the International Covenant on the Elimination of All Forms of Racial Discrimination (ICERD) provides that all persons have a right to public health, medical care, social services, and social security.

The African Charter affirms the right to every person to enjoy the best attainable state of physical and mental health,[66] which includes maternal health. It further obligates states to undertake steps aimed at ensuring that all persons receive medical attention whenever they are sick.[67] The African Commission has noted that preventable maternal mortality violates the rights to health, life, and dignity of all women in Africa, which includes affected Kenyan and Ugandan women living in rural areas.[68] Furthermore, Article 14(1) of the African Children's Charter provides that every child enjoys the right to enjoy the best attainable state of physical, mental, and spiritual health.

In *Purohit and Moore v. The Gambia*, the African Commission expressed that 'it is aware that millions of people in Africa are not enjoying the right to health maximally because African countries are generally faced with the problem of poverty which renders them incapable to provide the necessary amenities, infrastructure and resources that facilitate the full enjoyment of this right. Therefore, having due regard to this depressing but real state of affairs, the African Commission would like to read into Article 16 the obligation on part of States party to the African Charter to take concrete and targeted steps, while taking full advantage of its available resources, to ensure that the right to health is fully realized in all its aspects without discrimination of any kind'.[69] Clearly the notion of progressive realization within available resources must not be viewed as an excuse to defeat or deny economic, social, and cultural rights like the right to health.

Article 14 of the Maputo Protocol provides that all women have the right to health, which consists of sexual and reproductive health. The above position has been echoed by the African Commission.[70] Therefore, all women living in the rural areas of Kenya and Uganda enjoy the same entitlements. The protocol further requires member states to take measures geared towards ensuring that all women have access to adequate and affordable health services, especially those living in rural areas.[71]

From the above instruments, it can be concluded that every woman has the right to safe and respected maternal health care. Fundamental human rights are violated when pregnant and birthing women endure preventable suffering, including death, illness, injury, mistreatment, abuse, discrimination, and denials of information and bodily autonomy. The law advocates for provision of health care and ensuring equality between men and women, which are the fundamental objectives of treating health as a human right.

Specifically, states have to ensure that women in both urban and rural areas have access to adequate healthcare facilities, counselling, and services in family planning. Implicit in the above obligations is the requirement that states ensure women have appropriate services in connection with pregnancy, childbirth, and the post-natal period, including family planning and emergency obstetric care. The above translates into states ensuring safe motherhood and reducing maternal mortality and morbidity in both normal and abnormal times.

8.3.4 Kenyan and Ugandan domestic legal and policy frameworks that create a basis for enjoyment of maternal healthcare rights

8.3.4.1 The case of Uganda

The 1995 Constitution of Uganda does not explicitly recognize the right to health and access to maternal health care[72] but does contain a number of key provisions and constitutional objectives and directives geared towards the advancement and safeguarding of the right to health, which may be utilized towards the promotion of maternal healthcare rights in Uganda.[73] Objectives XIV (b) and XX of the National Objectives and Directive Principles of State Policy (NODSP) require the state to take all practical measures to ensure the provision of basic medical services to the population, which include maternal health-related services. A reading of Article 45 coupled with Article 8A of the Constitution and Objectives XIV and XX altogether leads to the conclusion that the right to health exists under the 1995 Constitution.[74]

Article 45 of the Constitution guarantees the protection of other human rights not expressly contained in the Constitution, which includes the right to maternal health care. It stipulates that '*the non-inclusion of some rights and freedoms in* Chapter 4 *does not exclude their existence*'. This implies that the right to maternal health care is indirectly guaranteed by the Constitution. In particular, Article 21(1) and (2) stipulates that all persons are equal before the law and shall not be discriminated based on their status, including sex, colour, ethnicity, race, and social or economic standing, among others. By curbing such forms of discrimination, the right to access maternal health care is guaranteed since any of the above grounds can hamper the women in Uganda from accessing and enjoying their right to maternal health care due to the vulnerable nature of African women when it comes to access and enjoyment of sexual and reproductive health rights, which include maternal health-related services.[75]

Furthermore, Article 21(4) obligates the parliament to enact laws that seek to implement programmes and policies that seek to reduce societal differences in the form of social, economic, educational, and other forms of inequities, thereby advancing the right to maternal health since gender disparities have played a key role in the high maternal mortality ratio in Uganda.[76] Article 24 guarantees the right to human dignity and forbids torture, cruel, inhumane, and degrading treatment. The above provision applies to pregnant women in Uganda, including those living in rural areas who are always at the risk of being detained for failure to clear their medical bills[77] and also encounter cruel and degrading treatment while accessing maternal health-related services.[78] Despite this provision, pregnant women continue to be treated in cruel, inhumane, or degrading ways, even at the hands of health service providers. In *Joyce Nakacwa v. Attorney General and 2 others*[79], the petitioner delivered a baby by the roadside near Naguru Hospital. She proceeded to the maternity clinic with the baby still attached to her after birth to complete the birth process but received no medical care and was instead referred to Mulago Hospital without a referral letter. She lost her baby and sued the hospital, claiming that the hospital's denial to offer her a decent place to complete the birth process violated her right to freedom from torture and cruel, inhuman, and degrading treatment. The court acknowledged that the medical worker's omissions contributed to the death of the child. Nakacwa's case highlights the torturous situations that pregnant women are confronted with in the healthcare system.

Another judicial intervention on the right to maternal health was espoused in the case of *CEHURD and Others v. Nakaseke District Local Administration*,[80] where the plaintiffs sued on behalf of a woman who had died at the defendant' hospital due to lack of emergency obstetric care. It was alleged by the plaintiffs that the deceased had an obstructed labour condition but did not receive the appropriate medical care and attention due to the absence of a doctor assigned to her. The judge visited the hospital in locus to assess the evidence and held that the deceased's right to basic medical care was violated when the government hospital failed to provide a mother with access to emergency obstetric care. The defendant was also found to have breached Article 33(3) of the Constitution because the doctor on duty was absent without explanation to conduct the caesarean operation when needed. As a result of the patient waiting in pain for eight hours without medical attention, she died due to a ruptured uterus. The state was found to have breached its duty to protect women's rights given their unique status and natural maternal functions in society.

One of Uganda's oldest and perhaps one of the most important pieces of legislation for the preservation and management of public health is the 'Public Health Act', which commenced on 15 October 1935. Under section 29 of the Act, the relevant minister is empowered to make rules for the prevention of spread of a specific disease through issuance of a statutory order. Section 36 of the same Act, also empowers the same minister with powers to enforce precautions aimed at preventing the introduction of an infectious disease into Uganda through regulating, restricting, or prohibiting entry into Uganda or any part of Uganda of any person or persons of any specified class or description or from any specified country, locality, or area and even impose specific requirements or conditions regarding the medical examination, detention, quarantine, disinfection, vaccination, isolation, or medical surveillance or otherwise of persons entering, or the examination, detention, or disinfection or otherwise of such persons as aforesaid or of articles or things introduced into Uganda or any part of Uganda. One would have expected this particular legislation to lay down specific provisions that stipulate how generally the right of health can be realized, but unfortunately it is silent in this regard.

The National Drug Policy and Authority Act 1993 (National Drug Authority Act 2016) creates the National Drug Policy and National Drug Authority (NDA), which is responsible for regulating the use of drugs in Uganda, while the National Drug Policy stipulates the guidelines followed by the NDA in ensuring that the required drugs, which are cost-effective drugs, are available in Uganda.[81] This legislation is pivotal in the advancement of maternal healthcare services in Uganda by ensuring that pregnant women living in rural areas have access to the required medication when sick. However, the above law is outdated and may not depict the current realities of maternal health, such as accessing maternal health services during pandemics like COVID-19.

Other important legislations include the following: The Local Government Act (Cap 243) establishes district councils which are mandated to provide medical services, including maternal and child healthcare services.[82] However, there is no clear provision regulating the provision of maternal and child healthcare services. The Domestic Violence Act of 2010 prohibits domestic violence by prescribing penalties which the perpetrators of domestic violence will face. However, the implementation of the act has been delayed by limited government funding.[83] The Penal Code Act (Cap 120) forbids the killing of an unborn child.[84] However, it criminalizes abortion,[85] which has greatly contributed to the rampant cases of maternal deaths in Uganda.[86]

In a bid to enhance the promotion and protection of maternal healthcare rights in Uganda, a number of policies have been adopted by the government of Uganda, as elaborated later.

Under Uganda Vision 2040, it is envisioned that Uganda will transform from a peasantry to a modern and prosperous society within a period of 30 years.[87] Part of the anticipated strategies include instituting 'a paradigm shift from facility-based to a household based health delivery system' and efforts driven to 'reduce the number of maternal deaths by over 6,000 and child deaths by over 16,000 every year'.[88] It is the goal of the government of Uganda to 'design, pilot and implement appropriate service delivery models for hard-to-reach areas and disadvantaged population groups', such as rural women.[89]

Furthermore, with regard to rural women and other vulnerable groups, it is proposed that the national policy on health shall be guided by, among others, placing emphasis on the government exploring alternative, equitable, and sustainable options for health financing and health service that target the poor and other vulnerable groups, which include for instance rural women.[90]

The 2004 National Adolescent Sexual and Reproductive Health Policy seeks to promote access to cheap and good-quality healthcare services and information among adolescents to promote the inclusion of adolescents' health needs in the country's development process county and to eliminate gender disparity and violence.[91] This policy is pivotal in advancing the right to maternal health care of Ugandan women living in rural areas by ensuring that they also have access to cheap and good-quality health care, which they may not ordinarily have access to due to lack of financial resources.

The government has also adopted the Uganda Gender Policy, which seeks to promote the emancipation of all Ugandan women, stimulate gender equality, and reduce the gender-related disparities related to socio-cultural discrimination, gender-based violence, and maternal and child mortality.[92] It further aims at promoting community sensitization regarding the rights of both women and men.[93] The above policy is very pivotal in the improvement of maternal healthcare rights of rural Ugandan women since it can be used by the government as a key tool to eradicate the causes of gender inequality in Uganda.

The Second National Development Plan aims at promoting the well-being of all persons regardless of age in Uganda and ensuring they enjoy healthy lives,[94] by ensuring all persons have access to sexual and reproductive healthcare services,[95] which include maternal health care. It also seeks to reduce the high maternal mortality rate in Uganda,[96] eliminate the gender-based causes of maternal and neonatal mortality, ensure availability of and access to ANC and postnatal care, and promote skilled birth attendance and the use of health facilities.[97] This policy also applies to Ugandan women living in rural areas.

8.3.4.2 The case of Kenya

The domesticlegal framework governing maternal healthcare services in Kenya is stipulated under numerous national laws and policies passed and adopted by the government of Kenya, as elaborated later.

Kenya's 2010 Constitution explicitly recognizes the right to health under Article 43(1)(a), wherein it is stipulated that every person has the right to the highest attainable standard of health, which includes the right to healthcare services, including reproductive health care. Furthermore, Article 43(2) of the Constitution provides for the right of access to emergency treatment, which includes maternal healthcare-related services such as access to safe abortion. The above provision can be relied upon to advance the maternal healthcare rights of Kenyan women living in rural areas, which are a key component of reproductive health care.

Article 28 of the Constitution also recognizes the right to dignity of all persons in Kenya, which includes pregnant women in rural areas of Kenya. The above provision is key in the promotion and protection of maternal healthcare rights in Kenya since the enjoyment of maternal healthcare rights is dependent upon other rights including the right to dignity.[98] The same Constitution further provides for the right to access information,[99] which includes maternal healthcare-related information. It is important to note that access to sexual and reproductive health information enables women to access sexual and reproductive health services whenever the same are required,[100] while lack of access to sexual and reproductive health-related information may lead to maternal morbidities and mortalities and unsafe abortions.[101]

Article 56 of the 2010 Kenya Constitution obliges the government to adopt and implement affirmative action-related programmes aimed at ensuring that minorities and marginalized groups have reasonable access to water, infrastructure, and health services. This provision applies to women living in rural areas of Kenya, including pregnant women in such areas. In the matter of the enforcement of the Bill of Rights under Article 22(1) of the Constitution of Kenya (2010) *John Mathenge v. Attorney General and 2 Others*,[102] the court stated that the Constitution of Kenya (2010) through Article 22(1) vests the power of enforcing the Bill of Rights to the Judiciary and indicates that any claim that a fundamental right has been denied, violated, infringed, or threatened may be brought before the court.

The right to the highest attainable standard of health is included in the Bill of Rights in Article 43(1) and the powers of the court to enforce fundamental rights established the justiciability of socio-economic rights beyond doubt.[103] In the case of *Kenya Society for the Mentally Handicapped v. Attorney*

General and Others,[104] the court gave guidance on its role in enforcing the right to health as required by Article 22:

> *[T]he Court's purpose is not to prescribe certain policies but to ensure that policies followed by the State meet constitutional standards and that the State meets its responsibilities to take measures to observe, respect, promote, protect and fulfill fundamental rights and freedoms and to a party who comes before the Court.*

The right to health under the Kenyan Constitution, 2010, finds expression in Article 43(1)(a), which states that 'every person has the right to the highest attainable standard of health, which includes the right to health care services, including reproductive health care'. In the case of *P.A.O. and 2 Others v. Attorney General*,[105] the high court affirmed that the right to health is 'a fundamental human right indispensable for the exercise of other human rights', and '[e]very human being is entitled to the enjoyment of the highest attainable standard of health conducive to living a life in dignity'. It further noted that the right to health encompasses '. . . not only the positive duty to ensure that its citizens have access to health care services and medication but must also encompass the negative duty not to do anything that would in any way affect access to such health care services and essential medicines'.

In the John Mathenge case,[106] the high court stated that Kenya thus has a constitutional and international law obligation with respect to ensuring that its citizens have access to the highest attainable standard of health. The right to health is also recognized in regional and international law, which by virtue of Article 2(5) and (6) of the Constitution forms part of the Kenyan law. Kenya is bound by the provisions of the International Covenant on Civil and Political Rights (ICCPR) and the ICESCR.[107] To provide guidance on the normative content of the right to health, the CESCR developed General Comment No. 14 on Article 12, wherein it is highlighted that the normative content of this right requires that 'the right to health in all forms and at all levels contains the following interrelated and essential elements', availability, accessibility, and acceptability on quality. While the General Comments are not binding, they do have persuasive authority and give states guidance on the normative content of the rights enshrined in relevant instruments.[108] General Comment No. 14, arguably, forms part of the law in Kenya because its principles formed part of the binding dictum.

In *Maimuna Awour and another v. The Attorney General and Others*,[109] while elaborating on the right to health in Kenya, the court was guided by the CESCR, and it was noted that:

> In this regard, the CESCR states that ICESCR requires state parties to ensure that health services are available, accessible, acceptable, and of good quality. It interprets availability to encompass 'not only . . . timely

> and appropriate health care but also . . . the underlying determinants of health such as access to safe and potable water and adequate sanitation, an adequate supply of safe food, nutrition and housing, healthy occupational and environmental conditions and access to health-related . . . information'.

Under sections 5 and 6, the 2017 Health Act of Kenya recognizes the right of every person to realize the highest attainable standard of health, which encompasses having access to reproductive health services and being informed about reproductive health services such as affordable, safe, and acceptable family planning services. Other important Kenyan legislations include the Access to Information Act, which requires the government to always keep its citizenry informed in case of any danger to public health or safety.[110] Furthermore, the 2012 County Governments Act obligates county governments to use the media to conduct advocacy regarding key developmental issues such as health.[111]

The above provisions are vital in the advancement of maternal healthcare rights in Kenya since they recognize the citizens' right to access reproductive health services, which consists of maternal healthcare-related services.

In 2013, the Ministry of Health launched the Kenya National Patients' Rights Charter which recognizes the right to access health care that comprises reproductive health care, among others, the right to dignity, the right to the highest attainable quality of healthcare products and services, and the right to receive emergency treatment in any health facility irrespective of the ability to pay.[112]

The Kenya Health Policy 2014–2030 seeks to enable all persons in Kenya to enjoy the highest standard of health depending on their respective needs.[113] In a bid to achieve the above, the policy proposes the implementation of the Kenya Essential Package for Health (KEPH), which consists of a variety of healthcare interventions affecting a number of key clusters including maternal and child health, among others.[114] It also aims at the integration of gender during the planning and implementation processes of all health programmes[115] and promoting access to reproductive health services including maternal- and neonatal-related services.[116] The above policy is a key tool in the advancement of maternal healthcare rights of rural women in Kenya.

Another important policy is the National Adolescent Sexual and Reproductive Health Policy, 2015, which aims at promoting the progressive realization of sexual and reproductive health of Kenyan adolescents; incorporation of adolescent sexual and reproductive health and rights issues during the national planning process; and addressing the social, cultural, economic, and demographic factors that affect sexual and reproductive health of adolescents.[117]

In the Kenya Health Sector Strategic Plan July 2018–2023 (KHSSP 2018–2023), the government seeks to enhance the universal health coverage in

Kenya by ensuring that all Kenyans have access to affordable, equitable, and high-quality health care.[118] In a bid to achieve the above, the plan proposes the implementation of key policies and programmes including improved reporting and raising of the number of maternal and perinatal death audits so as to address the loopholes in the quality of care,[119] as well as promoting the access to and use of reproductive, maternal, and newborn health services, such as focused ANC, skilled delivery, postnatal care, and family planning.[120]

In 2006, Kenya adopted the Kenya Community Health Strategy 2020–2025, which is a community-based approach where it is envisioned that the country will adopt primary health care as the approach to deliver universal health coverage, and this is well articulated in the Kenya Primary Care Strategic Framework 2019–2024, which gives prominence to community-based primary health care.

8.4 Impact on maternal healthcare rights of Kenyan and Ugandan COVID-19 mitigation measures

In a bid to contain the spread of COVID-19, Kenya imposed strict curfews and lockdown rules. The government also banned international flights, large social gatherings, large weddings and funerals, and church gatherings, and closed schools in a bid to prevent the hastened transmission of the virus.[121] Furthermore, the government imposed a 30-day lockdown,[122] a national lockdown, and curfews that restricted movement between 7.00 p.m. and 4.00 a.m. – the time was subsequently changed from 9.00 p.m. to 5.00 a.m.[123] The above instituted government directives interrupted access to health services by pregnant mothers, thereby posing a huge impasse. Although the CESCR has noted that the right to health obliges states to ensure that all persons including marginalized groups such as children, older persons, and women have access to health facilities, goods, and related services which must be within their safe physical reach regardless of one's racial, social, or economic status,[124] the curfews and nation-wide lockdowns imposed by both states violated this key component of the right to health of the rural women in Kenya and Uganda.

Similarly, in March 2020, the government of Uganda rapidly undertook a number of measures aimed at preventing the spread of COVID-19. These included closing schools and places of worship, banning public gatherings and the use of public transport, closing entry points into the country, and declaring a national lockdown and curfew.[125] The Ugandan government also issued special travel permits to patients and healthcare workers across the country, recruited more than 200 additional health workers to reduce pressure on the existing health workers, printed and distributed nationwide COVID-specific informational materials in local languages, and ensured continued provision of routine and emergency health services, including family planning, immunization, and delivery care.[126]

Despite the above proactive measures, a lasting impact was created on the realization of maternal health rights in Kenya and Uganda since women and child mothers experienced psychological, mental, physical, and emotional harm resulting from the enforcement of such measures, especially the imposition of curfews, restrictions on movements outside homes, and the total ban on both public and private transport, yet some emergencies happened at night which made it hard to access maternal healthcare-related services, as will be elaborated later.

8.4.1 Suspension of private and public transport

On 25 March 2020, President Museveni of Uganda suspended private and public transport in Uganda in a bid to contain the spread of coronavirus.[127] This was later extended by another 21 days until 5 May 2020, which was further extended for another 14 days to allow for an expert review of the situation with a view of informing the government's decision on whether to lift or maintain the lockdown.[128] In June 2021, another ban on public transport was issued prohibiting interdistrict movements, which made it impossible to move from one district to another.[129] Kenya, on the other hand, identified and placed high-risk counties under total lockdown to curb the spread of COVID-19.[130]

The above restrictions hampered access to maternal healthcare services of Ugandan women, especially of those living in rural areas who had to resort to either walking on foot despite the distant location between their homes and the health facilities, or use motorcycles (Boda bodas) to access the health facilities, while those unable to use the above methods had to seek permission from the Resident District Commissioner (RDC) to allow them to be driven or taken to the health facilities.[131] For example, it was reported that in the Teso region, pregnant mothers resorted to using boda bodas (motorcycles) which later became expensive, thereby causing some mothers to deliver from home while others shunned seeking ANC services due to the transport burden involved in the early stages of the pandemic as a result of the travel bans imposed.[132]

There was also the case of Scovia Nakawooya, aged 39 years, who died in labour as she walked to the hospital after public transport was suspended, not knowing whom to call for permission.[133] Uganda's ambulance system is not accessible and reliable in most rural areas and is not effective in such situations. Her husband reportedly tried to look for a boda boda transport, but the operators feared arrest because boda bodas had been suspended. She tried to walk to a nearby health centre. By the time she reached, the baby had died, undelivered. She also died shortly thereafter. By 8 April 2020, at least seven women in labour had reportedly died on their way to hospitals, according to media reports.[134]

The ban on public and private transport undermined the accessibility component of the right to health of rural women in Kenya and Uganda since the CESCR Committee has noted that health facilities, services, and goods must be accessible to everyone, especially the most vulnerable or marginalized sections of the population, such as women, ethnic minorities and indigenous populations, children, older persons, adolescents, persons with disabilities, and persons with HIV/AIDS without discrimination.[135] Thus, both governments violated their duties to protect the right to health of its citizens in rural areas of Kenya and Uganda through the imposition of the ban on public and private transport, which made it difficult for vulnerable women in rural Kenya and Uganda to access the necessary maternal health-related services.

Furthermore, the above measures resulted in home deliveries due to an increased preference for traditional birth attendants (TBAs) as the women shunned health facilities.[136]

States are obligated to respect the right to health by refraining from denying or limiting equal access for all persons, including prisoners or detainees, minorities, asylum seekers, and illegal immigrants, to preventive, curative, and palliative health services.[137] The African Commission has noted that the duty to respect rights prohibits states from hindering, directly or indirectly, women's rights and ensures that women are duly informed on family planning/contraception and safe abortion services, which should be available, accessible, acceptable, and of good quality.[138] Thus, the imposition of a travel ban on private and public transport in both countries which led to the resentment of public health facilities was an indirect interference with the enjoyment of maternal health of the women in rural Kenya and Uganda.

There was also limited access to sexual and reproductive health services, including family planning services, since the travel restrictions made it difficult to access and ship in emergency contraceptives.[139] The Maputo Protocol obliges states to respect and promote the right to health of women, including their sexual and reproductive health, by providing adequate, affordable, and accessible health services to women, especially those in rural areas, as well as establishing and strengthening the existing pre-natal, delivery, and post-natal health and nutritional services for women during pregnancy and while they are breast-feeding.[140]

The African Commission on Human and Peoples' Rights has also called upon states to ensure that their citizens have free access to antenatal and obstetric services.[141] It has also noted that preventable maternal mortality infringes women's right to health, dignity, and life, including that of those living in rural areas.[142] Therefore, both governments violated the above obligations since the ban on private and public transport hampered women in rural Kenya and Uganda from accessing sexual and reproductive health services, including family planning services.

Relatedly, in a bid to counter the challenges related to the suspension of private and public transport, the Ugandan president gave additional guidance requiring that for any emergent case dealing with pregnant women, they had to seek permission from RDCs to be allowed to move. This requirement was later removed on 19 April 2020.[143] Unfortunately, this implied that women had to incur an extra cost of calling for and waiting for RDCs' permission, and while some lacked the confidence to contact the RDCs for permission or could not easily access the RDCs, some could not access their contacts, and those who called could not get through to the RDC, thus hampering access to health facilities, which in the long run led to delays in accessing medical services.

The African Commission has noted that the right to health care without discrimination obliges states to remove impediments to the health services reserved for women.[144] The CEDAW Committee has called upon states to place a gender perspective at the centre of all policies and programmes affecting women's health and to involve women in the planning, implementation, and monitoring of such policies and programmes and in the provision of health services to women.[145]

Therefore, the requirement to first seek permission from specific government officials or offices such as the RDCs prior to being allowed to move to and from healthcare facilities hindered women in the rural areas of Kenya and Uganda from accessing maternal health-related services when needed; and it is to be noted that this state measure did not consider the impact on women's right to accessing healthcare services in rural areas of Kenya and Uganda. Meanwhile, others could not access ambulances to take them to facilities since ambulances were not readily available and motorcycles could not carry passengers, forcing some to resort to the use of TBAs,[146] leading to a decline in the utilization of standard maternal healthcare-related services such as delivery, ANC attendance, child immunization, and advanced equipment in patients with high-risk pregnancies.

It is also important to note that women living in rural areas tend to be illiterate, and some can barely speak English, so communication with the RDCs became difficult. They therefore choose to suffer in silence since they could not easily seek the required RDC's permission, which was necessary before expectant women could travel to health facilities.[147] Similarly, while some Kenyan pregnant women could not access emergency transport to the health centres due to fear of being beaten by police or as a result of limited or no movement during the outbreak of the pandemic, others resorted to the use of TBAs for fear of contracting COVID-19 and due to a decline in the provision of primary healthcare services including health facility deliveries.[148] Article 16 of the African Charter provides that every individual has the right to enjoy the best attainable state of physical and mental health, and this includes women in rural areas.

Furthermore, both governments violated Article 12 of the CEDAW, which obliges states to ensure that women have access to appropriate services in connection with pregnancy, confinement, and the post-natal period since some women had no means of transportation to health facilities, thereby hindering their access to pregnancy-related services, which in the long run violated their right to health during this period.

8.4.2 Imposition of nation-wide curfews

Both countries imposed nation-wide curfews which restricted movement in Kenya, for example, between 7.00 p.m. and 4.00 a.m., which was subsequently changed from 9.00 p.m. to 5.00 a.m.,[149] while in Uganda the curfew ran from 7 p.m. to 6:30 a.m. in March 2020[150] but was later changed to run from 9.00 p.m. to 5:30 a.m.[151]

Due to the above measure, transportation to health facilities during the curfew hours became difficult since transport means were cut off, yet pregnancy emergencies knew no curfew hours, and some women in Uganda and Kenya could not easily travel to and access maternal healthcare-related services.[152]

The CEDAW Committee in its General Recommendation No. 24 on Article 12 has called upon states to remove all the barriers to women's access to health services including sexual and reproductive health, and reduce maternal mortality rates by ensuring access to safe motherhood and prenatal services.[153] The imposition of curfews in Kenya and Uganda which limited women's access to health facilities amounted to an unnecessary barrier towards the access to health facilities and violation of the right to health including maternal health of women in rural areas of Kenya and Uganda.

Furthermore, Ugandan women experienced both physical and psychological harassment at the hands of the authorities or law enforcement agencies like the Local Defence Units (LDUs) when accessing maternal healthcare-related services. For example, some experienced harassment in the form of physical beatings under the guise of enforcing the presidential guidelines regarding the curfew.[154] In Kenya, there was a 25% decline in hospital attendance and immunizations in the first quarter of 2020, which was partly attributed to the fear of pregnant women and their companions of being arrested and harassed by police during the enforcement of the curfew and other lockdown-related measures.[155]

The CESCR Committee has noted that the realization of women's right of health is also dependent on the removal of all barriers interfering with access to health services, education, and information, including in the area of sexual and reproductive health.[156] Thus, both states of Uganda and Kenya were obligated to curb the harassment experienced by both Kenyan and Ugandan women since they later hampered women in rural areas from accessing maternal health-related services.

Although expectant mothers had been allowed to seek medical services during emergencies, the location of healthcare centres necessitated long trekking to hospitals, leaving devastating effects on women and child mothers including wayside deliveries, unattended births, stillbirths due to birth-related complications, haemorrhaging, and transfer of HIV/AIDS viruses from mother to child in some cases. Recent evidence has shown that women face access challenges that are both structural, such as transportation to health facilities, and social, such as fear of healthcare workers. These settings also have already existing challenges with regard to the quality of maternal healthcare services, and women report receiving maternal health services of varied quality.[157]

An example of the earlier challenges can be seen from the case of Katukore of Katete Ward, Nyamitanga Division in Mbarara Municipality, who gave birth to baby on the roadside as she was walking to the hospital due to the transport ban.[158] Quite similar happenings occurred in Kenya, where it was reported at least three deaths of women during childbirth, while others gave birth by the roadside or in other unsanitary public places due to delays in accessing transportation resulting from government COVID-19 containment measures such as a ban on all public and private passenger transport.[159]

The right to health requires that health facilities, services, and goods must be within the safe physical reach for all sections of the population, especially vulnerable or marginalized groups, such as women, adolescents, and children, among others.[160] Thus, as the location of healthcare centres required long trekking to hospitals by pregnant women in rural areas of Kenya and Uganda, this was a violation of their right to health since the health facilities ought to have been easily accessible, which was not the case. As a result of curfew, some women in Kenya lost their sources of income,[161] which hampered their ability to access healthcare services including maternal health care due to the financial hardships during the lockdown, since priority was geared towards purchasing food and other household items as opposed to seeking medical care as some lacked transportation to the health facilities.[162]

8.5 Governments' prioritization on containing COVID-19

Governments' prioritization on containing COVID-19 while ignoring the provision of other healthcare-related services, including maternal health, left a number of women in need of maternal health services unattended to.

In the wake of COVID-19, all efforts were geared towards containment of COVID-19, thereby diverting all resources meant for the promotion of maternal health-related components and aggravating maternal mortality and morbidity,[163] yet women need unlimited access to ANC during pregnancy, skilled care during childbirth and support in the weeks after childbirth (postnatal care), and access to contraceptives.[164] This was a violation of their duty to fulfil women's sexual and reproductive rights, which obligates states to adopt relevant laws, programmes, and policies aimed at the fulfilment of women's sexual and reproductive rights, including the allocation of sufficient and available resources for the full realization of those rights.[165]

Furthermore, the above measure amounted to a violation of their duty to respect women's sexual and reproductive rights, which prohibits states from hindering the enjoyment of women's rights either directly or indirectly.[166] Therefore, the diversion of all state resources including those meant for the promotion of maternal health rights towards the containing of the COVID-19 pandemic hampered the enjoyment of maternal health-related rights of rural women in Kenya and Uganda since they could not access the services related to their sexual and reproductive rights when required.

In Uganda, some hospitals stopped providing contraceptives under the guise of avoiding crowding in health facilities.[167] For example, between 23 March 2020 and 21 April 2020, non-essential visits to Kawempe National Referral Hospital were banned, while clinics offering services of ANC and childhood immunization were temporarily closed.[168] The CESCR has noted that states must ensure that functioning public health and healthcare facilities, goods, and services, as well as programmes, are available in sufficient quantity within their states.[169] Therefore, lack of access to maternal health-related services due to the prioritization of the containment of COVID-19 violated the right to health, including maternal health of rural women in Kenya and Uganda.

In Uganda, at least 12 people were allegedly killed by security officers enforcing measures to restrict the spread of coronavirus.[170] Many others suffered severe injuries when they landed in the hands of law enforcement agencies.[171] There is also the incident in Rubaga Division in Uganda, where a seven-month pregnant woman named Mercy Nakate was beaten on 27 March 2020 by a group of policemen and members of LDU conducting patrol. They accused her of disobeying presidential guidelines on non-movement and non-congregation, for apparently, she and other people had sought shelter in a makeshift structure. She had moved out of her house to buy some herbs, reportedly one of those ethno-botanical products that pregnant women use. Rain forced her to seek shelter in a makeshift facility used by residents. The patrol team found them. Others ran away, leaving her behind. '. . . it was then that the policemen who were on patrol found us and immediately began beating us. The other people ran away but given my condition, I could not run. They descended on me, hitting and kicking me despite my cries for mercy'.[172]

The CESCR has also noted that the realization of women's right to health requires the removal of all barriers interfering with access to health services, education, and information, including in the area of sexual and reproductive health.[173] Furthermore, states are obliged to ensure that third parties do not limit people's access to health-related information and services,[174] including maternal health-related services. Thus, the failure to control the rampant behaviour of its state agents that led to some women shying away from accessing maternal health-related services shows the government violated its duty to protect the right to health of its citizens. The African Commission has also noted that the duty to protect requires state parties to take the necessary measures to prevent third parties from interfering with the enjoyment of women's sexual and reproductive rights.[175]

The lack of access to contraceptives increased the risk of unwanted pregnancies, and the pregnant women living in rural areas could not easily access the health facilities due to the ban on private and public transport.[176] It is estimated that disruptions in access to family planning services, including access to contraception and safe abortions, will result in an additional rise in maternal deaths and abortion-related complications.[177] Furthermore, due to the lockdown restrictions, access to contraceptives greatly reduced as was seen in the districts of Kapchorwa and Mbarara where patients could not easily access contraceptives since medical suppliers of contraceptives could not easily import emergency contraceptives due to the travel restrictions in place.[178]

Meanwhile in Kenya, some health facilities and health workers in Kilifi County focused all their attention towards the containment of COVID-19, which in the long run led to the diversion of resources necessary for the provision of maternal healthcare services, thereby making it difficult to provide adequate maternal health care to pregnant women in Kenya.[179] For example, since some health facilities in Kilifi County were temporarily closed while health workers were reallocated duties related to the containment and treatment of COVID-19, the poor expectant women in rural Kenya chose to deliver with the aid of TBAs, who were not only the cheaper but also the only available option to them.[180] In Uganda, between April and May 2020, some doctors from Kawempe National Referral Hospital were reallocated to COVID-19 centres to offer acute care due to the expectation of a huge increase in the COVID-19 cases.[181] The African Commission has noted that states must ensure that their women have access to good-quality reproductive health care, which must be available and be provided free from any coercion, discrimination, and violence.[182]

The CESCR has called upon states to avoid limiting access to contraceptives and other means of maintaining sexual and reproductive health.[183] Therefore, the limited access to contraceptives of Kenyan and Ugandan rural women violated their right to health since access to contraceptives is a key component of the right to health.

8.6 Future pandemics and the way forward

The COVID-19 pandemic has been a wake-up call for the global community, underscoring the need for preparedness and effective responses to future pandemics. Understanding the link between the impact of COVID-19 on the enjoyment of the right to health and potential future pandemics is crucial in shaping the way forward for African countries in general and Kenya/Uganda in particular. The subject matter discussed in this chapter holds significant importance in tackling future pandemics, and its implementation or application will be critical in safeguarding the right to health. As part of the way forward coming from this study, it is recommended that African governments (Kenya and Uganda inclusive) should take several steps to ensure that women in need of maternal healthcare services continue to receive them even during pandemic times, by taking into consideration the following:

8.6.1 Strengthening health infrastructure and preparedness

Investments in responsive and adaptable health infrastructure, warning systems, and crisis/emergency preparedness are vital in mitigating the impact of future pandemics in African countries. African countries must prioritize strengthening their healthcare systems, including training and recruiting adequate staffing, expanding hospital capacities, improving diagnostic capabilities, and ensuring an adequate supply of medical equipment and essential medicines. To this end, building resilient health systems that can effectively respond to emerging health crises is crucial for protecting the right to health during future pandemics.

Connected with strengthening health infrastructure and preparedness, it is proposed that the Kenyan and Ugandan governments should ensure that they come up with policies that promote access to quality and equitable medical services for all with special consideration on women and child mothers. It is apparent that proper responses increase populations' trust in the government, reduce fear, promote uptake of health services and quality health care, and save lives. This can also be done through strengthening collaborative maternal health services, by capacitating village health teams (VHTs) and TBAs to conduct births in cases of national emergency or pandemics to can reduce the burden on staff at health facilities, and this may increase the promotion and uptake of preventive health behaviours. Connected with this study, it is proposed that the government of Uganda will need to revise and/or enact a public health act that is in line with the recognized access to right to health standards or best practices that respond to even the pandemic times.

8.6.2 Maintaining essential healthcare services

The disruption of routine healthcare services during the COVID-19 pandemic demonstrated the need to prioritize the continuity of essential health services, even during health crises. African countries should develop robust contingency plans that ensure the provision of critical healthcare services, such as pre/post ANC, immunizations, reproductive health services, and management of chronic diseases. It is proposed that African governments should fast-track the development and instruction of a national health emergency response policy and strategy, in order to ensure that when future pandemic outbreaks occur, health facilities are able to respond to maternal health services (MHS) needs. Also, governments, through a multi-stakeholder approach, should ensure that maternal health services remain as a priority available to the most vulnerable sections of the population, especially those in rural areas, whether or not the country is in crisis. By maintaining these services, the right to health can be protected, even in the midst of a pandemic.

8.6.3 Addressing socio-economic inequalities

Future pandemics are likely to exacerbate existing socio-economic inequalities, making it imperative to address these disparities proactively. African governments should implement comprehensive social protection measures, such as income support programmes, food security initiatives, and access to quality education. It is proposed that African governments should lay focus on employing post-national or regional pandemic responsive measures and strategies that work towards the reduction of health inequalities, which may mean the discontinuation of or modification of current programmes or actions that have driven socio-economic inequalities.

There is also an important role for national agencies, including public and third sector organizations, to support local delivery through advocacy and evidence building. By addressing socio-economic inequalities, vulnerable populations can be better protected, and the right to health can be upheld during future pandemics.

8.6.4 Enhancing community engagement and empowerment

Community engagement and empowerment play a crucial role in effectively responding to pandemics. Encouraging active community participation in public health decision-making, disseminating accurate and timely information, and promoting health literacy can help ensure a coordinated and effective response. Empowering communities to actively participate in their own healthcare and decision-making processes is essential for protecting the right to health in future pandemics.

8.6.5 Embracing technological innovations

The COVID-19 pandemic highlighted the potential of technological innovations in healthcare delivery. Based on this study, it is proposed that African governments should optimize modern day service delivery settings and platforms, including the use of technological solutions such as telemedicine and ensuring the establishment of effective risk screening, triage, and patient flow for all. They should equally maintain or increase resources for continuation of maternal health services with a functional referral system, including emergency obstetric and newborn care and linkage with higher-level hospitals. To realize the above, the proposal is that African countries should invest in digital health infrastructure, such as telemedicine, mobile health applications, and data analytics, to enhance healthcare access and delivery. These innovations can help bridge gaps in healthcare services, improve surveillance and early detection, and facilitate efficient resource allocation during future pandemics.

8.6.6 States should facilitate health workers to do their jobs

Sick healthcare providers strain an already under-resourced healthcare system. Handling of safety concerns of healthcare providers has been poor, putting their lives and those of patients at risk. Consequently, healthcare providers have threatened to go on strike due to lack of PPE and poor working conditions on several occasions since the first case of COVID-19 was reported. Moreover, community-based health workers (CHWs) are poorly remunerated, equipped, and facilitated to support formal healthcare providers to reduce the healthcare burden. More advocacy is needed at the national and regional levels to ensure that all healthcare providers, including community health workers, have PPE and are trained on COVID-19 infection prevention and control, equipped, and facilitated to ensure the well-being of pregnant women and mothers, and society at large.

8.6.7 Future pandemic response measures and strategies

Future responses to pandemics should be balanced with reproductive and maternal health services by giving special consideration to women in all responses; creating a special task force decentralized to a village/cell to handle MHS-related emergencies; and using an already-created database of women seeking MHSs and using the same to track down and follow such women. Taking the example of Kakamega County of Kenya, local administrators have registered pregnant women so as to facilitate their movement when in labour during night curfew hours.[184] Pregnant women in labour during curfew hours can call the local administrators, who link them with licensed boda boda riders (motorbike taxis) from their location and issue slips allowing transportation, so the riders can take the women to health facilities. Most women use boda boda riders as the few available ambulances serve a vast area.[185]

As a way forward, it is therefore proposed that future responses to pandemics should be balanced with reproductive and maternal health services by

(i) giving special consideration to women in all responses;
(ii) creating a special task force decentralized to a village/cell to handle the MHS-related emergencies; and
(iii) using an already-created database of women seeking MHSs and using the same to track down and follow such women.

8.7 Conclusion

The subject matter discussed in this chapter is critical in tackling future pandemics and protecting the right to health in Africa. In this study, it has been shown that both international treaties and domestic legislations/policies of Kenya and Uganda impliedly recognize the right to maternal healthcare rights of women in both pandemic and non-pandemic times. The governments of both states have committed themselves to protecting and promoting this right through international declarations and their domestic legislation and policies, and at international conferences.

There is no doubt that throughout sub-Saharan Africa, the COVID-19 pandemic had an incontrovertible negative impact on the maternal healthcare rights/welfare landscape, with one of its most troubling effects being its lop-sided impact on vulnerable groups like rural women. Learning from how Kenya and Uganda responded to the challenges posed by the COVID-19 pandemic, by strengthening health infrastructure and preparedness, maintaining essential healthcare services, addressing socio-economic inequalities, enhancing community engagement, and embracing technological innovations, African countries can be better equipped to respond effectively to future pandemics. Kenya's and Uganda's experiences and lessons learned from the COVID-19 pandemic provide a blueprint for proactive and comprehensive action to protect the right to health for all, ensuring a healthier and more resilient Africa in the face of future pandemics.

In this study, it has been shown that just like in many sub-Saharan African countries, the rural women of Kenya and Uganda have borne the brunt of the harmful effects of the COVID-19 pandemic, leading to numerous deaths, complicated pregnancies, injuries, and losses. This was a result of limited and heavily restricted access to essential maternal and child health services for a significant time period of lockdowns as a result of COVID-19 restrictions and scarce resources in already overstretched hospitals and health centres. It is evident that the COVID-19 pandemic impacted maternal health care (rights) both directly and indirectly as a consequence of drastic state-driven interventions to contain its spread, hence leading to dire negative health, social, and economic consequences.

It is very important that African governments learn from the challenges that the COVID-19 pandemic posed to each state as a blueprint for future health crises, and institute adequate and relevant response plans as a countermeasure for emerging diseases of public health importance. In order to avoid a future 'vicious cycle' of repetitive pandemic impacts on vulnerable groups like rural women, it is recommended that African states must adopt new adaptable healthcare policies, strategies, and measures that are inclusive to the needs, standards, and expectations of those that require maternal healthcare services during pandemics. It is evident that without African governments introducing all-inclusive measures that respond to the pandemic's gendered impacts, there is every possibility that future pandemics will always reverse hard-won battles for realizing women's rights.

Notes

1 World Health Organisation 'Coronavirus disease (COVID-19) pandemic' available at https://www.who.int/europe/emergencies/situations/covid-19 (accessed 4 January 2024).
2 World Health Organization 'WHO-convened global study of origins of SARS-CoV-2: China part joint WHO–China study joint report' (2021) 116, available at https://www.who.int/publications/i/item/who-convened-global-study-of-origins-of-sars-cov-2-china-part (accessed 13 October 2023).
3 MR Gordon & WP Stroppel 'Lab leak most likely origin of COVID-19 pandemic, energy department now says' *The Wall Street Journal* February 2023 available at www.wsj.com/articles/covid-origin-china-lab-leak-807b7b0a (accessed 13 October 2023). See also A Kasprak 'DOE and FBI say lab origin of COVID is 'most likely' – but won't say why' *Snopes* March 2023 available at www.snopes.com/news/2023/03/03/fbi-doe-covid-origin/ (accessed 13 October 2023).
4 World Health Organization 'Origin of SARS-CoV-2' *World Health Organisation* (2020) 26, available at https://iris.who.int/bitstream/handle/10665/332197/WHO-2019-nCoV-FAQ-Virus_origin-2020.1-eng.pdf (accessed 13 October 2023).
5 World Health Organization 'Statement on the second meeting of the International Health Regulations (2005) emergency committee regarding the outbreak of novel coronavirus (2019-nCoV)' available at www.who.int/news/item/30-01-2020-statement-on-the-second-meeting-of-the-international-health-regulations-(2005)-emergency-committee-regarding-the-outbreak-of-novel-coronavirus-(2019-ncov) (accessed 13 April 2022). See A Gallegos 'WHO declares public health emergency for novel coronavirus' *Medscape Medical News* (2020) available at www.medscape.com/viewarticle/924596 (accessed 21 December 2021); See also SL Wee et al 'W.H.O. declares global emergency as Wuhan Coronavirus spreads' *The New York Times* 30 January 2020 available at www.nytimes.com/2020/01/30/health/coronavirus-world-health-organization.html (accessed 1 December 2021).
6 MC Neil et al 'Coronavirus has become a pandemic: WHO says' *The New York Times* 11 March 2020 available at www.nytimes.com/2020/03/11/health/coronavirus-pandemic-who.html (accessed 21 December 2021).
7 World Health Organization 'Classification of omicron (B.1.1.529): SARS-CoV-2 variant of concern' (2021) available at www.who.int/news/item/26-11-2021-classification-of-omicron-(b.1.1.529)-sars-cov-2-variant-of-concern (accessed 21 December 2021).
8 The Independent 'Uganda confirms first COVID-19 case' *The Independent* 22 March 2020 available at www.independent.co.ug/uganda-confirms-first-covid-19-case/ (accessed 13 October 2023).
9 World Health Organization 'The Coronavirus disease 2019 (COVID-19) strategic preparedness and response plan for the WHO Africa region: 1 February 2021–31 January 2022' (2021) available at www.afro.who.int/sites/default/files/2021-04/WHO%20AFR%20Covid-19%202021%20SRP_Final_16042021.pdf (accessed 10 December 2021).
10 Johns Hopkins University & Medicine 'Uganda-COVID-19 overview' (2021) available at https://coronavirus.jhu.edu/region/uganda (accessed 21 December 2021).
11 Ministry of Health 'Coronavirus (pandemic) COVID-19'available at www.health.go.ug/covid/ (accessed 13 October 2023).

12 S Colombo et al 'COVID-19 in Africa: The little we know and the lot we ignore' (2020) 44 *Epidemiol Prev* 408–422, 146.
13 F Margini et al 'Case study: The initial COVID-19 response in Uganda' *Think Well and Ministry of Health Uganda* (2020) available at https://thinkwell.global/wp-content/uploads/2020/09/Uganda-COVID-19-Case-Study-_18-Sept-20201.pdf (accessed 8 January 2020).
14 M Nanyingi 'The evolution of the COVID-19 pandemic in Kenya' *Royal Society of Tropical Medicine and Hygiene* (2020) available at https://rstmh.org/news-blog/news/the-evolution-of-the-covid-19-pandemic-in-kenya (accessed 22 December 2021).
15 World Health Organization 'WHO (COVID-19) Home Page-Kenya' https://covid19.who.int/region/afro/country/ke (accessed 13 October 2023).
16 National Geographic Encyclopedia 'Rural area' available at www.nationalgeographic.org/encyclopedia/rural-area/#:~:text=Encyclopedic%20Entry%20Vocabulary,A%20rural%20area%20is%20an%20open%20swath%20of%20land%20that,very%20close%20to%20one%20another (accessed 20 January 2022).
17 United Nations 'Social protection in rural areas: Achieving universal access for all' (2021) available at https://www.un.org/development/desa/dspd/2021/05/social-protection-in-rural-areas/ (accessed 4 January 2024).
18 Worldometer 'Africa Population' available at https://www.worldometers.info/world-population/africa-population/#google_vignette (accessed 4 January 2024).
19 Women Watch 'The UN system: Working together to empower rural women' (2012) available at www.un.org/womenwatch/feature/ruralwomen/index.html (accessed 14 January 2022).
20 As above.
21 Ecologia Youth Trust 'Empowering rural women in Kenya' (2016) available at www.ecologia.org.uk/2016/10/empowering-rural-women-kenya/(accessed 15 January 2022).
22 Trading Economics 'Matrix' available at https://tradingeconomics.com/matrix (accessed 15 January 2022).
23 As above.
24 Constitution of the World Health Organization, 1.
25 World Health Organization 'Maternal health' (2016) available at www.who.int/maternal-health/en/ (accessed 20 December 2021).
26 Rural Health Information Hub 'Defining maternal health' available at www.ruralhealthinfo.org/toolkits/maternal-health/1/definition (accessed 20 December 2021).
27 UN Human Rights Council 'Report of the Special Rapporteur on the right of everyone to the enjoyment of the highest attainable standard of physical and mental health' para 17 available at https://digitallibrary.un.org/record/584517?ln=en (accessed 13 April 2022).
28 D Kifle et al 'Maternal health care service seeking behaviors and associated factors among women in rural Haramaya district, Eastern Ethiopia: A triangulated community-based cross-sectional study' (2017) 14(6) *Reproductive Health* 2.
29 T Firoz et al 'Measuring maternal health: Focus on maternal morbidity' (2013) 91 *Bulletin of the World Health Organization* 794.
30 World Health Organization 'Recommendation 2: Health indicators' available at www.who.int/woman_child_accountability/progress_information/recommendation2/en/ (accessed 21 December 2021).
31 TR Edward et al 'Hunter's tropical medicine and emerging infectious diseases' (2020) 138 [journal]
32 Ministry of Health 'National guidelines for quality obstetrics and perinatal care' (2011) 11 available at http://guidelines.health.go.ke:8000/media/

National_Guidelines_for_Quality_Obstetrics_and_Perinatal_Care.pdf (accessed 22 December 2021).

33 UNICEF 'Maternal mortality' (2019) available at https://data.unicef.org/topic/maternal-health/maternal-mortality/ (accessed 22 December 2021); See also MC Hogan et al 'Maternal mortality for 181 countries, 1980–2008: A systematic analysis of progress towards millennium development goal 5' (2010) 375 *The Lancet* 1609.

34 World Health Organization 'Maternal health' available at www.who.int/health-topics/maternal-health#tab=tab_1 (accessed 13 October 2023).

35 Uganda Bureau of Statistics 'Uganda demographic and health survey (UDHS) 2022' September 2023 available at www.ubos.org/wp-content/uploads/publications/09_2023UDHS_2022_Key_Findings_Presentation_B.pdf (accessed 13 October 2023).

36 World Health Organization 'Maternal and child health: Uganda' (2011) 1 available at www.who.int/pmnch/media/membernews/2011/ugandabackgroundpaper.pdf (accessed 21 December 2021).

37 UNFPA Kenya 'Maternal Health' available at https://kenya.unfpa.org/en/topics/maternal-health-16 (accessed 13 October 2023).

38 As above.

39 World Health Organization 'Maternal and child health: Kenya' (2011) 2 available at www.who.int/pmnch/media/membernews/2011/20121216_kenyaparliament.pdf (accessed 21 December 2021).

40 UNFPA 'Maternal Health and HIV' available at https://kenya.unfpa.org/en/topics/maternal-health-and-hiv (accessed 21 December 2021).

41 Ministry of Health 'Roadmap for accelerating the reduction of maternal and neonatal mortality and morbidity in Uganda' (2007–15) 11 available at http://library.health.go.ug/sites/default/files/resources/Road%20map%20for%20accelerating%20the%20reduction%202007-15.pdf (accessed 20 December 2021).

42 World Health Organisation 'Everybody business: Strengthening health systems to improve health outcomes: WHO's framework for action' (2007) 3 available at https://www.who.int/publications/i/item/everybody-s-business----strengthening-health-systems-to-improve-health-outcomes (accessed 4 January 2024).

43 World Health Organization 'Health inequities and their causes' 22 February 2018 available at www.who.int/news-room/facts-in-pictures/detail/health-inequities-and-their-causes (accessed 21 July 2023).

44 National Academies of Sciences, Engineering, and Medicine; Health and Medicine Division; Board on Population Health and Public Health Practice; Committee on Community-Based Solutions to Promote Health Equity in the United States; A Baciu, Y Negussie, A Geller et al editors *Communities in action: Pathways to health equity* (2017 January 11). '3 The root causes of health inequity' available at www.ncbi.nlm.nih.gov/books/NBK425845/ (accessed 28 July 2023).

45 OO Olebire et al 'Identifying key challenges facing healthcare systems in Africa and potential solutions' (2019) 12 *International Journal of General Medicine* 395–401.

46 As above.

47 World Health Organization 'Global expenditure on health: Public spending on the rise?' (2021) 3 available at https://apps.who.int/iris/handle/10665/350560 (accessed 21 July 2023).

48 GA Tessema 'The COVID-19 pandemic and healthcare systems in Africa: A scoping review of preparedness, impact and response' 2021 *BMJ Global Health* 1.

49 As above.

50 SCA Anyangwe et al 'Inequities in the global health workforce: The greatest impediment to health in sub-Saharan Africa' (2007) 4(2) *International Journal of Environmental Research Public Health* 93.

51 The Africa-Europe Foundation 'The unequal distribution of workforces between Africa and Europe' 10 November 2022 available at www.africaeuropefoundation.org/stories/health-addressing-the-health-workforce-crisis-in-africa-and-in-europe/ (accessed 24 July 2023).
52 World Health Organization 'Health workforce' available at www.who.int/data/gho/data/themes/health-workforce (accessed 24 July 2023).
53 BSC Uzochukwu 'Health care financing in Nigeria: Implications for achieving universal health coverage' (2015) 18(4) *Nigerian Journal of Clinical Practice* 437–444.
54 AP Fenny 'Social health insurance schemes in Africa leave out the poor' (2018) 10(1) *Internal Health Journal* 1–3.
55 As above.
56 World Health Organization 'Out-of-pocket expenditure as percentage of current health expenditure (CHE) (%)' 14 April 2023 available at www.who.int/data/gho/data/indicators/indicator-details/GHO/out-of-pocket-expenditure-as-percentage-of-current-health-expenditure-(che)-(-) (accessed 24 July 2023).
57 Arts 12(2) (a)-(c).
58 UN Committee on Economic, Social and Cultural Rights (CESCR Committee) 'General Comment No. 14: The right to the highest attainable standard of health' E/C.12/2000/4, para 14.
59 As above, para 21.
60 Art 24 of the CRC.
61 Art 12.
62 Art 5(b).
63 Art 11(2).
64 Committee on the Elimination of Discrimination against Women (CEDAW Committee), General Recommendation 24: Women and Health, A/54/38/Rev.1, para 1.
65 Art 25.
66 Art 16.
67 Art 16(2).
68 ACHPR/Res.135 (XXXXIIII) 08: Resolution on Maternal Mortality in Africa, para 1.
69 African Commission on Human and Peoples' Rights Communication 241 of 2001.
70 General Comment No. 2 on Art 14 (1) (d) and (e) of the Protocol to the African Charter on the Rights of Women, para 5.
71 As above, para 29.
72 BK Twinomugisha 'Exploring judicial strategies to protect the right of access to emergency obstetric care in Uganda' (2007) 7 *African Human Rights Law Journal* 285.
73 Arts 21, 23, 24, 45.
74 See also CEHURD and Others Versus Attorney General, Constitutional Appeal No. 1 of 2013, at p. 53, where the Supreme Court held that the 1995 Constitution guarantees the citizens right to access medical care.
75 V Balogun and E Durojaye 'The African commission on human and peoples' rights and the promotion and protection of sexual and reproductive rights' (2011) 11 *African Human Rights Law Journal* 380.
76 R Morgan et al 'Gender dynamics affecting maternal health and health care access and use in Uganda' (2017) 32 *Health Policy and Planning* 13–14.
77 A Wesaka 'It is illegal for hospitals to detain patients for failure to pay hospital bills' *Daily Monitor* 22 November 2016 available at www.monitor.co.ug/Magazines/HealthLiving/Illegal-hospitals-detain-patients-bills/689846-3458948-11spvftz/index.html (accessed 12 December 2021).

78 Centre for Human Rights and Development (CEHURD) and EQUINET 'EQUINET case study report: Review of constitutional provisions on the right to health in Uganda' (2018) 16.
79 Constitutional Petition No. 2 of 2001.
80 High Court Civil Suit 111, 2012.
81 Sec 3(1) a.
82 Second schedule part 2(c).
83 Civil Society Budget Advocacy Group 'Quarter 1 FY 2018/19 gender-based violence monitoring report: Kaberamaido district' November 2018, 9 available at http://csbag.org/wp-content/uploads/2018/03/CSBAG_Funding-Analysis-of-the-Domestic-Violence-Act-.pdf (accessed 2 December 2021).
84 Secs 212 and 213.
85 Secs 141–143.
86 CECSR Committee 'Concluding observations on the initial report of Uganda' (E/C.12/UGA/CO/1) 8 July 2015, para 35.
87 Uganda Vision 2040, 4.
88 As above, 89–90.
89 Uganda National Health Policy of 2010, 44.
90 Draft National Health Policy, 4.3.
91 Ministry of Health 'National adolescent sexual and reproductive health policy' (2015) 8 available at https://platform.who.int/docs/default-source/mca-documents/policy-documents/policy/ken-ad-17-02-policy-2015-eng-national-adolescent-srh-policy.pdf (accessed 2 December 2021).
92 Ministry of Health 'Uganda gender policy 2007 (2007) 14 & 19.
93 As above, 14–15.
94 Ministry of Health 'Second national development plan (NDPII) (2015/16–2019/20) 188.
95 As above, 272.
96 As above, 188 and 125.
97 As above, 126.
98 B Odallo et al 'Litigating to ensure access to quality maternal health care for women and girls in Kenya' (2018) 26(53) *Reproductive Health Matters* 123; See also Republic Vs Minister for Home Affairs and 2 Others Ex-parte Leonard Sitanize Misc. Civil Case 1652 of 2004 (2008) eKLR, 11.
99 Art 35.
100 Center for Reproductive Rights and the Trust for Indigenous Culture and Health 'Access to SRHR information by women and girls in Kenya: Assessment of Nairobi, Homabay, Kericho and Kilifi Counties' (2021) 1 available at https://reproductiverights.org/kenya-access-to-srhr-information-women-girls/. (accessed 2 December 2021).
101 JL Morris and H Rushwan 'Adolescent sexual and reproductive health: The global challenges' (2015) S40–S42 *International Journal of Gynecology and Obstetrics* 40–42.
102 Constitutional Petition No 147 of 2015.
103 GM Musila 'Realizing the transformative promise of the 2010 constitution and new electoral laws' in GM Musila (ed) *Handbook on election disputes in Kenya: Context, legal framework, institutions and jurisprudence* (2013) 120.
104 Petition No. 155A of 2011.
105 PAO and others v Attorney General Petition No. 409 of 2009; Okwanda v Minister of Health Services and 3 others Petition 94 of 2012; L.N and 21 others v Ministry of Health and 2 others Petition No. 218 of 2013; W.J & another v Astarikoh Henry Amkoah & 9 others Petition No. 331 of 2011; and Maimuna Awour and another v the Attorney General and others Petition No. 562 of 2012.
106 John Mathenge (n 102 above).

107 Acceded to by Kenya on 1 May 1972 and provides that the state parties undertake to guarantee that the rights enunciated in the Covenant will be exercised without discrimination of any kind as to race, colour, sex, language, religion, political or other opinion, national or social origin, property, birth, or other status. 22 In General Comment No. 20 the CESCR confirmed that the "other status" listed in ICESCR Article 2(2) includes sexual orientation and gender identity.
108 C Blake 'Normative instruments on international human rights law: Locating the general comment' *Centre for Human Rights and Global Justice Working Paper No. 17* (2008) 3.
109 Petition No. 562 of 2012.
110 Sec 5(2).
111 Sec 94.
112 Ministry of Health 'The Kenya national patients'*Rights Charter* (2013).
113 Ministry of Health 'Kenya health policy 2014–2030' (2014) 5.
114 As above, 30.
115 Kenya Health Policy 2014–2030, Objective viii.
116 As above, Objective 4(iv).
117 Ministry of Health (n 91 above) 6.
118 Ministry of Health-Kenya 'Kenya health sector strategic plan' (2018) ix.
119 As above, 58–59.
120 As above, 59–60.
121 C Tanui 'Church services, mosque gatherings banned as govt moves to contain COVID-19'*Capital News* 22 March 2020 available at www.capitalfm.co.ke/news/2020/03/22 (accessed 13 January 2022).
122 Africa News 'Kenya imposes new lockdown – what are the restrictions?'*Africa News* 26 March, 2020 available at www.africanews.com/2021/03/26/kenya-imposes-new-lockdown-what-are-the-restrictions// (accessed 13 January 2022).
123 Tanui (n 121 above).
124 CESCR (n 58 above) para 12(b).
125 Margini (n 13 above).
126 Ministry of Health 'Update on the COVID19 response in Uganda, press release' (2020) available at www.health.go.ug/covid/2020/04/02/update-on-the-covid19-response-in-uganda/ (accessed 13 January 2022).
127 Garda World 'Uganda: Authorities suspend public transport as of March 25/update 2' *Garda World* 26 March 2020 available at www.garda.com/crisis24/news-alerts/326696/uganda-authorities-suspend-public-transport-as-of-march-25-update-2 (accessed 14 January 2022).
128 J Kiiza 'Uganda relaxes coronavirus lockdown measures' *New Vision* 15 April 2020 available at www.newvision.co.ug/new_vision/news/1518485/-live-coronavirus-lockdown-ugandas (accessed 14 January 2022).
129 K Kazibwe 'Public, private transport banned as Museveni announces total lockdown' *Nile Post* 18 June 2021 available at http://nilepost.co.ug/2021/06/18/public-private-transport-banned-as-museveni-announces-total-lockdown/ (accessed 14 January 2022).
130 Reuters and G Obulutsa et al 'Kenya's president orders new lockdown to curb COVID-19 wave' *Reuters* 26 March 2021 available at www.reuters.com/world/middle-east/kenyas-president-orders-new-lockdown-battle-covid-19-wave-2021–03–26/ (accessed 15 January 2022).
131 AM Tusingwire 'COVID-19 in Uganda: The fates and futures of maternal health' April (2020) *Konrad Adenauer Stiftung*8.
132 The Independent 'Antenatal visits, deliveries drop in health facilities in Teso' *The Independent* 14 May 2020 available at www.independent.co.ug/antenatal-visits-deliveries-drop-in-health-facilities-in-teso/ (accessed 15 January 2022).

133 E Biryabarema 'In Uganda, mothers in labour die amidst coronavirus lockdown' *Reuters* April 9 2020 https://www.reuters.com/article/us-health-coronavirus-uganda-idUSKCN21R2FA/ (accessed 4 January 2024).
134 Ibid.
135 CESCR (n 58 above).
136 A Kyolatengerire 'Why March registered upsurge in pregnant women deaths' *New Vision* (2020) available at www.newvision.co.ug/news/1522709/march-registered-upsurge-pregnant-women-deaths (accessed 15 January 2022).
137 CESCR (n 58 above) para 34.
138 General Comment No. 2 on Article 14.1 (a), (b), (c) and (f) and Article 14. 2 (a) and (c) of the Protocol to the African Charter on Human and Peoples' Rights on the Rights of Women in Africa, para 42.
139 Tsvangirayi Mukwazi 'Coronavirus lockdowns mean millions of women can't access birth control' *Associated Press* 9 April 2020 available at *www.marketwatch.com/story/coronavirus-lockdowns-mean-millions-of-women-cant-access-birth-control-2020–04–09* (accessed 15 January 2022).
140 Maputo Protocol, art 14(1) and 2(a & b).
141 ACHPR/Res.135 (XXXXIIII) 08: Resolution on Maternal Mortality in Africa, para 1.
142 As above, preamble; para 2.
143 A Masake 'Gendered impacts of COVID-19: Proposed interventions for vulnerable groups' *Policy Brief* (2020) 9 available at https://cepa.or.ug/wp-content/uploads/2020/06/COVID-Policy-Brief-UPDATED.pdf. (accessed 15 January 2022).
144 African Commission, General Comment No. 2, para 25.
145 CEDAW General Recommendation No. 24: Article 12 of the Convention (Women and Health), para 31(a).
146 E Pallangyo 'The impact of COVID-19 on midwives' practice in Kenya, Uganda and Tanzania: A reflective account' (2020) 89 *Midwifery* 102774.
147 Tusingwire (n 131 above).
148 SO Ombere 'Maternal health services and COVID-19' (2021) (6) *Frontiers in Sociology* 3–4.
149 Tanui (n 121 above).
150 *H Kyeyune 'Uganda declares curfew to curb spread of COVID-19' Anadolu Agency 31 March 2020* available at *www.aa.com.tr/en/africa/uganda-declares-curfew-to-curb-spread-of-covid-19/1785775* (accessed 15 January 2022).
151 M Oduor 'Uganda imposes new lockdown – what are the restrictions?' *Africa News* 7 June 2020 available at www.africanews.com/2021/06/07/uganda-imposes-another-lockdown-what-are-the-restrictions// (accessed 15 January 2022).
152 *E Ateva 'COVID-19 curfew restrictions impact reproductive, maternal, and newborn health and rights worldwide' The White Ribbon Alliance (2020)* available at *www.whiteribbonalliance.org/2020/06/08/covid-19-curfew-restrictions-impact-women-and-newborns-worldwide/* (accessed 15 January 2022).
153 Para 31 (b & c).
154 Tusingwire (n 131 above) 9.
155 JM Mwobobia 'The repercussions of COVID-19 fight' *Standard Newspaper* 1 June 2020 available at www.standardmedia.co.ke/health/article/2001373476/the-repercussions-of-covid-19-fight; See also A Oketch 'Hospital births, vaccination visits drop as Kenya battles virus' *All Africa* (2020) available at https://allafrica.com/stories/202005280235.html (accessed 15 January 2022).
156 Para 21.
157 V Naanyu et al 'Why do women deliver where they had not planned to go? A qualitative study from peri-urban Nairobi Kenya' (2020) 20(30) *BMC Pregnancy Childbirth* 2.

158 New Vision 'Mother delivers baby from roadside toilet' *New Vision* 18 May 2020 available at https://www.newvision.co.ug/news/1518983/mother-delivers-baby-toilet-hospital (accessed 4 January 2024).
159 A Gordon, 'In Kenya, these interventions are decreasing maternal mortality' *Aljazeera* 13 December 2022 available at https://www.aljazeera.com/features/2022/12/13/in-kenya-these-interventions-are-decreasing-maternal-mortality (accessed 4 January 2024).
160 CESCR (n 58 above) para 12(b).
161 M Quaife et al 'The impact of COVID-19 control measures on social contacts and transmission in Kenyan informal settlements' (2020) 18(4) *BMC Medicine* 316.
162 J Oluoch-Aridi et al 'COVID-19 and maternal health in Kenya' 2020(1) *Frontiers in Global Women's Health* 6; M Shupler et al 'COVID-19 lockdown in a Kenyan informal settlement: Impacts on household energy and food security' (2020) *medRxiv* 9.
163 United Nations 'Policy brief: The impact of COVID-19 on women' *United Nations* (2020) 10 available at www.un.org/sexualviolenceinconflict/wp-content/uploads/2020/06/report/policy-brief-the-impact-of-covid-19-on-women/policy-brief-the-impact-of-covid-19-on-women-en-1.pdf (accessed 15 January 2022).
164 UNFPA 'Providing emergency obstetric and newborn care' *UNFPA* (2012) 2 available at www.unfpa.org/sites/default/files/resource-pdf/EN-SRH%20fact%20sheet-Urgent.pdf (accessed 15 January 2022).
165 African Commission, General Comment No. 2 (n 70 above) para 45.
166 Ibid, para 42.
167 *Mukwazi (n 139* above).
168 JF Burtet al'Indirect effects of COVID-19 on maternal, neonatal, child, sexual and reproductive health services in Kampala, Uganda' (2021) (6) *BMJ Global Health*2.
169 CESCR (n 58 above) para 12(a).
170 BBC 'Uganda – where security forces may be more deadly than coronavirus' *BBC* 23 July 2020 available at https://www.bbc.com/news/world-africa-53450850 (accessed 4 January 2024).
171 New Vision'10 Police officers held for 'torturing' women over breaking curfew' *New Vision* 7 April 2020 available at https://www.newvision.co.ug/news/1517669/ugandan-police-held-torturing-women-breaking-curfew (accessed 4 January 2024).
172 Daily Monitor 'Coronavirus curfew: Police officers detained for torturing woman' *Daily Monitor* 4 April 2020 available at www.monitor.co.ug/uganda/news/national/coronavirus-curfew-police-officers-detained-for-torturing-woman-1883928?view=htmlamp (accessed 15 January 2022).
173 CESCR (n 58 above) para 21.
174 As above, para 35.
175 African Commission, General Comment No. 2 (n 70 above) para 43.
176 Tusingwire (n 131 above) 9.
177 T Riley et al 'Estimates of the potential impact of the COVID-19 pandemic on sexual and reproductive health in low- and middle-income countries'(2020) 46 *International Perspective on Sexual and Reproductive Health* 73–76.
178 *Mukwazi (n 139* above).
179 Ombere (n 148 above) 3.
180 As above, 4–5.
181 Burt (n 168 above).
182 African Commission, General Comment No. 2 (n 70 above) para 53.
183 CESCR (n 58 above) para 35.

184 NTV Kenya 'Plight of expectant women during curfew' (2020) available at www.youtube.com/watch?v=yxuzt_iV4ec (accessed 24 December 2020).
185 D Oluoch 'Free emergency transport for expectant women during curfew hours' *The Standard* (2020) available at www.standardmedia.co.ke/evewoman/article/2001369581/free-emergency-transport-for-expectant-women-during-curfew-hours (accessed 24 December 2021).

9

IMPACT OF COVID-19 ON THE SEXUAL AND REPRODUCTIVE HEALTH AND RIGHTS OF WOMEN IN ESWATINI

Simangele Mavundla and Ann Strode

9.1 Background

The COVID-19 pandemic has had a significant impact on the enjoyment of the right to health in Africa, including Eswatini. In particular, the COVID-19 pandemic has affected access to contraception and sexual and reproductive health and rights (SRHR). This chapter discusses in depth the right to health, particularly access to contraception, and presents strategies to avert future pandemics from interfering with the rights of women and girls in Eswatini to access contraception.

This chapter focuses on the SRHR of women and girls, although the definitions and services discussed later should be made available to all genders. Scholars and advocates of SRHR have made many attempts to define what SRHR are. The Guttmacher–Lancet Commission defines SRHR as 'a state of physical, emotional, mental and social wellbeing about all aspects of sexuality and reproduction, not merely the absence of disease, dysfunction or infirmity'.[1] According to the International Conference on Population and Development (ICPD) Programme of Action, reproductive health is

> a state of complete physical, mental and social wellbeing and not merely the absence of disease or infirmity in all matters relating to the reproductive system and its functions and processes.[2]

Thus, reproductive health implies that people can have a satisfying and safe sex life and that they can reproduce and have the freedom to decide if, when, and how often to do so.[3] On the other hand, reproductive health care is a collection of methods, techniques, and services that contribute to

DOI: 10.4324/9781032671437-12

reproductive health and well-being by preventing and solving reproductive health problems.[4]

This includes sexual health, which aims to improve lives and personal relationships, not just counselling and care related to reproduction and sexually transmitted diseases.[5] The World Health Organization (WHO) defines sexual and reproductive health as 'a state of physical, emotional and social wellbeing about sexuality'.[6] It recognizes individuals' right to reproductive autonomy and access to reproductive healthcare services.[7]

This chapter focuses on access to contraceptives in Eswatini during the COVID-19 pandemic. This is an important issue, as the United Nations 2030 Agenda for Sustainable Development identifies access to SRHR as a cornerstone for development.[8] The pandemic has created economic and logistical challenges to accessing contraceptives and other sexual and reproductive health (SRH) services for people of all ages, but women have been disproportionately affected. There are numerous rights that have been violated by the partial or complete loss of the right to access SRHR services, particularly contraceptives, in Eswatini. These rights include the right to access information (age-appropriate comprehensive sexuality education), the right to physical integrity, the right to dignity, the right to life, the right to reproductive health, and the right to attain the highest standard of health.

9.2 COVID-19 response in Eswatini

The COVID-19 pandemic was first identified in Wuhan, China, but its origins remain uncertain, and WHO declared it a pandemic on 11 March 2020.[9] Many countries, including Eswatini, adopted measures to effectively deal with the pandemic through the declaration of the coronavirus disease (also known as COVID-19) a national disaster. As a result of these declarations, lockdowns and restrictions on people's movement were put in place to stop the rapid spread of the coronavirus, which seemed to be spreading at an unprecedented rate, leaving a trail of devastation, fear, and death in its wake.

In Eswatini, following a confirmed case of COVID-19, King Mswati III directed the then Prime Minister of Eswatini to invoke Section 29 of the Disaster Management Act 2006 and declare a national state of emergency for two months.[10] This occurred on 17 March 2020. The prime minister later died on 13 December 2020, after testing positive for COVID-19 on 15 November 2020.[11] These events led to the implementation of strict lockdown measures, which were monitored and enforced by the police and army. Travel restrictions were imposed, and public transport, which is the most commonly used mode of transportation in the country, was closed and reserved only for essential workers. Many industries and sectors that were deemed non-essential were ordered to close their doors. People were generally afraid and feared that visiting healthcare centres would increase their risk of contracting the virus.

According to Shongwe, Eswatini's response to the COVID-19 pandemic has been reactive.[12] In fact, the country is said to have been among the least prepared in Africa to deal with the virus.[13] This was exacerbated by the fact that the country has a weak health system that has long struggled with shortages of life-saving and basic medical supplies.[14] For example, it was reported that there was a shortage of contraceptives in Eswatini hospitals during the period of strict and partial lockdown, while antiretroviral drugs (ARVs) were reportedly available.[15] Shongwe vehemently argues that it is the duty of the Eswatini government to protect the constitutional rights of citizens in a national emergency, including their right to access health services.[16]

9.3 SRHR and COVID-19

Despite the challenges posed by COVID-19, access to contraception has many benefits for society, such as reducing safe and unsafe abortions, unintended pregnancies, maternal mortality, poverty, child mortality and premature births, and gender inequality. Through access to contraception, women have the power to take control of their bodies and make informed decisions about their reproductive health. They can choose whether or not to become pregnant, when to become pregnant, and how often to become pregnant. This means safe pregnancy, safe delivery, and appropriate antenatal and postnatal care. It also means access to family planning counselling and a range of modern contraceptive methods.

Although the term 'contraceptive' is almost synonymous with pregnancy prevention, it does more than simply prevent pregnancy. Some forms of contraceptives, such as condoms, can help prevent both pregnancy and sexually transmitted infections (STIs), including the human immunodeficiency virus (HIV). There are modern and traditional forms of contraception available to women and men.[17] Modern forms of contraception are highly effective because they are scientifically based. In contrast, traditional contraceptive methods may not be scientifically validated and include withdrawal methods.[18] Access to contraception is important for women because it allows them to choose whether or not to become pregnant, avoid unwanted pregnancies and abortions, avoid common STIs, and plan for pregnancy.

However, a study that looked at contraceptive use and accessibility during the pandemic found that many women had an unmet need for modern contraceptive methods.[19] The study found that about more than 47 million women could lose access to contraception, leading to seven million unintended pregnancies as a result of the COVID-19 crisis.[20] Prior to the advent of COVID-19, it was reported that there were about 121 million unintended pregnancies worldwide, resulting in 73 million abortions per year between 2015 and 2019.[21] In percentage terms, the study found that 48% of pregnancies that occurred were unwanted and that 61% of unwanted pregnancies ended in abortion.[22]

However, for low- and middle-income countries (of which Eswatini is one), the study found that there were a number of unintended pregnancies which ended in abortion.[23] According to Riley et al., the estimates of the potential impact of the COVID-19 pandemic on SRH in low- and middle-income countries are high, as access to SRHR services has been severely curtailed.[24]

On the other hand, access to age-appropriate, comprehensive sexuality education (CSE) enables young people and adolescents to learn about and understand their bodies and relationships. CSE also helps them make informed choices about their sexuality and resist exploitation, sexual harassment, and abuse.[25] COVID-19 regulations' restrictions and closures have hampered the provision of contraceptives and other reproductive health products, including menstrual products, which are essential for women's health and sustainable development. Below, the chapter zooms into women's and girls' access to contraceptives in the context of the COVID-19 pandemic in Eswatini.

9.4 Access to contraceptive in Eswatini in the era of COVID-19

A plethora of studies have looked at how COVID-19 has impacted access to health and SRH services in the Kingdom of Eswatini. However, very few studies have looked holistically at access to contraceptives by women and girls in the context of Eswatini.

In the COVID-19 era, Eswatini began to experience an unmet need for contraceptives and an increase in unintended pregnancies and other women-related problems such as violence against women and children. This unmet need can be seen in the sudden decline in contraceptive use. For example, the proportion of women using modern methods was 97.8% in 2019.[26] In 2020, the use of modern contraceptives among all women in Eswatini dropped to 52%.[27] Prior to COVID -19, the fertility rate in Eswatini in 2018 was 3.2, a significant decline from the 1990 figure of 5.1.[28] It remains to be seen how the pandemic has dealt with the fertility issue.

It is clear from the above statistics that COVID-19 regulations in Eswatini have negatively impacted access to contraceptives and family planning services, including through structural challenges, movement problems, family planning issues, and sexual and gender-based violence (SGBV) resulting from exclusive compliance with the regulations.

9.4.1 Infrastructural challenges

The infrastructural challenges addressed here are some of the COVID-19 measures that affected the normal functioning of hospitals, schools, and non-essential services, such as many non-governmental organizations (NGOs), some government offices, and public centres that are central to SRHR services, especially contraceptive, counselling, and distribution. According to a study conducted by the International Treatment Preparedness Coalition (ITPC) in selected countries in Southern and Eastern Africa, including Eswatini, the infrastructural challenges stem from the fact that the main hospitals were converted into COVID-19 centres, some HIV clinics were closed, and community health services were curtailed and restricted by regulations on gatherings and activities.[29]

In Eswatini, the Regional Referral Hospital in the Lubombo region was designated as a COVID-19 isolation and treatment centre.[30] As a result, the hospital was unable to attend to the health needs of the general population as usual, which meant that women and girls who needed access to contraceptives were not able to receive care. This meant that women and girls now had to rely on other clinics and hospitals that may not have been easily accessible or available to them.

The WHO has emphasized that states must ensure a minimum level of access to essential material components of the right to health, such as the provision of essential medicines and maternal and child health services.[31] This obligation exists to ensure that in the event of a crisis or a state of disaster, countries like Eswatini integrate SRH needs, such as contraception, antenatal care, and cervical cancer screening, into the management of the disaster. This ensures that women with disabilities, young women, and women in general have easy access to contraceptives. In Eswatini, it is common to go to public hospitals and find that there are no drugs available. Every now and then it is reported that essential medicines are not in stock, and the disruption of the supply chain by the COVID-19 pandemic has exacerbated the unavailability of essential medicines in hospitals, including contraceptives.

Due to the social distancing rules in place in Eswatini and the priority given to the fight against coronavirus, access to contraceptives in hospitals was difficult. A simple visit to the hospital to refill contraceptives was faced with long queues for COVID-19 screening in public hospitals. In most of the hospitals, for example, a COVID-19 test was mandatory before anyone could access health services, which discouraged women and girls who could not afford the COVID test from seeking treatment.[32] Also, waiting for the COVID-19 test result and the financial costs associated with the test (as it was expensive) made access to health facilities the biggest structural challenge for women and girls.[33]

Schools are another vital infrastructure that came to a standstill due to the provisions of COVID-19 regulations and later due to the political unrest that occurred in Eswatini from June to July 2021. The prolonged school closures in the country due to the COVID-19 pandemic have led to an increase in teenage pregnancies and girls going to school.[34] As a result, UNICEF, UNESCO, and WHO issued a joint press statement expressing concern to the Eswatini government that schools had been closed for a period of more than 13 months.[35] The prolonged and extended school closure in Eswatini deprived students of the opportunity to benefit from valuable lessons such as CSE. The most serious consequence of this prolonged school closure is that many girls were unable to return to school due to teenage pregnancies. Studies have already shown that it is taboo for many parents in Eswatini to talk to their children about sex.[36] The joint press statement from the UN agencies correctly portrayed the lacuna that was faced by Eswatini learners as follows:

> *Continued school closures expose children to more violence, increased teenage pregnancy, greater likelihood of permanent learner dropout and threaten to reverse any progress made in improving educational outcomes.*[37]

Public buildings such as libraries and government offices where free condoms might be available were also inaccessible to the general public due to social distancing rules, which meant that condoms, the most commonly used contraceptive among young people, were withheld from those who really needed them. For example, one of the findings of the ITPC report is that during the COVID-19 pandemic, there was a major shortage of condoms – so much so that women and girls who wanted to use a condom could not get one and use it for safer sex.[38] This meant that women and girls who used condoms to prevent pregnancies and other STIs could not plan their pregnancies and were vulnerable to STIs, including HIV.

9.4.2 Movement challenges

Many countries restricted people's freedom of movement in various ways. Eswatini restricted movement, including personal contact, due to the pandemic. Severe restrictions and movement controls through hard and partial lockdowns and domestic quarantine may have prevented many women and girls who wanted to access contraceptives from receiving any form of assistance. Although this situation is not unique to Eswatini, Eswatini took drastic measures to ensure that movement was restricted. As some clinics and hospitals were converted into COVID-19 centres and mobile clinics in the communities were discontinued, women and girls had to travel long distances to access contraceptives, with the usual means of transport severely restricted by the government.[39]

In Eswatini, for example, the government demanded that all public transport stop operating. At least 90% of the population in Eswatini rely on public transportation.[40] As public transport is overcrowded, the Eswatini government later allowed public transport operators to operate at 70% capacity after the initial closure, with all passengers wearing masks. It should be noted that due to the high operating costs of public transport, public transport charges were also drastically increased. These costs exacerbated the problem of free movement for women and girls as it became expensive. The restricted public transport system, although introduced to combat the spread of the virus, also contributed to making access to contraceptives difficult, as many women and girls could not travel to family planning clinics. It is therefore not far-fetched to suggest that the obstruction of transport significantly contributed to the cycle of perpetual unplanned pregnancies, as people could not easily get to family planning centres. The UN Population Fund (UNFPA) also reported that in Eswatini, since the start of the lockdown, there have been increased cases of women giving birth either at home or on the way to the facility, indicating the problems with restricted movement.[41]

In addition, the COVID-19 regulations introduced the issuance of travel permits so that people could move from A to B. One could not exercise the right to move as they please in the Kingdom of Eswatini. Anyone who wanted to travel had to obtain a permit from the chiefdoms and the police. People needed travel permits to move from one place to another, including women and girls. According to the findings of the ITPC report, the issue of permits was overridden by confidentiality, as women and girls had to disclose why they needed a permit to travel where.[42]

The most significant impact of the COVID-19 regulations in Eswatini on women and girls is the requirement for travel permits, which resulted in forced disclosure and breaches of confidentiality.[43] Women and girls living with HIV and AIDS faced serious privacy and confidentiality concerns due to these permits, especially at checkpoints or roadblocks where police enforced compliance with COVID-19 regulations.[44] It is essential to ensure that COVID-19 responses align with human rights norms by respecting the privacy and confidentiality of women and girls, particularly for those living with HIV.

This is mainly because studies conducted in the past have shown that women and girls are stigmatized and discriminated against because of their HIV-positive status by family members, community members, and also by some health professionals.[45] In this study, Mavundla discovered that women and girls experience emotional, sexual, physical, and financial violence solely because they are HIV positive.[46] Hence, if the government and stakeholders are not cautious, COVID-19 responses that fail to prioritize women and girls could exacerbate gender inequalities and, in turn, place a greater burden on the healthcare system and other systems, undoing the progress achieved over the years in terms of gender equality.

Another strategy to contain the COVID-19 virus that tampered with the right to freedom of movement is social distancing. This strategy impacted service delivery by non-governmental organizations (NGOs) and other public sectors. To enable social distancing measures, stakeholders such as NGOs that provide services and information on SRHR to youth and women had to operate at reduced capacity or take other measures to ensure that their services reached their clientele. Many organizations have had to use social media platforms to access their clients and members. It is reported that UNFPA developed technologies to reach women and girls with information about SRH that they needed during COVID-19. For example, in Eswatini, a youth-friendly application called 'TUNEME APP' was developed and used by youth as a safe place to talk about their problems without being judged.[47]

9.4.3 Family planning challenges

A participant in the ITPC study noted as follows:

> *access to family planning was not the priority of the facility – COVID-19 was; and emergency services were more prioritised. So, if you come for family planning, they said please go home – we only do it once a week, and on that day they only take a certain number, so if you fall off the wagon you won't get it. If you do, you don't get a choice.*[48]

Women and girls have been vulnerable to the impact of the COVID-19 pandemic on various fronts, particularly concerning family planning. According to UNFPA, the number of women unable to access family planning services during the COVID-19 era has steadily increased.[49] According to the 2017 National Housing and Population Census report, Eswatini has a fertility rate of 3.2 children per woman, as mentioned earlier.[50] However, this gain in reducing the fertility rate might be reversed if access to family planning services is hindered due to the impact of COVID-19. The pandemic has further disrupted antenatal, skilled birth, and postnatal family planning services, which could have significant consequences for maternal health and family planning in the country.[51]

According to UNFPA Eswatini, the use of family planning services decreased by 47% between January and May 2020 compared to that in the same period last year.[52] This means that more women and girls than usual had unintended pregnancies during the period of hard and partial lockdown in Eswatini. Indeed, the COVID-19 regulations and restrictions have increased the number of women with unmet need for modern contraceptives in the Kingdom. Unintended pregnancies also lead to an increased need for abortions.

In Eswatini, abortion is illegal except in a few exceptional circumstances. Since abortion on demand is not permitted in the country, there is a strong likelihood of an increase in unsafe street abortions. Unfortunately, this situation also contributes to a higher maternal mortality rate, which is already elevated compared to that in other countries in the region. Indicators suggest that the maternal mortality rate in the Kingdom will continue to be high due to the impact of the COVID-19 pandemic. This is evident from the latest report of the Kingdom of Eswatini on the implementation of the Millennium Development Goals (MDGs). The report reveals that concerning the fifth MDG aimed at reducing maternal mortality, the maternal mortality rate remains high at 593 per 100,000 live births. Although the percentage of skilled births increased from 82% in 2010 to 88.3% in 2014, the overall maternal mortality rate continues to be a concerning issue.[53]

The Constitution provides for a restricted right to abortion in section 15(5), which states that it is unlawful except where pregnancy endangers a woman's life or where pregnancy results from violence, such as rape or incest, or may be allowed on grounds that the parliament deems necessary. There were no regulations to advise health workers and women seeking abortion on how to access it in practice; as a result, many women have been unable to obtain the necessary service. According to Mavundla and Ngwena, even though rape is one of the grounds for accessing legal abortion under section 15 of the Constitution, the lack of transparency in abortion laws that would operationalize the provision of the Constitution denies women substantive equality.[54] The authors contend that

> denying survivors of sexual violence access to safe abortion constitutes a violation of the woman's human rights, including cruel, inhumane and degrading treatment.[55]

Whether in time of crisis or not, access to safe, voluntary family planning remains a human right. As UNFPA points out, family planning is a key factor in reducing poverty while remaining central to the attainment of gender equality and women's enfranchisement.[56]

9.4.4 Sexual and gender-based violence

Much research has indicated that the COVID-19 pandemic interacts with existing inequalities, including gender inequalities, violence against women and girls, and economic injustice.[57] One area where such inequalities have been identified is in the vulnerability of women and girls to SGBV in the Kingdom of Eswatini. Unfortunately, it has been shown that women who experience SGBV have little opportunity to negotiate the use of condoms or even contraceptives in that circumstance.

Many countries, including Eswatini, reported that SGBV has increased dramatically during the COVID-19 pandemic, which is facilitated by socio-economic factors.[58] SGBV was found to have contributed to the increase in teenage and adolescent pregnancies in Eswatini.[59] Sexual violence, including incest, leads to unwanted pregnancies and STIs if victims are not supported and treated.

The law in Eswatini protects adolescents from sexual exploitation through the statutory rape offence and the Sexual Offences and Domestic Violence Act of 2018, but cases of rape and rape/sexual assault are not reported to the police for investigation so that the apparatus of the criminal justice system can be invoked. This is partly because the perpetrators are known to the victim's family, who then decide to settle the matter by other means.

An International Commission of Jurists (ICJ) study in 2021 reported that in Eswatini, 41% of lower secondary school dropouts and 52% of upper secondary school dropouts were due to teenage pregnancy.[60] Also, studies on gender-based violence (GBV), especially violence against women and girls, have shown that SGBV prevents women and girls from negotiating safer sex in their relationships and makes it difficult to take medication because violent partners were found to have taken medication such as ARVs and thrown them away.[61]

It is important to note that violence against women and girls, whether in a state of peace or disaster, remains a life-threatening human rights issue and violates international, regional, and national human rights law and gender equality principles.[62] Eswatini continues to grapple with the problem of SGBV despite its commitment under international human rights instruments, including the Maputo Protocol, to ensure the protection of women and girls from all forms of violence, including sexual violence, and at the national level.

9.5 International norms on SRHR binding on Eswatini

There are international instruments binding on Eswatini that deal directly or indirectly with the promotion of SRHR and to which Eswatini is a party. Despite the existence of international standards to promote and protect the rights of women and girls, reports from international human rights agencies have highlighted some of the negative impacts that the COVID-19 pandemic has had on women and girls. These atrocities included 'increased domestic violence, sexual violence, femicide, harmful practices, sex trafficking, including sexual harassment, and, in some cases, coercion by landlords to vacate houses, denial of access to Gender-Based Violence (GBV) and reproductive health services, stigmatization, and attacks on healthcare workers, 70 per cent of whom are women'.[63]

Most of these negative impacts of the COVID-19 pandemic on women and girls were already the subject of international human rights law before COVID-19 regulations were introduced. These instruments have binding standards sufficient to allow women and girls to access family planning services in times of disaster and peace. Two of the instruments are universal human rights: One is child-specific, that is catering only for persons under 18 years, and the other is women-specific. The UN instruments include the Convention on the Rights of the Child (CRC), the Convention on the

Elimination of All Forms of Discrimination against Women (CEDAW), the International Covenant on Civil and Political Rights (ICCPR), and the International Covenant on Economic, Social, and Cultural Rights (ICESCR).

Eswatini ratified the CRC in 1995. The CRC recognizes rights that promote SRH services and acknowledges the state's obligation to eliminate and reduce infant and child mortality. It should be noted that the CRC links infant rights to women's rights to SRH, as read in Article 24 of the CRC. The proviso obligates state parties like Eswatini to 'ensure appropriate pre-natal and post-natal health care for the mothers'.[64]

It also states that states like Eswatini are to adopt or develop preventive health care to provide guidance for parents and family planning education and services.[65] It must be noted that the family planning referred to is at the instance of the parents and not the child. The CRC indirectly addresses SRHR regarding those little humans below the age of 18 by prohibiting the sexual abuse of children. The CRC has issued General Comment No. 4 on adolescent health and development to clarify SRHR in relation to adolescents.[66]

In addition, in 2013, the CRC Committee adopted General Comment No. 15 on the rights to health of children and adolescents. The Committee endeavoured to formulate children's rights from a child rights perspective. According to this general comment, children from all walks of life have the right 'to opportunities to survive, grow and develop within the context of physical, emotional, and social well-being'.[67]

In the general comment, the Committee directly addresses the issue of teenage pregnancy by recommending that states like Eswatini 'ensure that public health systems and services are extended to meet the specific sexual and reproductive health needs of adolescents, including family planning and safe abortion services'.[68]

The Committee also called on state parties to work towards ensuring that 'girls can make autonomous and informed decisions about their reproductive health'.[69] The Committee warned against taking drastic measures to discriminate on the basis of adolescent pregnancy, such as exclusion from school and opportunities availed for continuous education ensured.[70]

Eswatini is also a state party to the CEDAW, which it ratified without reservations in 2004.[71] Article 12 of the Convention deals with women's rights to health, including SRHR. It provides for access to family planning and calls on states to provide free reproductive health services to women where appropriate.[72] The CEDAW Committee adopted General Comment No. 24 on women and health. The Committee recognized the interrelation between women's right to health during pregnancy and childbirth and in relation to family planning.[73] The Committee reaffirmed the link between the right to be free from discrimination in the health care and the right to be free from discrimination in all matters relating to marriage and family relations (in the short interaction between Articles 12 and 16).[74]

Another international instrument that addresses the state's obligation to promote and fulfil SRHR is the ICCPR.[75] Eswatini ratified the ICCPR in 2004 without any reservations or declarations. The ICCPR protects women's SRHR indirectly through the right to life. This right is provided for in Article 6, which states

> *Every human being has the inherent right to life. This right shall be protected by law. No one shall be arbitrarily deprived of his life.*[76]

The Human Rights Committee (HRC), the body that monitors the implementation of the ICCPR, has observed that the right to life protected in Article 6 of the ICCPR is undermined by the consequences of unsafe abortions and preventable maternal deaths, as it interferes with the right to life of the mother/woman.[77] This is outlined in the HRC's General Comment No. 36, paragraph 8.[78]

The UN ICESCR was also ratified by Eswatini in 2004.[79] SRHR are protected directly by the ICESCR in Article 12, which guarantees the right to health. Article 10(2) of the covenant also addresses the need for 'special protection for mothers during a reasonable period before and after childbirth'.[80] This provision specifies that working mothers should be granted paid leave or leave with adequate social security benefits during this period.[81]

The CESCR has opined in General Comment No. 14 that SRH is included in the right to health. This means that women have the right to have access to health-related education and to decide whether or not to fall pregnant, through access to family planning methods of their choosing.[82]

WHO has developed the 'Consolidated Guideline on sexual and reproductive health and rights of women living with HIV' of 2017. These guidelines are not binding on states, but they set out policy directives for states. They call for a women-centred approach to health service delivery. This approach envisages women as active participants and beneficiaries of a health system that responds to their needs and rights.[83] It is also seen as an approach that promotes and emphasizes gender equality as central to the achievement of SRHR of all women, among other things.[84]

9.6 Regional instruments on SRH binding on Eswatini

Eswatini is a member state of the African Human Rights system. The country ratified the African Charter on Human and Peoples' Rights (ACHPRs) in 1995.[85] Article 16 of the ACHPRs provides that states must ensure the highest attainable standard of physical and mental health.[86] Moreover, in 2012, the country ratified the Maputo Protocol,[87] which is specifically focused on women and addresses SRHR comprehensively for women and girls.

The Maputo Protocol directly and indirectly provides for SRHR for women and girls. Article 4 of the protocol indirectly safeguards women's SRHR, as it includes provisions for women's rights to life, integrity, and security of person. These provisions are crucial in protecting and promoting the overall well-being and health of women and girls. It states as follows:

> *Every woman shall be entitled to respect for her life and the integrity and security of her person. All forms of exploitation, cruel, inhuman or degrading punishment and treatment shall be prohibited.*

This means that conducts that violate women's bodily integrity, such as violence against women and sexual violence, are outlawed, and state parties are to adopt laws and other measures to punish and eradicate such conduct.[88]

The protocol addresses women's health and reproductive rights in Article 14, which imposes obligations on countries like Eswatini to promote and uphold women's rights to health, including SRHR. Article 14 guarantees women's rights to control their fertility, make decisions about having children, and determine the spacing and number of their children. It also ensures the right to choose any method of contraception and the right to protect themselves against STIs, including HIV/AIDS.[89]

Additionally, Article 14 provides for the right to family planning education and being informed about their partner's health status regarding STIs and HIV.[90] States are further obligated to protect women's reproductive rights, if necessary, by ensuring access to medical abortion while ensuring women have affordable and adequate health services.[91]

The African Commission on Human and Peoples' Rights has adopted two general recommendations to clarify the meaning of Article 14 concerning women's health and sexual and reproductive rights. In 2012, the Commission adopted General Comment No. 1 on Article 14(1)(d) and (e).[92] The Commission highlighted the state obligations stemming from Article 14(1)(d) to be the adoption of laws and policies that ensure women can claim and exercise their right to protection. Additionally, Article 14(1)(e) emphasizes women's rights to access adequate, reliable, non-discriminatory, and comprehensive information about their health.

Furthermore, the Commission emphasized the significance of the right for women to be informed about the health status of their partner, recognizing its importance in safeguarding women's health and reproductive rights. General Comment No. 2 on Article 14(1)(a), (b), (c), and (f) and Article 14(2)(a) and (c) of the Maputo Protocol strengthens and reinforces women's SRHR in Africa. This comment urges states to take decisive actions to eliminate all administrative laws, policies, procedures, practices, and attitudes or stereotypes that hinder women from fully enjoying their SRHR. By doing so, it seeks to ensure that women have unhindered access to comprehensive and quality sexual and reproductive healthcare and services.[93]

9.7 Domestic legal framework on SRHR in Eswatini

The domestic legal framework of the Kingdom of Eswatini provides for SRHR. At the apex of the legal framework is the Constitution of 2005,[94] and it is where the right to basic healthcare services is stipulated in section 60(8). This section establishes the state's responsibility to promote free and compulsory basic health education and the provision of healthcare services for all citizens. However, it is important to note that this provision is listed under the directive principles of state policy rather than the bill of rights. As a result, it is considered non-justiciable, meaning it cannot be enforced through legal action in court.

Section 15(5) of the Constitution provides for a restricted right to abortion. Abortion is unlawful except where pregnancy endangers a woman's life or where pregnancy results from violence, such as rape or incest. Abortion may also be allowed on grounds that the parliament deems necessary. However, there are no regulations in place to advise health workers and women seeking abortion on how to access it in practice. As a result, many women have been unable to obtain the necessary service.

The Healthcare Act and Regulations No. 5 of 1969 are relatively old and primarily address how the healthcare sector handles communicable and non-communicable diseases. Notably, the term SRHR is not mentioned anywhere in the Act.

On the other hand, the Sexual Offences and Domestic Violence Act of 2018 specifically prohibits GBV and sexual violence. It focuses on addressing issues related to sexual offenses and domestic violence in the country.

Furthermore, the Children's Protection and Welfare Act contains Section 244, which explicitly states that children must not be denied information on reproductive healthcare, devices, and technologies related to reproductive health care. Additionally, in cases where a child is a victim of sexual abuse and exploitation, the Act mandates the provision of emergency contraception as soon as feasible.

It is evident that while the Healthcare Act of 1969 may not explicitly address SRHR, other legislations like the Sexual Offences and Domestic Violence Act and the Children's Protection and Welfare Act play crucial roles in promoting and safeguarding reproductive health and rights in Eswatini, particularly for women and children.

Other crucial soft law policy documents in Eswatini include the Kingdom of Eswatini multisectoral guidelines to facilitate adolescents' access to services related to HIV and SRH of 2019,[95] and the national policy on SRH of 2013. The 2019 guidelines highlight concerning statistics, revealing that youth in the country aged 15–24 years account for 45% of all new HIV infections, with girls aged 15–19 years being five times more likely to contract HIV than boys.[96] Moreover, the comprehensive knowledge among adolescents about HIV and condom use is decreasing, which raises concerns about their SRH.[97] To address these challenges, the guidelines propose strategies that focus on empowering and engaging young people.

The guidelines further emphasize the importance of partnering with young people to put them at the centre of services. This can be achieved by supporting them as activists and advocates, enabling them to promote greater access to health information, products, and interventions for HIV and SRH prevention and treatment. The strategies include providing life skills and comprehensive sexuality education, promoting condom and contraceptive use, and facilitating economic empowerment among the youth.[98] By involving young people in this process, the guidelines aim to alleviate some of the challenges faced by the youth of Eswatini in the realm of HIV and SRH.

The 2013 National Policy on Sexual and Reproductive Health serves as a guiding framework for the government's efforts and initiatives concerning SRHR issues. The primary objective of this policy is to facilitate, support, and deliver integrated and well-coordinated services related to SRH.[99] The policy is premised on the acknowledgement of the human rights and freedoms of all citizens (Emaswati). It explicitly recognizes the right to health, which includes SRH rights, without any form of discrimination based on sex, gender, culture, religion, age, race, disability, HIV status, or economic status.[100]

The SRHR policy is backed by a national SRH strategy for the year 2014–2018. This strategy provides a roadmap for the provision of SRH services in the country, outlining specific goals and actions to be undertaken during that time frame. Together, the policy and the strategy aim to advance and promote SRH rights, ensuring access to comprehensive and quality healthcare services for all citizens in Eswatini.

The following are some of the key limitations of the domestic legal framework on SRHR in Eswatini:

- The right to basic healthcare services is not justiciable.
- The right to abortion is restricted, and there are no regulations in place to facilitate access to abortion services.
- There is a lack of awareness of SRHR rights among women and health workers.
- Failure to implement policies in full.

These limitations have a significant impact on the health and well-being of women in Eswatini. They restrict women's access to essential healthcare services and can lead to unsafe abortions. The government of Eswatini should take steps to address these limitations and ensure that all women have access to comprehensive SRHR services.

Given the existing legislative and other measures that Eswatini has at its disposal, at both the international and national levels, there is substantial evidence suggesting that the country could have been better equipped to mitigate the negative impact of the COVID-19 pandemic on access to contraceptives and family planning services. By effectively implementing the legal norms, provisions, and all the measures that are already in place, both binding and non-binding, the country could have taken significant steps towards ensuring that individuals continue to have access to essential SRH services during the pandemic.

Effective implementation of these measures could have facilitated the promotion and protection of SRHR, enabling women and girls to access vital contraceptives and family planning services without interruption. By upholding these existing legal norms and provisions, Eswatini could have demonstrated its commitment to safeguarding the well-being and rights of its citizens, even in times of crisis, and made strides in mitigating the impact of COVID-19 on SRHR in the country.

9.8 Averting future pandemics in Eswatini

There are certain strategies which Eswatini can pay attention to in order to avert future pandemics from interrupting access to health service, in particular access to contraceptive. These will include strengthening the healthcare infrastructure, establishing contingency plans, and stockpiling essential supplies, among other things. These strategies could enable Eswatini to promote and fulfil access to contraceptives for women and girls, only if the government shows sufficient political will and budgetary commitments.

In order to strengthen healthcare infrastructure, Eswatini would need to invest in a robust healthcare system to ensure its capacity to respond effectively to future pandemics. As suggested by Berawi, governments must focus on increasing the number of health facilities.[101] Creating effective contingency plans becomes crucial to minimize disruptions to contraceptive access. These contingency plans should encompass measures to ensure an uninterrupted supply chain of contraceptives, maintain service provision, and safeguard the rights of women and girls. By having well-structured and proactive plans in place, Eswatini can better protect the SRHR of its population during times of crisis.

In stockpiling essential supplies, Eswatini would need to maintain a strategic reserve of essential contraceptive supplies to help mitigate potential shortages during pandemics. While Roer and Globus Harris suggest that acquiring and maintaining a large stockpile of medical supplies could be costly for governments and public or private entities, this argument does not hold true when it comes to access to contraceptives.[102] In fact, ensuring an adequate supply of contraceptives becomes even more critical during times of crisis to meet the heightened demand and protect the SRH of women and girls.

By adopting these strategies, Eswatini can enhance its preparedness and response capabilities, thereby better safeguarding the right to health of its population in the event of future pandemics. Moreover, by integrating SRHR services and ensuring access to contraceptive services becomes a core component of emergency response strategies, Eswatini can effectively protect the SRHR of its population during pandemics. This proactive approach will not only mitigate potential disruptions but also uphold the well-being and rights of women and girls in times of crisis.

9.9 Conclusion and recommendations

Like many other countries around the world, Eswatini responded to the COVID-19 pandemic by invoking the National Disaster Management Act, which allowed for the implementation of regulations such as lockdowns and movement restrictions. Consequently, these measures resulted in the suspension and violation of many rights of the citizens. This chapter specifically focused on investigating the right of access to SRHR services, particularly access to contraceptives. The significance of this right is underscored by its recognition as a cornerstone of development at the UN level.

In the case of Eswatini, some challenges that hindered the right to access contraceptives during COVID-19 were not adequately addressed, particularly concerning key infrastructure closures and movement restrictions that negatively affected women's and girls' rights. The government did not implement measures to ensure that during the lockdown, SGBV would be prevented and prosecuted effectively. This oversight is concerning, given that GBV has been an ongoing issue in the country, leading to the enactment of the Sexual Offences and Domestic Violence Act of 2018.

The government should have foreseen that stringent measures to tackle COVID-19 could lead to a higher prevalence of GBV, given the existing problem in the country. To protect the rights of women and girls, it was crucial to put in place comprehensive plans and support systems during the lockdown period.

Indeed, there is a growing concern that the COVID-19 outbreak may soon be followed by future pandemics that could pose significant threats to human existence.[103] It is crucial for the global community to be vigilant and prepared to face such challenges in the future. Eswatini's state of preparedness for future pandemics will play a vital role in ensuring that women and girls do not face interruptions in accessing essential SRHR services, including contraceptives. By proactively planning and implementing measures to strengthen healthcare infrastructure, develop comprehensive contingency plans, and integrate SRHR services into emergency response strategies, Eswatini can effectively protect the SRHR of its population during pandemics.

9.10 Recommendations

It is crystal clear that the COVID-19 pandemic has brought to the forefront opportunities that can ensure that access to SRHR and, in particular, access to family planning for women and adolescents are improved. It is in this vein that the following recommendations are addressed to the government of Eswatini and its stakeholders:

- It is recommended that whenever the Disaster Management Act is evoked in the country, it should be evoked in a non-arbitrary manner so as not to violate the rights that are considered to be a cornerstone of development. There was so much overreach in the use of discretionary powers by the government to the extent that schools were closed for a period exceeding a year.
- It is recommended that in the future, regulations on disaster management (regardless of the kind) should be formulated with the input of the citizens, including women's groups in the country, so that they would factor in incidences peculiar to women's experiences, such as SGBV and access to family planning.
- The country can adopt the WHO consolidated guideline on SRHR of women living with HIV as it promotes a women-centred approach to health care and access to SRHR.
- Launch a research study on a national scale to investigate the challenges and problems that women and adolescents face during the implementation of hard lockdowns and partial lockdowns, which continue to be in effect two years after the outbreak landed on Eswatini's shores.
- Ensure that hospitals with restrictions on SRH services provision are removed so that everybody who has a need may have access.
- Ensure that the problem that has been recurring over the years of shortages of essential medicines is dealt with head-on so that women and girls' rights to access contraceptives are met.
- The government should fund public hospitals adequately in light of the fact that a number of people have lost their livelihoods and jobs due to the lockdowns restrictions and are not in a position to afford private hospital services.
- Promulgate the law that would regulate legal abortion as stipulated in the Constitution of Eswatini of 2005 so that rape victims may access their right to SRH services and care.
- Ensure that adolescents who drop out of school due to pregnancy are given the necessary support so that they return to school to finish their schooling because doing otherwise would amount to discrimination.
- It is recommended that the country be in a state of high preparedness and adopt high-level response plans in order to avert future pandemics akin to the COVID-19 pandemic.
- Civil society organizations have a duty to lobby the government of Eswatini and advocate for the fulfilment of SRHR services in view of the fact that there are no political parties in the country that would act on behalf of their members.

Notes

1 Lancet 'From accelerate progress – sexual and reproductive health and rights for all: Report of the Guttmacher–Lancet Commission report' (2018) available at https://www.thelancet.com/commissions/sexual-and-reproductive-health-and-rights.
2 International Conference on Population and Development Programme of Action (ICPD Programme of Action) in 1994, para 7.2–7.3.
3 UN ICPD 1994, para 7 6. See also LB Pizzarossa 'Here to stay: The evolution of sexual and reproductive health and rights in international human rights law' (2018) 6 *MDPI Laws* 1–29.
4 E Durojaye 'Evolution of sexual and reproductive health as human rights under international law' *Dullar Omar Institute* (undated) available at https://dullahomarinstitute.org.za/socio-economic-rights/Workshops/2018/colloquium-unpacks-sexual-and-reproductive-health-and-rights-in-africa/ebenezer.pdf (accessed 13 January 2022).
5 As above.
6 As above.
7 As above.
8 N Kanem *Sexual and reproductive health rights: The cornerstone of sustainable development* available at www.un.org/en/chronicle/article/sexual-and-reproductive-health-and-rights-cornerstone-sustainable-development (accessed 30 November 2021).
9 WHO *Press release* 11 March 2020 available at www.who.int/director-general/speeches/detail/who-director-general-s-opening-remarks-at-the-media-briefing-on-covid-19–11-march-2020#:~:text=WHO%20has%20been%20assessing%20this,to%20use%20lightly%20or%20carelessly (accessed 19 May 2022).
10 The Government of the Kingdom of Eswatini *Declaration of national emergency in response to Coronavirus* available at latest Press Statement (gov.sz) (accessed 19 May 2022).
11 BBC *Ambrose Dlamini: Eswatini's PM dies after testing positive for COVID-19* 14 December 2020 available at www.bbc.com/news/world-africa-55297472 (accessed 19 May 2022).
12 MN Shongwe 'Eswatini's legislative response to COVID-19: Whither human rights?' (2020) 20 *African Human Rights Law Journal* 412–435, 413.
13 As above.
14 As above.
15 International Treatment Preparedness Coalition (ITPC) *Confined by COVID-19: Women and girls, HIV and SRHR – the challenges, the responses and calls to action report* (December 2020).
16 Shongwe (n 12 above) 423.
17 There are different types of modern methods of contraception that people can use. These include female and male sterilization, the intra-uterine device (IUD), implants, injectables, oral contraceptive pills, male and female condoms, vaginal barrier methods (including the diaphragm, cervical cap and spermicidal foam, jelly, cream, and sponge), lactational amenorrhea method (LAM), emergency contraception, and other modern methods not reported separately (e.g. the contraceptive patch or vaginal ring).
18 Traditional methods of contraception include rhythm (e.g. fertility awareness-based methods and periodic abstinence), withdrawal, and other traditional methods not reported separately.
19 J Aly, KO Haeger, A Christy et al 'Contraception access during the COVID-19 pandemic' (2020) 5 *Contraception and Reproductive Medicine* 17 available at https://doi.org/10.1186/s40834-020-00114-9. See also the United Nations 'Impact of the COVID-19 pandemic on family planning and ending gender-based violence, female genital mutilation and child marriage' in *Interim technical note* (2020) 1–7.

20 Aly et al (n 19 above).
21 JM Bearak et al 'Unintended pregnancy and abortion by income region, and the legal status of abortion: Estimates from a comprehensive model for 1990–2019' (2020) *Lancet Global Health* e1152–e1161 available at www.thelancet.com/journals/langlo/article/PIIS2214-109X(20)30315-6/fulltext
22 As above, e1157.
23 As above.
24 T Riley, E Sully, Z Ahmed & A Biddlecom 'Estimates of the potential impact of the COVID-19 pandemic on sexual and reproductive health in low- and middle-income countries' (2020) 46 *International Perspectives on Sexual and Reproductive Health* 73–76.
25 S Mavundla 'Comprehensive sexuality education in Swaziland schools' (2015) 16 *Economic and Social Rights in South Africa ESR Review* 6–10.
26 Un World Fertility and Family Planning 2020: Highlights, 30.
27 As above, 15.
28 As above, 30.
29 International Treatment Preparedness Coalition (ITPC) (n 15 above) 4.
30 Eswatini Government Gazette no. 53, Coronavirus (Covid-19) Regulations, 2020 (Legal Notice 72 of 2020).
31 WHO, The Right to Health Fact Sheet No. 31, 5.
32 International Treatment Preparedness Coalition (ITPC) (n 15 above).
33 As above.
34 As above.
35 UNICEF Eswatini, UNESCO Eswatini and WHO Eswatini 'UNICEF, UNESCO and WHO are concerned over school closures in Eswatini' 29 July 2021 available at www.unicef.org/eswatini/press-releases/unicef-unesco-and-who-concerned-over-school-closures-eswatini (accessed 28 May 2022).
36 Mavundla (n 25 above).
37 As above.
38 International Treatment Preparedness Coalition (ITPC) (n 15 above).
39 As above.
40 S Padidar, Sm Liao, S Magagula, TAM Mahlaba, NM Nhlabatsi et al 'Assessment of early COVID-19 compliance to and challenges with public health and social prevention measures in the Kingdom of Eswatini, using an online survey' (2021) *PLoS One* 1–28, 2.
41 UNFPA *New innovative app enables family planning in Eswatini, even during the COVID-19 pandemic* 21 July 2020 available at https://esaro.unfpa.org/en/news/new-innovative-app-enables-family-planning-eswatini-even-during-covid-19-pandemic (accessed 29 May 2022).
42 International Treatment Preparedness Coalition (ITPC) (n 15 above).
43 As above.
44 As above, 15.
45 S Mavundla 'Battered, dejected, ejected and rejected: The rights of HIV positive women to be protected from violence in Eswatini' Unpublished PhD thesis, UKZN, 2020.
46 Mavundla (n 45 above).
47 UNFPA 'Hear her . . . stories of hope and resilience East and Southern Africa' (2021) 28.
48 International Treatment Preparedness Coalition (ITPC) (n 15 above) 6.
49 UNFPA (n 47 above) 35.
50 As above, 35.
51 EK Ameyaw, BO Ahinkorah, AA Seidu et al 'Impact of COVID-19 on maternal healthcare in Africa and the way forward' (2021) 79 *Arch Public Health* 1–5.
52 UNFPA (n 47 above) 35.
53 Swaziland 'Millennium development goals 2015 report' 61.

54 S Mavundla & C Ngwena, Access to legal abortion for rape as a reproductive health right: A commentary on the abortion regimes of Swaziland and Ethiopia in C Ngwena & E Durojaye (eds) *Strengthening the protection of sexual and reproductive health and rights in the African region through human rights* (2014) 61–78.
55 Mavundla & Ngwena (n 54 above).
56 UNFPA (n 47 above) 50.
57 International Treatment Preparedness Coalition (ITPC) (n 15 above).
58 The Global Fund, *In Eswatini, young women are leading the fight against HIV and COVID-19* 21 July 2021 available at www.theglobalfund.org/en/blog/2021-07-21-in-eswatini-young-women-are-leading-the-fight-against-hiv-and-covid-19/ (accessed 29 May 2022).
59 As above.
60 ICJ 'Swazi women's right to health during the time of COVID-19 recommendations to ensure the enjoyment of the highest attainable standard of physical and mental health' (2021) 27.
61 SD Mavundla, A Strode & Z Essack 'Access to justice for women in Eswatini: HIV-positive women as a vulnerable population' in A Budoo-Scholtz & EC Lubaale (eds) *Violence against women and criminal justice in Africa* (2022) 339–370, 353.
62 UN Women 'COVID-19: Ending violence against women and girls – key priorities and interventions for effective response and recovery' (2020) 2.
63 As above.
64 UN International Convention on the Rights of the Child (CRC) 1990, article 24(2)(d).
65 As above, article 24(1)(f).
66 CRC 'General comment no. 4: Adolescent health and development in the context of the convention on the rights of the child' 2003.
67 CRC 'Committee general comment no. 15 (2013) on the right of the child to the enjoyment of the highest attainable standard of health' (art. 24) available at https://globalhealth.usc.edu/2013/04/17/convention-on-the-rights-of-the-child-draft-general-comment-no-15-the-right-of-the-child-to-the-enjoyment-of-the-highest-attainable-standard-of-health-article-24/ (accessed 30 May 2022).
68 As above, para 56.
69 As above.
70 As above.
71 UN International Convention on the Elimination of All Forms of Discrimination Against Women (CEDAW) 1981.
72 As above, article 12(1) & (2).
73 UN Committee on CEDAW General Recommendation No. 24: Article 12 of the Convention (Women and Health) 1999.
74 Pizzarossa (n 3 above) 8.
75 UN International Covenant on Civil and Political Rights (ICCPR) 1966.
76 As above, article 6.
77 Pizzarossa (n 3 above).
78 Human Rights Committee 'General comment no. 36 (2018) on article 6 of the international covenant on civil and political rights on the right to life' (CCPR/C/GC/36).
79 UN International Covenant on Economic, Social and Cultural Rights (CESCR) 1966.
80 As above.
81 As above.
82 UN Committee on ICESCR 'General comment no. 14 on the right to the highest attainable standard of health (article 12)' 2000 (E/C.12/2000/4) para 8.

83 World Health Organization (WHO) 'Consolidated guideline on sexual and reproductive health and rights of women living with HIV' (2017) 4.
84 As above.
85 African Charter on Human and Peoples' Rights (ACHPRs) of 1981.
86 As above, Article 12.
87 The Protocol to the African Charter on Human and Peoples' Rights on the Rights of Women in Africa (Maputo Protocol) 2003.
88 As above, article 4(2)(a)-(d).
89 As above, article 14(1).
90 As above.
91 As above, article 14(2).
92 The African Commission on Human and Peoples' Rights General Comments on Article 14 (1) (d) and (e) of the Protocol to the African Charter on Human and Peoples' Rights on the Rights of Women in Africa 2012.
93 African Commission on Human and Peoples' Rights General Comment No. 2 on Article 14.1 (a), (b), (c) and (f) and Article 14. 2 (a) and (c) of the Protocol to the African Charter on Human and Peoples' Rights on the Rights of Women in Africa 2012.
94 Swaziland Constitution 1 of 2005, entry into force in 2006.
95 Eswatini Government Multisectoral Guidelines to Facilitate Adolescents' Access to Services Related to HIV and Sexual Reproductive Health of 2019.
96 As above, 1.
97 As above, 3.
98 As above. 4.
99 Eswatini 'National policy on sexual and reproductive health' (2013) 14.
100 As above, 15.
101 MA Berawi 'Empowering healthcare, economic, and social resilience during global pandemic COVID-19' (2020) 3 *International Journal of Technology* 436–439.
102 EH Roer & I Globus-Harris 'A mechanism to reduce medical supply shortfalls during pandemics' (2020) available at www.rand.org/pubs/perspectives/PEA187-1.html (accessed 22 July 2023).
103 United Nations Environment Programme *Preventing the next pandemic – zoonotic diseases and how to break the chain of transmission* (2020) available at https://unsdg.un.org/sites/default/files/2020-07/UNEP-Preventing-the-next-pandemic.pdf (accessed 31 May 2022).

10

PROTECTION OF THE RIGHT TO HEALTH OF MINORITIES AND VULNERABLE GROUPS DURING THE COVID-19 PANDEMIC

Mansha Mohee

10.1 Introduction

The COVID-19 pandemic has shed new light on health disparities and inequities amid public health crises.[1] Studies conducted since the outbreak have provided ample empirical evidence of its disproportionate health impacts, including higher rates of infection and fatality among minority groups,[2] explained by an interplay of factors, primarily, differential exposure, a greater incidence and predisposition to underlying health conditions, and a heightened vulnerability to loss of income and employment.[3] In the early months of the pandemic, the United Nations Human Rights Council (UNHRC) stressed upon the uneven adverse effects of the pandemic towards compounding existing inequalities.[4] Yet, public health measures have been assessed to largely exacerbate discrimination and to fail to apply a gender and social inclusion lens in their design and implementation.[5] In the African context, studies have highlighted the marked results of the dearth of a human rights-based approach in government-led responses to vulnerable groups, particularly the poor,[6] persons with disabilities,[7] women,[8] refugees,[9] persons living with HIV/AIDS,[10] and rural communities.[11]

The protection of the right to health is severely compromised during public health crises due to the propensity for health system failures.[12] These challenges are conflated in low- and middle-income countries where there is a chronic lack of investment in healthcare infrastructure,[13] and more crucially in the case of minorities and vulnerable groups as a result of their stymied access to medication, health services, and health-related education and information. In addition, health marginalization is typically multilayered, aggravated by the effects of the social, economic, political, and legal determinants

DOI: 10.4324/9781032671437-13

of health, which include a range of non-medical circumstances affecting health outcomes, such as employment and income, access to adequate housing, clean water and healthy food, education, language and culture, and representation in the governance processes and structures shaping health policy. While these challenges have been recognized in the context of the COVID-19 pandemic,[14] they warrant a more thorough examination in African countries. Understanding these links is critical to elaborating multisectoral and inclusive processes and responses to the pandemic and its health risks, in a given region, and ensuring the effectiveness and equity of interventions.

This chapter assesses the state of protection of the right to health of minorities and vulnerable groups in Africa in the face of the COVID-19 pandemic, focusing on three of the most severely affected groups, namely, poor communities, women and girls, and sexual minorities, and advances focus areas for its enhanced protection. First, it examines the paradigmatic underpinning for differential experiences of minorities and vulnerable groups amid the COVID-19 pandemic. It sets out the conceptual framework on health marginalization in the context of the pandemic in order to identify the distinct structural drivers of health disparities and inequities. It then outlines relevant standards in international and regional normative frameworks on the right to health relating specifically to minorities and vulnerable groups. It also identifies state obligations in the backdrop of health crises. Secondly, an audit of human rights reports provides an overview of the impact of the pandemic on the protection of the right to health of poor communities, women and girls, and sexual minorities across the African continent. The third section of the chapter proposes focus areas at the national and regional levels for enhancing the protection of the right to health in Africa amid the pandemic. The chapter concludes with some salient lessons and prospects for recovery and better preparedness in future health crises.

10.2 Minorities and vulnerable groups and the right to health amid pandemics

Marginalization is defined as 'a multidimensional and dynamic phenomenon reflecting a complex interplay between every person's vulnerability and political, economic, social and cultural features'.[15] While marginalization is prevalent across fields and countries, the indicators of marginalization vary in different settings and regions and are informed by the historical and socio-economic context of a society.[16] Minorities and vulnerable groups face higher risks of marginalization in a society, since they are inherently distanced from power and resources that enable their self-determination. The relationship between marginalization and health is well established in literature.[17] Significantly however, the pandemic has given rise to new forms of marginalization.

This section provides an understanding of the peculiar nature of health marginalization amid the pandemic, examines state duties as established in international human rights law in the protection of the right to health of minorities and vulnerable groups, and analyses those obligations in the context of public health emergencies.

10.2.1 Conceptualizing health marginalization during the COVID-19 pandemic

Health marginalization, within and between countries, can be understood by its underlying upstream determinants, notably the 'conditions in which people grow, learn, live and age' which are fashioned by social, economic, and political forces.[18] A broad range of social theories of health inequality have come to be recognized in public health science, shifting its focus from individual behaviour to structural and fundamental theories of health. These include, in particular, structural violence, the political economy of health, critical race theory, and the fundamental cause theory, which seeks to explain the social gradient in health.[19] Law is also a key determinant of health, which if not based on evidence or human rights can entrench or perpetuate the underlying conditions for health inequity.[20] The result of poor social policies, unfair economic programmes and bad politics, health marginalization adversely affects health outcomes.

The socio-economic impacts of the pandemic and COVID-19 containment measures have amplified existing vulnerabilities while also creating new ones.[21] The UN Sustainable Development Group has highlighted the broad-ranging characteristics of vulnerabilities in the context of the pandemic, which include among others, personal situation or status, occupation, location, and legal status.[22] Personal situation or status alludes to marginalized or excluded populations that exhibit reliance on the informal economy for livelihood; face inadequate access to social services; lack voice, representation, and access to technologies; or who live in conflict-affected areas. These vulnerabilities are often not singular but intersectional. The UN Development System Immediate Development Response has identified a wide-ranging list of at-risk populations requiring specific attention amid the pandemic. It includes women; older persons; adolescents, children, and youth, especially girls and young women; persons with disabilities; indigenous peoples; migrants; refugees; stateless and internally displaced persons; conflict-affected populations; minorities; persons in detention or in institutionalized settings; slum dwellers; homeless persons; people living with HIV/AIDS and other people with pre-existing medical conditions; people living in remote rural areas; the food insecure, people in extreme poverty, or those facing insecure and informal work and incomes; and groups which are not protected from discrimination and exclusion by laws, policies, and practices.[23]

It is also noteworthy that occupation can also be a vulnerability. Frontline health workers, social workers, those working in production and supply chains, and those in the informal or service sector may not be sufficiently protected in responses to the pandemic. Moreover, vulnerabilities are exacerbated in fragile locations, such as refugee camps, prisons and immigration detention centres, and slums, which have limited access to social services. In addition, legal status is also a vulnerability. Refugees, migrants, and stateless persons are intrinsically susceptible to risks as they do not benefit from the same legal entitlements and protection mechanisms as citizens.

Aside from exposing pre-existing vulnerabilities, the COVID-19 pandemic has also provoked novel ones. One of the most significant emerging forms of vulnerability is digital disadvantage. The digital divide caused by accelerated technological change has been shown to influence health outcomes.[24] The digitally disadvantaged are more at risk since they have less access to digital resources and services for work, consumption, and communication and to meet their needs and those of their families.[25]

10.2.2 The normative and institutional framework on the protection of the right to health of minorities and vulnerable groups in Africa

10.2.2.1 Normative framework

Health is described as the 'state of complete physical, mental and social well-being and not merely the absence of disease or infirmity'.[26] The right to health, defined as 'the enjoyment of the highest attainable standard of health'[27] is recognized under international human rights law. The Universal Declaration of Human Rights refers to 'the right to a standard of living adequate for the health and well-being of himself and of his family, including food, clothing, housing and medical care and necessary social services'.[28] The right to health is enshrined in Article 12 of the International Covenant on Economic, Social, and Cultural Rights.[29] At the regional level, Article 16 of the African Charter on Human and Peoples' Rights entrenches the right to health.[30] Importantly, the normative content of the right to health has been broadly understood, in light of its social, economic, and political determinants. General Comment no. 14 states as follows:

> . . . an inclusive right extending not only to timely and appropriate health care but also to the underlying determinants of health,[31] such as access to safe and potable water and adequate sanitation, an adequate supply of safe food, nutrition and housing, healthy occupational and environmental conditions, and access to health-related education and information, including on sexual and reproductive health. A further important aspect is

> the participation of the population in all health-related decision-making at the community, national and international levels.[32]

The right to health relies on four interrelated and essential elements, namely availability, accessibility, acceptability, and quality.[33] In particular, accessibility refers to non-discrimination, physical accessibility, economic accessibility, and information accessibility. It is recognized that

> health facilities, goods and services must be accessible to all, especially the most vulnerable or marginalized sections of the population,[34] in law and in fact, without discrimination on any of the prohibited grounds.[35]

The recognized grounds for discrimination are extensive and include race, colour, sex, language, religion, political or other opinion, national or social origin, property, birth, physical or mental disability, health status (including HIV/AIDS), sexual orientation, and civil, political, social, or other status, which has the intention or effect of nullifying or impairing the equal enjoyment or exercise of the right to health.[36] In addition, most pertinently, states are required to protect vulnerable members of a society even in times of severe resource constraints through the adoption of relatively low-cost targeted programmes.[37]

The right to health of specific groups is enshrined in other international human rights instruments, such as the Convention on the Elimination of All Forms of Discrimination against Women,[38] the Convention on the Rights of the Child,[39] and the Convention on the Rights of Persons with Disabilities.[40] At the regional level, the African Charter on the Rights and Welfare of the Child,[41] the Protocol to the African Charter on Human and Peoples' Rights on the Rights of Women in Africa,[42] and the African Youth Charter[43] establish the right to health of the child, women, and youth. States also have obligations to ensure women's access to health services, education, and information, including in the area of sexual and reproductive health.[44]

Health equity and the social, economic, and political determinants of health have also been highlighted in international instruments. The 2011 Rio Political Declaration on Social Determinants of Health focused on five critical action areas, notably to adopt better governance for health and development, to promote participation in policymaking and implementation, to further reorient the health sector towards reducing health inequities, to strengthen global governance and collaboration, and to monitor progress and increase accountability.[45] More recently, World Health Organization (WHO) has highlighted the need for a multisectoral approach to policy decisions encompassing various spheres affecting health, such as housing, education, and transport for COVID-19 recovery.[46] At the regional level, the Principles and Guidelines on the Implementation of Economic, Social, and Cultural Rights in the African Charter on Human and Peoples' Rights (the Nairobi Principles) also emphasize the need for national plans and policies to account for the determinants of health and ensure equitable access by vulnerable groups.[47] Furthermore, state duties in this regard have been corroborated in jurisprudence. In *Free Legal Assistance Group & Others v Zaire*, the African Commission on Human and Peoples' Rights (ACHPR) drew the link between the social determinants of health and the right to health by holding that the failure by the state to provide basic services such as potable water, electricity, and essential medicines constituted a violation of the right to health.[48]

10.2.2.2 Institutional framework

The protection of the right to health of minorities and vulnerable groups in Africa is characterized by several institutional frameworks and special initiatives and interventions. At the international level, the WHO Department of Social Determinants of Health leads efforts in tackling the social, economic, and political determinants of health. The secretariat supports countries and health partners in addressing health inequities. The WHO Division of Data, Analytics, and Delivery for Impact maintains the Health Equity Monitor Database, a regularly updated database containing disaggregated health data.[49] It also developed the Health Equity Assessment Toolkit to enable countries to assess inequalities at national or subnational levels as well as tools to build the capacity for collecting, analysing, and reporting on health inequality data for global and national monitoring.[50]

At the regional level, the African Union (AU) Health Strategy 2016–2030 highlights the need for multisectoral partnerships addressing socio-economic and environmental determinants of health and enabling better health sector performance.[51] In furthering this objective, the African Union Commission (AUC) is mandated to undertake advocacy, resource mobilization, and dissemination of best practices at the continental level in support of the implementation of the Strategy. The African Union Development Agency (AUDA-NEPAD) is responsible for mobilizing and directing technical expertise and financial resources to implement regional and national programmes and projects, supporting research and knowledge management and providing technical support to the AUC's policy processes and activities. The Regional Economic Communities (RECs) are mandated to provide technical support to member states, advocate for increased resources for health systems strengthening, harmonize the implementation of national action plans, monitor and report progress, and identify and share best practices.

Civil society, the private sector, and development partners are also recognized as key players in supporting countries in addressing the social, economic, and political determinants of health. The African Development Bank's (AfDB's) Strategy for Quality Health Infrastructure in Africa 2022–2030 provides for technical and financial support interventions towards improved access to quality health services across the continent, including addressing challenges to uneven distribution in rural areas.[52] Research institutes as well as non-governmental and community-based organizations such as the African Population and Health Research Center (APHRC),[53] the African Medical and Research Foundation (AMREF),[54] and the Africa Health Organization (AHO)[55] conduct policy-relevant research on health-related issues facing Africa and lead programmes to promote health equity on the continent.

10.2.3 Protection of the right to health in pandemics

States are required to take steps to realize the right to health, subject to the principles of progressive realization and maximum available resources.[56] States however have core minimum obligations that they must fulfil immediately to realize the right to health, regardless of their economic and human resources, as follows:

(a) *To ensure the right of access to health facilities, goods, and services on a non-discriminatory basis, especially for vulnerable or marginalized groups;*[57]
(b) To ensure access to minimum essential food that is nutritionally adequate and safe, to ensure freedom from hunger to everyone;
(c) *To ensure access to basic shelter, housing, and sanitation, and an adequate supply of safe and potable water;*[58]
(d) To provide essential drugs, as from time to time defined under the WHO Action Programme on Essential Drugs;
(e) *To ensure equitable distribution of all health facilities, goods, and services;*[59]
(f) To adopt and implement a national public health strategy and plan of action, on the basis of epidemiological evidence, addressing the health concerns of the whole population.[60]

States also have obligations of comparable priority to the core obligations, which include

i) Ensuring reproductive, maternal . . ., and child health care;
ii) Providing immunization against major infectious diseases occurring in the community;
iii) Taking measures to prevent, treat, and control epidemic and endemic diseases;
iv) Providing education and access to information concerning the main health problems in the community, including methods of preventing and controlling them; and
v) Providing appropriate training for health personnel, including education on health and human rights.[61]

It should be highlighted that these core obligations are non-derogable, to which states cannot justify non-compliance.[62] The adoption of any retrogressive measures incompatible with the core obligations under the right to health constitutes a violation of the right to health.[63]

The normative components constituting the minimum core obligations amid pandemics have not been sufficiently elaborated in international law. The European Committee of Social Rights adopted a Statement of Interpretation on the Right to Protection of Health in Times of Pandemics in 2020.[64] In its guidance, the Committee highlights the state obligation to ensure adequate implementation of measures to prevent and limit the spread of the virus, which includes testing and tracing, physical distancing and self-isolation, the provision of adequate masks and disinfectant, as well as the imposition of quarantine and lockdown arrangements. It also underlines state obligations to ensure the treatment of all those falling ill in a pandemic, including the availability of a sufficient number of hospital beds, intensive care units, and equipment as well as the deployment of a sufficient number of healthcare professionals. It further provides the obligation to ensure that the working conditions of healthcare workers are healthy and safe. There is also a duty to ensure health education about the risks posed by the disease and to prevent those risks or other factors on human health. The statement further highlights that health care in a pandemic must be effective and affordable to everyone and for health care to adequately protect groups at particularly high risk.

It is noteworthy that the ACHPR has not provided similar interpretive guidance which could be most relevant to African states. While the guidelines of the European Committee of Social Rights are useful, they are not exhaustive and do not include other potentially relevant duties critical to the protection of the right to health of marginalized groups, such as duties to publish disaggregated data that would help identify discrimination on grounds such as ethnicity, and socio-economic status, to ensure the regular flow of food supplies with a particular attention to deprived households, and to control the spread of misinformation and fake news about viruses and the diseases they cause, including racial blame and victimization.[65]

In December 2021, state parties to the WHO decided to begin the process of drafting and negotiating a convention on strengthening pandemic prevention, preparedness, and response.[66] It remains to be seen if this instrument will address health equity in the context of pandemics and provide further guidance on state duties.[67]

10.3 Impact of the pandemic on the protection of the right to health of minorities and vulnerable groups

The pandemic has largely amplified existing health inequities and adversely affected some groups more than others. This section studies the impact of the pandemic on the protection of the right to health of minorities and vulnerable groups in the African context, focusing on three severely affected groups, notably the poor, women and girls, and sexual minorities.

10.3.1 The poor

Africa has one of the highest levels of poverty and disease burdens[68] as well as income inequality and health inequities caused by socio-economic factors globally.[69] The pandemic has worsened poverty and hunger and widened income inequality in the continent, halting progress made towards the Sustainable Development Goals and Agenda 2063 in the last two decades.[70] It was estimated that 58 million people were vulnerable to falling into poverty in Africa in 2021 due to the effects of the pandemic.[71] The latter has also had significant detrimental effects on the functioning of health systems, of which the poor have mostly borne the brunt.[72] Due to limited fiscal capacity, countries in the region have not been able to offer adequate financial support to individuals, households, and businesses through social protection programmes.[73] The dearth of data on populations and living standards resulted in assistance failing to reach the poorest and most vulnerable.[74] Importantly, in lockdowns and curfews, physical distancing and control strategies based on assumptions about household structures have proven to be inadequate or counterproductive in such environments.[75] As poor communities mostly live in informal settlements where housing density is high, with poor sanitation and ventilation, they have been more susceptible to disease transmission.[76] Similarly, access to food was severely reduced due to the limited capacity for storing food in informal settlements.

10.3.2 Women and girls

Women's health has been severely impacted by the pandemic. Women have been more exposed to the virus as a result of constituting a much larger proportion of the workforce worst affected by the crisis, notably that of frontline and essential services, tourism, and hospitality industries.[77] Furthermore, women have also been more vulnerable to the pandemic as a result of their economic and employment status. Women are generally paid less and face poorer working conditions than their male counterparts. In 2019, 90% of women in sub-Saharan Africa were estimated to work in the informal economy sector, with no social protection.[78] Women faced more difficulties in obtaining government palliatives or aid during the pandemic.[79] The prioritization of COVID-19 and a significantly burdened healthcare system limited critical services for women. WHO surveys conducted over the course of the pandemic consistently indicated disruptions to sexual, reproductive, maternal, newborn, child, and adolescent health services, with studies in 2021 indicating continuing disruptions in 40% of African countries.[80] In 6 out of 11 African countries surveyed in the latter surveys, maternal deaths in health facilities had risen by 16% and by 11% on average between February and May 2020 compared with that in the same period in 2019. While sexual violence increased during the pandemic,[81] services for women who have experienced sexual violence declined in 56% of African countries between November and December 2021, compared with that in the period before the pandemic.[82] Moreover, the use of contraceptives fell in 48% of African countries, while teenage pregnancies increased in 2020.[83]

10.3.3 Sexual minorities

While public health data on the impacts of COVID-19 on sexual minorities is starkly wanting given the absence of national data collection on sexual orientation,[84] LGBTQ+ communities are known to have faced stigmatization during past infectious disease outbreaks[85] and to have higher incidences of underlying conditions likely to lead to severe COVID-related illnesses.[86] Global evidence has demonstrated the compounding effect of the pandemic on LGBTQ+ communities' access to basic necessities such as employment, insurance, medical care, and loans.[87] A higher prevalence of anxiety, psychological distress, and mental health conditions was also highlighted within sexual minority communities as a result of social isolation.[88] The pandemic also reduced access to HIV testing and medication as well as to HIV providers via telemedicine, especially for those without access to technology.[89] Similar evidence is, however, scarce in the African context where reports have underscored the human rights implications of government measures on sexual minorities, albeit not focusing on health disparities.[90]

10.4 Opportunities and challenges for enhanced protection

The pandemic has prompted an inquiry into new strategies for offsetting and mitigating the socio-economic impacts of health crises. In Africa particularly, the need for various immediate and long-term interventions has been identified, ranging from diversifying economies and limiting dependence on external funding,[91] strengthening disease surveillance systems[92] to incorporating mental health and psychosocial support in national responses,[93] decolonizing global health research,[94] and advocating prison reform.[95] This section adds to such policy recommendations, in view of strengthening the protection of the right to health of minorities and vulnerable groups in Africa. Since health marginalization is characterized by the interplay of social, economic, political, and legal determinants as outlined in Section 10.2 of this chapter, enhanced protection calls for a combination of normative, governance, economic, and public health interventions.

10.4.1 Evidence-based, tailored, and inclusive decision-making

COVID-19 policies and public health interventions in Africa have not sufficiently integrated human rights-based approaches.[96] Top-down strategies failed to address the specific needs of minorities and vulnerable groups, especially the poor, women and girls, and sexual minorities.[97] Moreover, national pandemic plans did not adequately incorporate priority setting processes, very rarely identifying equity as a factor for priority setting.[98] Blanket regulatory standards, ill-suited to the context and realities of marginalized communities, not only exacerbate health inequities, as highlighted in Section 10.3 of this chapter, but are also less likely to be complied with.[99] Significantly, they have proven to be especially impractical in the African setting.[100] Incorporating human rights-based approaches into the design and implementation of remedial measures requires equitable representation in decision-making and extensive consultations with at-risk populations for better insight into community and cultural practices and structures, living conditions, and local knowledge and capacities.[101] Policies and programmes also need to be multi-sectoral rather than restricted to the health sector, and involve a broad array of actors such as the media, religious institutions, community leaders, the private sector, and individuals. In addition, for policies to be targeted and effective, they need to be built on basic demographic, spatial, and economic data, to improve preparedness planning, programming, and evaluation of relief and assistance. The lack of reliable and disaggregated data systems and open data sharing in Africa have hindered national and continental efforts in designing and implementing pro-poor, inclusive and culturally responsive policies.[102] Going forward, African countries will also need to focus on strengthening their data collection and reporting along with their monitoring and evaluation systems. In addition, stakeholder mapping and coordination within countries and regions is also key to ensuring effective and efficient responses.

10.4.2 Improved normative guidance by regional human rights organs

The African Commission on Human and Peoples' Rights has the role of interpreting the rights in the African Charter on Human and Peoples' Rights.[103] Since the onset of the pandemic, the Commission has issued crucial guidance on legal standards, notably on a human rights-based response to the pandemic, as early as March 2020. Notably, it referred to the duty to ensure that special measures do not lead to discrimination and stigmatization.[104] It also highlighted that those measures need to be specific and responsive to the needs of vulnerable groups. In August 2020, the African Commission adopted a resolution on human rights standards in the recovery from the socio-political impacts of the pandemic. The resolution notably contains further guidance on the duties incumbent upon states in ensuring the right to non-discrimination in the context of the pandemic. It urges states to adopt affirmative measures for the protection of vulnerable groups; to establish mechanisms to prevent and remedy discriminatory applications of pandemic regulation measures; to ensure protection of non-nationals, refugees, asylum seekers, and migrants; and to ensure responses are gender-sensitive.[105] In another statement, it appealed to states to ensure equitable responses, affording special protection to women and girls through access to sexual and reproductive health services and providing support to women who are victims of gender-based violence and who have lost their sources of income.[106] In addition, the Women, Gender, and Development Directorate of the AUC has developed the AU Guidelines on Gender-Responsive Responses to COVID-19, which provides guidance on gender-sensitive approaches to COVID-19 in the continent. With regard to health, it emphasizes the need for including women in health leadership and decision-making, for furthering research on the gendered implications of health emergencies and disaggregated data in view of developing tailored preventive measures.[107] While the guidance provided thus far by the AUC and the African Commission is useful in illuminating the normative framework for states towards a human rights-based approach to the pandemic and recovery in the African setting, it has not delved sufficiently into the protection of the right to health, the structural determinants of health, and the governance and developmental aspects crucial to prompting states to adopt pro-poor and gender-sensitive interventions. Notably, it has not sufficiently drawn on the role, interplay, and coordination among the various regional human rights and development frameworks and institutional actors. Furthermore, it has not adequately delved into the relevant approaches for improved outcomes of national responses for specific groups, including poor communities and sexual minorities.

10.4.3 Increased budget prioritization and equity-promoting budgeting for resilient health systems

As a result of political instability, conflict, and poor governance, Africa has long-standing deficits in healthcare systems and infrastructure. In 2010, it was found that while the continent accounts for 25% of the global disease burden, it has only 3% of the world's health workers, 1% of the world's trained health workers, and less than 1% of the world's health expenditure.[108] In most countries of the region, the government's share of health spending stood at a mere 34% in 2020.[109] National systems are typically subsidized by donor funding. Moreover, in 2021, it was estimated that Africa only had 1.3 hospital beds per 1000 people, compared to 2.1 in Latin America and 6.1 in Europe.[110] These challenges have long been recognized by African states. In 2001, African governments, in the face of the rapid spread of HIV, tuberculosis, and other infectious diseases on the continent, committed to allocate at least 15% of their annual budget to the improvement of the health sector.[111] This target has not been reached in most African countries by the start of the pandemic and has instead been in decline. However, a country's wealth does not have an absolute incidence on the prioritization of health. Some lower-income countries including Ethiopia, the Gambia, and Malawi were among those having met the 15% Abuja target.[112] Across the continent, health infrastructure remains unevenly distributed and of poor quality, with grossly insufficient capital expenditure and dwindling donor support.[113] Since the onset of the pandemic, the African Commission on Human and Peoples' Rights has called upon states to step up efforts to meet the Abuja target and increase their budget allocations to the provision of the structural determinants of health, notably ensuring access to water, sanitation, social protection, education, and sustainable livelihood and addressing food insecurity and hunger.[114] In the recently adopted Call to Action on a New Public Health Order for Africa, the AUC and the Africa CDC called upon African states, the private sector, and civil society to invest in public health workforce and strong public health institutions and advance local vaccine and therapeutics production.[115] For African states to address health marginalization, they will also need to integrate a pro-poor and gender perspective and mainstream equity in their financing and debt management policies and their budget preparation and planning. Going forward, African states will need to increase resource allocation and investment in relevant institutions and civil society groups, promote corporate social responsibility, and create the platforms for enabling the engagement of women, sexual minorities, and gender experts in budgeting processes. In this respect, progress on gender-responsive and equity-promoting budgeting has been very slow and needs to be further prioritized in African states.[116]

10.4.4 Reparative approaches to global health equity

As highlighted in Section 10.2 of this chapter, health marginalization is prevalent both within and between countries. The COVID-19 pandemic has revealed stark global inequities in the context of international health crises. As of January 2022, only 9.5% of populations in low-income countries had been vaccinated. Of the 10 billion doses distributed worldwide, only 1% had been administered in low-income countries.[117] Vaccine inequity has had detrimental impacts on progress in development goals.[118] Research underscores the widening gap between countries in public health spending in the years to come in the face of the economic shocks from the pandemic and the impact of rising interest payments on public debt.[119] Most marginalized communities have paid the highest price of deepening global inequality.[120] States are subject to duties of international assistance and cooperation in helping developing countries fulfil their core obligations under the right to health:

> For the avoidance of any doubt, the Committee wishes to emphasize that it is particularly incumbent on States parties and other actors in a position to assist, to provide 'international assistance and cooperation, especially economic and technical' which enable developing countries to fulfil their core and other obligations indicated in paragraphs 43 and 44 above.[121]

For African states to address health marginalization in their COVID-related responses and long-term health responses, they need financial and technical assistance. Relevant international efforts however have fallen short of needs. The COVID-19 Vaccines Global Access (COVAX) and the COVID-19 Technology Access Pool have had underwhelming outcomes in advancing vaccine equity. The Coalition for Epidemic Preparedness Innovations (CEPI) replenishment summit, aimed at accelerating vaccine research and development for new infectious disease outbreaks, in March this year failed to meet the pledges requested.[122] As a result of the light shed by the pandemic on the power asymmetry in global health and its detrimental impact on the most vulnerable including poor communities, women and girls, and sexual minorities, the focus may need to shift to reparative justice models of equity instead of donor- and aid-based initiatives.[123] This would involve among others promoting calls for diversity and inclusion in global health organizations, for accountability for discriminatory policies, for local and indigenous knowledge, and for local decision-making in funding and research.[124]

10.4.5 Addressing fragility and conflict as drivers of health marginalization

The health impact of armed conflict is widely demonstrated.[125] It has notably been recently underlined as the WHO global initiative 'Peace for Health and Health for Peace' was launched on World Health Day in 2022, which aims to foster dialogue around health and peace.[126] Conflicts and violence typically lead to disruptions in access to clean water and shelter, poor sanitation, and the collapse of public health infrastructures. Significantly, vulnerable groups suffer worse health outcomes during conflict.[127] The COVID-19 pandemic has hindered conflict-resolution efforts and exacerbated existing conflict. Governments also capitalized on conflicts to crack down on human rights of vulnerable groups.[128] Given that most of the global conflict is concentrated within the African continent and, consequently, its significant impact on the health outcomes of the most vulnerable, further efforts need to be invested in conflict prevention using the frameworks of the AU.[129] Policy measures in health in Africa should also further address fragility and conflict, in light of their impact on health outcomes.[130]

10.5 Future pandemics and the way forward

In enhancing preparedness for future pandemics, targeted and tailored action is warranted to address the distinct and intersectional needs and impacts upon minorities and vulnerable groups, especially poor communities, women and girls, and sexual minorities. In this vein, it is critical to capitalize upon the heightened political attention to health and health marginalization generated by the COVID-19 pandemic for bolstering action and reform. Significantly, emerging research, data, and lessons learnt from the COVID-19 pandemic should be leveraged and consolidated in informing sustainable policy and interventions. First, the effects of poverty amid crises should be more profoundly factored into risk management and resilience measures. This involves ramping up labour market and business development programmes. It also requires public health reform, with a focus on universal health coverage and the deployment of contribution-based national health insurance schemes. African governments further need to strengthen institutional and human capacity as well as procure essential life-saving equipment. Moreover, gender-responsive pandemic planning should focus on systemic drivers of gender imbalances and discrimination and gendered impacts in health and health care, which will entail a spate of fiscal and economic, social protection and violence against women measures. For instance, since women face barriers in accessing health information, a diversity of channels such as women's groups and community leaders need to be prioritized in the dissemination of accurate information to women and girls during pandemics. It is also important that digital literacy programmes be deployed and sponsored given that health information campaigns are increasingly held online. Such information should be made available in local languages. Digital literacy is equally important to enhance women's access to e-commerce and business opportunities. In addition, governments ought to crucially confront pay structures and support within women-dominated sectors and unpaid child and family care as well as increase access to finance and livelihood relief to women in informal employment. Given the rise in gender-based violence observed during the pandemic, it is also crucial to further promote violence prevention efforts and strengthen law enforcement and justice responses to gender-based violence. Similarly, efforts should be stepped up in addressing the structural marginalization of sexual minorities in service delivery and sectoral initiatives, especially in health care. In-country systems should be put in place to monitor and advocate for inclusion and diversity within the health sector and advance service accessibility, especially in mental health and reproductive and sexual health. Furthermore, more attention is warranted to addressing the disproportionate poverty and unemployment levels among sexual minorities and the design of suitable social protection programmes.

10.6 Conclusion

This chapter has examined the impact of the COVID-19 pandemic on the right to health of minorities and vulnerable groups in Africa and suggested focus areas for enhanced protection at national and regional levels. A review of government-led responses indicates vulnerable groups, particularly poor communities, women and girls, and sexual minorities, have been disproportionately affected by government measures, which have exacerbated health marginalization. It is posited that five focus areas will be critical to the protection of the right to health of minorities and vulnerable groups in Africa in response to the pandemic and for preparedness to future health crises. These include the integration of human rights-based approaches in national responses to ensure inclusive and tailored policies that will account for the specific needs and contexts of various vulnerable groups. This also requires the strengthening of data collection, reporting, and sharing. Furthermore, it is suggested that the African Commission on Human and Peoples' Rights could extend its focus on vulnerable groups in pandemics and provide further normative guidance to states. Thirdly, a prioritization of health in national budgets and gender-responsive and equity-promoting budgeting is crucial for vulnerable populations to benefit from adequate health services. Moreover, alternate strategies for achieving global health equity may need to be pursued in view of closing on health disparities between high- and low- and middle-income countries. Finally, in light of the high incidence of conflict and violence across the continent and the nexus between fragility and poor health outcomes, regional mechanisms need to be further leveraged for conflict prevention. Lessons learnt and the invigorated political momentum on health equity brought about by the pandemic should be tapped into for enhancing fair, representative, and equitable health planning and management.

Notes

1 It has supplemented widely documented prior evidence of the unequal health impacts of past public health crises. For an overview, see notably C Bambra & others 'The COVID-19 pandemic and health inequalities' (2020) 74 *Journal of Epidemiol Community Health* 964–968.

2 An inquiry undertaken in the UK notably revealed a superior mortality rate from COVID-19 among Black, Asian, and minority ethnic (BAME) communities. See the Institute of Fiscal Studies 'Are some ethnic groups more vulnerable to COVID-19 than others?' May 2020 available at https://ifs.org.uk/inequality/are-some-ethnic-groups-more-vulnerable-to-covid-19-than-others/ (accessed 10 April 2022). Similarly, a study conducted in Chicago revealed the unevenly adverse health impacts of COVID-19 on marginalized populations. See MM

Ruprecht & others 'Evidence of social and structural COVID-19 disparities by sexual orientation, gender identity, and race/ethnicity in an urban environment' (2021) 98 *Journal of Urban Health* 27–40.

3 See notably, SV Katikireddi & others 'Unequal impact of the COVID-19 crisis on minority ethnic groups: A framework for understanding and addressing inequalities' (2021) 75 *Journal of Epidemiol Community Health* 970–974.

4 UNHRC 'Human rights implications of the COVID-19 pandemic' 43rd session, Geneva 2 June 2020, UN Doc. A/HRC/PRST/43/1.

5 See, for instance, World Health Organization (WHO) Regional Office for Europe 'Health inequity and the effects of COVID-19: Assessing, responding to and mitigating the socioeconomic impact on health to build a better future' (2020) available at https://apps.who.int/iris/bitstream/handle/10665/338199/WHO-EURO-2020-1744-41495-56594-eng.pdf?sequence=1&isAllowed=y (accessed 10 April 2022) 1.

6 J Mubangizi 'Poor lives matter: COVID-19 and the plight of vulnerable groups with specific reference to poverty and inequality in South Africa' (2021) 65 *Journal of African Law* 237–258.

7 EL McKinney, V McKinney & L Swartz 'Access to healthcare for people with disabilities in South Africa: Bad at any time, worse during COVID-19?' (2021) 63(1) *South African Family Practice* a5226.

8 U Effiong, UE Okeke & F Nwoko 'African women's health and the COVID-19 pandemic: Implications for policy and development' in O Adeola (ed) *Gendered perspectives on* COVID-19 *recovery in Africa: Towards sustainable development* (2021) 73–91.

9 VM Mutambara, TL Crankshaw & J Freedman 'Assessing the impacts of COVID-19 on women refugees in South Africa' (2022) 35(1) *Journal of Refugee Studies* 704–721.

10 OIO Adebisi & EE Lucero-Prisno 'Towards an inclusive health agenda: People who inject drugs and the COVID-19 response in Africa' (2021) 190 *Public Health* e7–e8.

11 J Visagie & I Turok 'Rural–urban inequalities amplified by COVID-19: Evidence from South Africa' (2021) 6(1) *Area Development and Policy* 50–62.

12 L Forman & JC Kohler 'Global health and human rights in the time of COVID-19: Response, restrictions, and legitimacy' (2020) 19(5) *Journal of Human Rights* 547–556.

13 Imperial College London 'Report 22 – equity in response to the COVID-19 pandemic: An assessment of the direct and indirect impacts on disadvantaged and vulnerable populations in low- and lower middle-income countries' (2020) available at www.imperial.ac.uk/mrc-global-infectious-disease-analysis/covid-19/report-22-equity/ (accessed 10 April 2022).

14 See notably L Paremoer 'COVID-19 pandemic and the social determinants of health' (2021) 372(129) *British Medical Journal* 1–5.

15 T Myhrvold 'Marginalisation as a possible health issue: An exercise in practice-based ethical education' (2012) *Nordic Journal of Applied Ethics* 42–57, at 46.

16 For a discussion of relevant issues in the African context, see EB Eshetu and SA Woldesenbet 'Are there particular social determinants of health for the world's poorest countries?' (2011) 11(1) *African Health Sciences* 108–115.

17 See notably M Marmot 'Social determinants of health: From observation to policy' (2000) 172(8) *Medical Journal of Australia* 379–382; MJ Lynam & S Cowley 'Understanding marginalization as a social determinant of health' (2007) 17(2) *Critical Public Health* 137–149 and DE Dawes *The political determinants of health* (2020).

18 WHO Commission on Social Determinants of Health 'Closing the gap in a generation: Health equity through action on the social determinants of

health' August 2008 available at www.who.int/publications/i/item/WHO-IER-CSDH-08.1 (accessed 27 April 2022).

19 M Harvey 'How do we explain the social, political and economic determinants of health? A call for the inclusion of social theories of health inequality within US-based public health pedagogy' (2020) 6(4) *Pedagogy in Health Promotion* 246–252.

20 LO Gostin & others 'The legal determinants of health: Harnessing the power of law for global health and sustainable development' (2019) 393(10183) *Lancet* 1857–1910.

21 WHO (n 5 above) at 1.

22 UN Sustainable Development Group 'A UN framework for the immediate socio-economic response to COVID-19' April 2020 available at https://unsdg.un.org/resources/un-framework-immediate-socio-economic-response-covid-19 (accessed 24 April 2022).

23 See as above, at 7.

24 International Labour Organization 'World employment and social outlook: Trends 2022' available at www.ilo.org/wcmsp5/groups/public/–dg reports/–dcomm/–publ/documents/publication/wcms_834081.pdf (accessed 24 April 2022) at 25.

25 L Robinson & others 'Digital inequalities in time of pandemic: COVID-19 exposure risk profiles and new forms of vulnerability' (2020) 25(7) *First Monday*.

26 Constitution of the World Health Organization (adopted 22 July 1946, entered into force 7 April 1948) 14 UNTS 185, Preamble.

27 See as above.

28 Universal Declaration of Human Rights (adopted and proclaimed 10 December 1948) UN General Assembly Resolution 217 A (III), article 25.

29 International Covenant on Economic, Social and Cultural Rights (adopted 16 December 1966, entered into force 23 March 1976) 999 UNTS 171, article 12.

30 African Charter on Human and Peoples' Rights (adopted 27 June 1981, entered into force 21 October 1986, 21 ILM 58, article 16). For an overview of the right to health under the regional human rights system, see E Durojaye 'An analysis of the contribution of the African human rights system to the understanding of the right to health' (2021) 21(2) *African Human Rights Law Journal* 751–781.

31 Emphasis added.

32 UN Committee on Economic, Social and Cultural Rights 'General comment no. 14: Article 12 of the convention' 22nd session, Geneva, 25 April–12 May 2000, UN Doc. E/C.12/2000/4, para 11.

33 See as above, para 12.

34 Emphasis added.

35 UN Committee (no. 32 above) para 12.

36 As above, para 18.

37 UN Committee on Economic, Social and Cultural Rights 'General comment no. 13: Article 2 of the convention' (1990)' 5th Session, Geneva, 14 December 1990, UN Doc. E/1991/23, para 12.

38 Convention on the Elimination of All Forms of Discrimination against Women (adopted 18 December 1979, entered into force 3 September 1981) 1249 UNTS 13, article 12.

39 Convention on the Rights of the Child (adopted 20 November 1989, entered into force e 2 September 1990) 1577 UNTS 3, article 24.

40 Convention on the Rights of Persons with Disabilities (adopted 13 December 2006, entered into force 3 May 2008) UN Doc. A/RES/61/106, article 25.

41 African Charter on the Rights and Welfare of the Child (adopted 11 July 1990, entered into force 29 November 1999) OAU Doc. CAB/LEG/24.9/49, article 14.

42 Protocol to the African Charter on Human and Peoples' rights on the Rights of Women in Africa (adopted 11 July 2003, entered into force 25 November 2005) available at https://au.int/sites/default/files/treaties/37077-treaty-charter_on_rights_of_women_in_africa.pdf (accessed 1 August 2023) article 14.
43 African Youth Charter (adopted 2 July 2006, entered into force 8 August 2009) available at https://au.int/sites/default/files/treaties/7789-treaty-0033_-_african_youth_charter_e.pdf (accessed 1 August 2023) article 16.
44 UN Committee on the Elimination of Discrimination Against Women 'General recommendation no. 24: Article 12 of the convention (women and health)' 20th session, Geneva, 20 August 1999, UN Doc. A/54/38/Rev.1.
45 'Rio political declaration on social determinants of health' 30th session of the World Conference on Social Determinants of Health, Rio de Janeiro, 21 October 2011, Doc. EB130/15. See also World Health Assembly 'Reducing health inequities through action on the social determinants of health' 62nd session, Geneva, 22 May 2009, Doc. WHA62.14 and World Health Assembly 'Outcome of the world conference on social determinants of health' 65th session, Geneva, 26 May 2012, Doc. WHA65.8.
46 WHO Executive Board 'Social determinants of health' 148th session, Geneva, 6 January 2021, Doc. EB148/24.
47 'The principles and guidelines on the implementation of economic, social and cultural rights in the African Charter on Human and Peoples' rights' 48th ordinary session of the African Commission on Human and Peoples' Rights, 10–24 November 2010, para 67.
48 (2000) AHRLR 74 (ACHPR 1995).
49 WHO *Health equity monitor database* available at www.who.int/data/health-equity/health-equity-monitor-database (accessed 20 April 2022).
50 WHO *Health equity assessment toolkit* available at www.who.int/data/health-equity/assessment_toolkit (accessed 20 April 2022).
51 African Union 'Africa health strategy 2016–2030, adopted at the ministers of health meeting' 26 May 2016 available at https://au.int/sites/default/files/pages/32895-file-africa_health_strategy.pdf (accessed 20 April 2022).
52 African Development Bank 'Strategy for quality health infrastructure in Africa 2022–2030' available at www.afdb.org/en/documents/strategy-quality-health-infrastructure-africa-2021-2030 (accessed 20 April 2022).
53 https://aphrc.org (accessed 20 April 2022).
54 https://amref.org (accessed 20 April 2022).
55 https://aho.org (accessed 20 April 2022).
56 International Covenant on Economic, Social and Cultural Rights (n 29 above), article 2.
57 Emphasis added.
58 As above.
59 As above.
60 UN Committee (n 32 above) para 43.
61 As above, para 44.
62 As above, para 47.
63 As above, para 48.
64 European Committee of Social Rights 'Statement of interpretation on the right to protection of health in times of pandemic' 21 April 2020 available at https://rm.coe.int/statement-of-interpretation-on-the-right-to-protection-of-health-in-ti/16809e3640 (accessed 1 August 2023).
65 L Montel & others 'The right to health in times of pandemic: What can we learn from the UK's response to the COVID-19 outbreak?' (2020) 22(2) *Health and Human Rights Journal* 227–241, at 239.

66 World Health Assembly 'The world together: Establishment of an intergovernmental negotiating body to strengthen pandemic prevention, preparedness and response' 5th plenary session, Geneva, 1 December 2021, Doc. SSA2/SR/5.
67 C Wenham, R Reisdorf & S Asthana 'Pandemic Treaty: A Chance to Level up on Equity' (2022) 377 *British Medical Journal* o1279.
68 ZA Bhutta & others 'Global burden, distribution and interventions for infectious diseases of poverty' (2014) 3 *Infectious Diseases of Poverty* 21.
69 O Okoi & T Bwawa 'How health inequality affect responses to the COVID-19 pandemic in sub-Saharan Africa' (2020) 135 *World Development* 105067.
70 UN Economic Commission for Africa 'Economic report on Africa 2021: Addressing poverty and vulnerability in Africa during the COVID-19 pandemic' (2021) available at https://repository.uneca.org/bitstream/handle/10855/47592/ERA%20 2021%20En%20%28b12002963%29.pdf?sequence=10&isAllowed=y (accessed 12 May 2022).
71 See as above.
72 H Amu & others 'COVID-19 and health systems functioning in sub-Saharan Africa using the "WHO building blocks": The challenges and responses' (2022) *Frontiers in Public Health* 10.
73 A Renzaho 'The need for the right socio-economic and cultural fit in the COVID-19 response in sub-Saharan Africa: Examining demographic, economic political, health, and socio-cultural differentials in COVID-19 morbidity and mortality' (2020) 17(10) *International Journal of Environmental Research and Public Health* 3445–3459.
74 OE Olayide 'Policy Milieu for combatting COVID-19 and sustainability of African economies' in P Carmody & others (eds) *COVID-19 in the Global South: Impacts and responses* (2020) 75–83, at 80.
75 Renzaho (n 73 above).
76 A Wilkinson 'The challenges of COVID-19 in informal urban settlements and the need for co-produced local responses' in P Carmody & others (eds) *COVID-19 in the Global South: Impacts and responses* (2020) 63–74, at 65.
77 International Labour Organization (n 24 above) at 28.
78 International Labour Organization 'Women and men in the informal economy: A statistical update' (2023) available at www.ilo.org/wcmsp5/groups/public/–ed_protect/–protrav/–travail/documents/publication/wcms_869188.pdf (accessed 1 August 2023) at 81.
79 UN Women, CARE International and Oxfam 'Rapid gender analysis: North East region, Nigeria' (2020) available at www.undp.org/africa/publications/covid-19-global-gender-response-tracker-fact-sheets (accessed 1 August 2023).
80 WHO 'Third round of the global pulse survey on continuity of essential health services during the COVID-19 pandemic: November-December 2021' 7 February 2022 available at www.who.int/publications/i/item/WHO-2019-nCoV-EHS_continuity-survey-2022.1 (accessed 12 May 2022).
81 See African Union Commission – Women, Gender and Development Directorate (AUC-WGDD), United Nations Entity for Gender Equality and the Empowerment of Women (UN Women), Office of the United Nations High Commissioner for Human Rights (OHCHR) and United Nations Population Fund (UNFPA) 'Gender-based violence in Africa during the COVID-19 pandemic' (2020) available at https://africa.unwomen.org/sites/default/files/Field%20Office%20 Africa/Attachments/Publications/2021/Policy%20Paper-%20GBV%20in%20 Africa%20during%20COVID-19%20pandemic_EN%2018%20Feb_compressed.pdf (accessed 12 May 2022).

82 WHO Regional Office for Africa 'COVID-19 takes a heavy toll on women's health' 3 March 2022 available at www.afro.who.int/countries/congo/news/covid-19-takes-heavy-toll-womens-health (accessed 12 May 2022).
83 See as above.
84 S Cahill & others 'Sexual and gender minority health in the COVID-19 pandemic: Why data collection and combatting discrimination matter now more than ever' (2020) 110(9) *American Journal of Public Health* 1360–1361.
85 NS Kline 'Rethinking COVID-19 vulnerability: A call for LGBTQ+ Im/migrant health equity in the United States during and after a pandemic' (2020) 4(1) *Health Equity* 239–242.
86 IW Holloway & others 'Associations between physical distancing and mental health, sexual health and technology use among gay, bisexual and other men who have sex with men during the COVID-19 pandemic' (2021) 68(4) *Journal of Homosexuality* 692–708.
87 Cahill (n 84 above).
88 S Wallach & others 'Address exacerbated health disparities and risks to LGBTQ+ individuals during COVID-19' (2020) 22(2) *Health and Human Rights Journal* 313–316.
89 JP Salerno, ND Williams & KA Gattamorta 'LGBTQ populations: Psychologically vulnerable communities in the COVID-19 pandemic' (2020) 12(S1) *Psychological Trauma* S239–S242.
90 See, for instance, 'Pandemic hits Rwanda's sexual minorities harder' *Rwanda Today* 16 December 2020 available at https://rwandatoday.africa/rwanda/news/pandemic-hits-rwanda-s-sexual-minorities-harder–3231252 (accessed 3 August 2022).
91 S Yaya, A Otu & R Labonté 'Globalisation in the time of COVID-19: Repositioning Africa to meet the immediate and remote challenges' (2020) 16 *Globalization and Health* 51.
92 AT Abodore & others 'Impact of poor disease surveillance system on COVID-19 response in Africa: Time to rethink and rebuild' (2021) 12 *Clinical Epidemiology and Global Health* 100841.
93 B Semo and SM Frissa 'The mental health impact of the COVID-19 pandemic: Implications for sub-Saharan Africa' (2020) 13 *Psychology Research and Behaviour Management* 713–720.
94 LJ Wallace & others 'COVID-19 in sub-Saharan Africa: Impacts on vulnerable populations and sustaining home-grown solutions' (2020) 111 *Canadian Journal of Public Health* 649–653.
95 VN Nweze & others 'Prison health during the COVID-19 era in Africa' (2021) 2 *Public Health in Practice* 100083.
96 See notably Mubangizi (n 6 above).
97 See notably H Tan & others 'How has Nigeria responded to the gendered impacts of COVID-19?' *Gender and COVID-19 Project* (2021) available at www.genderandcovid-19.org/wp-content/uploads/2021/09/PAC00467_Gender-and-Covid-19-Nigerias-Pandemic-Response.pdf (accessed 1 August 2023).
98 L Kapiriri & others 'Priority setting and equity in COVID-19 pandemic plans: A comparative analysis of 18 African countries' (2022) 37(3) *Health Policy and Planning* 297–309.
99 Wilkinson (n 76 above) at 71.
100 Renzaho (n 73 above) at 9.
101 O Obasesam & T Bwawa 'How health inequality affect responses to the COVID-19 pandemic in sub-Saharan Africa' (2020) 135 *World Development* 105067.
102 See for instance V Mueller & others 'COVID-19 policy modeling in sub-Saharan Africa' (2021) 43(1) *Applied Economic Perspectives and Policy* 24–38.
103 African Charter on Human and Peoples' Rights (n 30 above) article 45.

104 African Commission on Human and Peoples' Rights 'Press statement on human rights based effective response to the novel COVID-19 virus in Africa' 24 March 2020 available at www.achpr.org/pressrelease/detail?id=483 (accessed 3 June 2022).
105 African Commission on Human and Peoples' Rights 'Resolution on human and peoples' rights as central pillar of successful response to COVID-19 and recovery from its socio-political impacts' adopted virtually 7 August 2020, Doc. ACHPR/ Res. 449 (LXVI) 2020.
106 African Commission on Human and Peoples' Rights 'Press release of the special rapporteur on the rights of women in Africa on violation of women's rights during the COVID-19 pandemic' 6 May 2020 available at www.achpr.org/press release/detail?id=495 (accessed 9 November 2022).
107 African Union Commission 'Framework document on the impact of COVID-19 on gender equality and women's empowerment: AU guidelines on gender-responsive responses to COVID-19' 3 June 2020 available at https://au.int/en/documents/20200603/au-guidelines-gender-responsive-responses-covid-19 (accessed 9 November 2022) 10–11.
108 LN Crisp 'Global health capacity and workforce development: Turning the world upside down' (2011) 25 *Infectious Disease Clinics of North America* 359–367.
109 See Renzaho (n 73 above).
110 African Development Bank 'Strategy for quality health infrastructure in Africa 2021–2030' (n 52 above) at 1.
111 'Abuja declaration on HIV/AIDS, Tuberculosis and other related infectious diseases, adopted at the African summit on HIV/AIDS, Tuberculosis and other related infectious diseases' Abuja, 24–27 April 2007, Doc. OAU/SPS/ABUJA/3.
112 J Biegon '19 years ago today, African countries vowed to spend 15% on health' *African Arguments* 27 April 2020 available at https://africanarguments.org/2020/04/19-years-africa-15-health-abuja-declaration/ (accessed 15 June 2022).
113 African Development Bank, (n 52 above).
114 African Commission (n 105 above) at para 11.
115 'AU Call to Action: Africa's New Public Health Order' adopted by the AU Heads of State and Government and Heads of Delegations at the Special Side Event 'Africa's new public health order: Rejuvenating the global health security agenda' in the sidelines of the 77th session of the UN General Assembly, 21 September 2022 available at https://africacdc.org/news-item/call-to-action-africas-new-public-health-order/ (accessed 9 November 2022).
116 See the 'PEFA Gender responsive public financial management assessments' available at www.pefa.org/assessments?&f_ids[]=5941 (accessed 9 November 2022).
117 WHO *Global dashboard for vaccine equity* available at https://data.undp.org/vaccine-equity/ (accessed 15 June 2022).
118 K Salmon 'Africa's biggest economies will struggle in 2022' *The Economist* 8 November 2021 available at www.economist.com/the-world-ahead/2021/11/08/africas-biggest-economies-will-struggle-in-2022 (accessed 9 November 2022).
119 World Bank Group 'From double shock to double recovery – implications and options for health financing in the time of COVID-19: Technical update – widening rifts' September 2021 available at https://documents1.worldbank.org/curated/en/099414309202218567/pdf/IDU04f3c-5cd20bb9c045af0ac71072ea00a06cdb.pdf (accessed 9 November 2022).
120 Amnesty International 'Report 2021/22: The state of the world's human rights' 29 March 2022 available at https://reliefweb.int/report/world/amnesty-international-report-202122-state-worlds-human-rights-enar (accessed 9 November 2022).
121 UN Committee (n 32 above) para 45.

122 C Butler & E Ross 'New approaches needed to unlock global health funding' *Chatham House* 17 June 2022 available at www.chathamhouse.org/2022/06/new-approaches-needed-unlock-global-health-funding (accessed 9 November 2022).
123 See notably S Harman & others 'Global vaccine equity demands reparative justice – not charity' (2021) 6 *British Medical Journal* 1–4.
124 S Abimbola & others 'Addressing power asymmetries in global health: Imperatives in the wake of the COVID-19 pandemic' (2021) 18(4) *PLoS Medicine* e1003604.
125 Notably see MS Openshaw 'The health consequences of armed conflict in sub-Saharan Africa: How much do conflict intensity and proximity matter' (2012) 2(1) *African Conflict and Peacebuilding Review* 1–30.
126 WHO 'Conflict, climate crisis and COVID: World needs "peace for health and health for peace"' 7 April 2022 available at www.who.int/news-room/commentaries/detail/conflict–climate-crisis-and-covid–world-needs–peace-for-health-and-health-for-peace (accessed 9 November 2022).
127 O Ojeleke & others 'The impact of armed conflicts on health-care utilization in Northern Nigeria: A difference-in-difference analysis' (2022) *World Medical and Health Policy* 1–41.
128 Amnesty International 'Report 2020/21' (n 120 above).
129 African Union 'Continental structural conflict prevention framework' (2018) available at www.peaceau.org/uploads/01-cscpf-booklet-updated-final.pdf (accessed 15 June 2022).
130 See NA Oladayo 'The impact of conflict on health outcomes: A systematic evidence from sub-Saharan Africa' (2019) 8(1) *Journal of African Studies* 88–100.

11

THE NEXUS BETWEEN COVID-19 AND SEXUAL AND REPRODUCTIVE HEALTH OF ADOLESCENTS

Bringing adolescents 'home'

Godfrey Kangaude and Catriona Macleod

11.1 The impact of COVID-19

The major challenge of the coronavirus disease 2019 (COVID-19) pandemic for adolescents was not the disease itself but the secondary effects due to the measures governments took to contain the spread of the virus, including closing schools and restricting movement and social interactions.[1] These measures reduced adolescents' access to and utilization of sexual and reproductive health (SRH) services.[2] Under budgetary constraints, governments rerouted resources to contain the epidemic, neglecting SRH and social protection services. The reduced access to these services increased gender-based violence and unintended pregnancies.[3] The interruption of education closed spaces for skills development, learning, and social interaction with friends and contributed to social problems such as feelings of frustration, isolation, anxiety, and depression.[4]

The pandemic's impact was significant on already marginalized groups and exacerbated existing vulnerabilities and inequalities, especially in sub-Saharan Africa.[5] Adolescents, however, were most impacted by the secondary effects of COVID-19 and were disparately affected because of their unique identities and social locations. For instance, girls were uniquely affected because they could get pregnant. The inability of girls to access SRH services such as contraception and, therefore, to practise safe sex contributed to unintended pregnancies.

Furthermore, even if school closures negatively affected all learners, pregnancy meant that for some girls, schooling ended there as they had to drop out.[6] Teenage pregnancy is an important cause of early and child marriages. Apart from the disparate impact related to gender, the pandemic has

DOI: 10.4324/9781032671437-14

disproportionately impacted vulnerable girls and widened the existing disparities in access to health care, income, and education in sub-Saharan Africa.[7]

However, as Ahinkorah and others have observed, the obstacles to health care that adolescent girls face are not just physical barriers but also cultural norms, such as negative perceptions about the sexuality of girls.[8] An example of such norms is reflected in the disparaging views of parents about sexually active girls that were captured in a study to evaluate youth-friendly health services (YFHS) in Malawi. Researchers asked parents what they thought were the critical problems regarding health affecting the youth. In one focus group, the parents said, '[T]he youth of today are not scared of having relationships with old people – they sleep around with older men with the result that you have 13- or 14-year-olds having unwanted pregnancies'.[9]

In another focus group, parents expressed the following sentiments:

> *Today, girls go on their own to their boyfriends' houses. There are some old men who have sexual relationships with them and when they become pregnant the men abandon them. This is seen as a big problem because children's rights are being abused.*[10]

In yet another focus group, the parents thought this about girls:

> *[Sexual] problems arise from girls who put on miniskirts with the aim of seducing boys to have sex with them with this resulting in transmission of HIV/STIs. Government should introduce punishments for these girls and they should be jailed for one week.*[11]

These three quotes reflect negative views parents have about sexually active girls. Girls are not expected to express sexually agentic behaviours such as having boyfriends and engaging in premarital sexual conduct. Perceiving sexual agency through the lens of cultural norms, parents label sexually active unmarried girls as deviant and immoral. Nevertheless, even though social norms prohibit unmarried girls from having sex, boys and men pressure them into having sex.[12] Because of these double standards, girls have sex but avoid accessing SRH care, fearing that their communities would reprimand or label them sex workers.[13] Girls already faced such challenges during pre-pandemic times; the COVID-19 pandemic exacerbated their predicament.[14]

Governmental containment measures and individual responses to the threat of COVID-19 infection created a cascade of events and effects that contributed to reduced access to social, educational, and informational services for adolescents, including SRH. However, we argue that cultural prejudices towards adolescent sexuality negatively impacted adolescents' resilience to surviving the difficult circumstances initiated by governmental action.

A great deal of literature on the impact of the COVID-19 pandemic in middle- and low-income countries highlights the limitations of resources and services.[15] This book chapter focuses on cultural and psychosocial factors exacerbating adolescents' SRH experiences. In this book chapter, we use the notion of 'home' as where society meets the needs of the adolescent to feel safe and to belong, to argue for responses to promoting the well-being of adolescents that consider adolescent identity, especially their emerging sexualities. Adolescents would fare better in pandemics like COVID-19 not only because governments have maintained social and health services but also because adolescents have the emotional support to be resilient and, therefore, to enjoy sexual health and well-being even in the face of adversity.

11.2 Sexual and reproductive health and justice

The COVID-19 pandemic exacerbated existing injustices and inequities. For instance, girls already had challenges accessing SRH services because of cultural attitudes about the sexuality of unmarried girls.[16] Their sexual and reproductive health and rights (SRHR), such as contraceptive access, were already compromised before the pandemic. Therefore, the policy response to the challenges adolescents experienced because of the COVID-19 pandemic should address the resource, budgetary, and logistical challenges and tackle the social and cultural factors that affect adolescents' SRHR.

But firstly, it is critical to understand the meaning of SRHR. The Guttmacher–Lancet Commission created a comprehensive description from different definitions and sources:

> *Sexual and reproductive health is a state of physical, emotional, mental, and social well-being in relation to all aspects of sexuality and reproduction, not merely the absence of disease, dysfunction, or infirmity. Therefore, a positive approach to sexuality and reproduction should recognise the part played by pleasurable sexual relationships, trust, and communication in the promotion of self-esteem and overall well-being. All individuals have a right to make decisions governing their bodies and to access services that support that right. Achievement of sexual and reproductive health relies on the realisation of sexual and reproductive rights, which are based on the human rights of all individuals to:*
>
> - *have their bodily integrity, privacy, and personal autonomy respected;*
> - *freely define their own sexuality, including sexual orientation and gender identity and expression;*
> - *decide whether and when to be sexually active;*
> - *choose their sexual partners;*
> - *have safe and pleasurable sexual experiences;*
> - *decide whether, when, and whom to marry;*

- *decide whether, when, and by what means to have a child or children, and how many children to have;*
- *have access over their lifetimes to the information, resources, services, and support necessary to achieve all the above, free from discrimination, coercion, exploitation, and violence.*[17]

If adolescents could decide about their bodies, define their sexuality and identity, decide whether to be sexually active, freely choose sexual partners, and have safe and pleasurable sexual experiences, it would significantly contribute to their sexual health and sexual well-being. But now imagine the context in which some adolescents find themselves, where they are not accepted as sexual beings because, according to social and cultural norms, they should be sexually inert until they are married. It means that adolescents cannot even begin to realize these rights.

An SRHR framework does not explicitly address these intersecting social and cultural barriers. The SRHR framework envisages an atomized and autonomous individual positioned to exercise choice when the government does its part, for instance, when it has provided SRH services. However, a sexual and reproductive justice (SRJ) framework is better suited to engage these social, cultural, and political determinants than the individual rights paradigm.[18] The SRJ approach is built upon the concepts of reproductive justice coined by women of colour in the US in the 1990s. It constitutes three principles: The right to have a child, the right not to have a child, and the right to parent children in safe and healthy environments.[19] A fourth principle, sexual autonomy and gender freedom, completes the sexual justice dimension. This framework has been taken up and further developed in sub-Saharan African spaces.[20]

The SRJ framework's strength is that it pays attention to the gendered power dynamics and social, cultural, and political factors that shape the lives and experiences of the group in question.[21] In its 2022 report, the High-Level Commission on the Nairobi Summit on ICPD25 Follow-up endorsed the SRJ framework to realize sexual and reproductive rights commitments countries made at the International Conference on Development and Population (ICPD) of 1994 and renewed at the Nairobi Summit in 2019. The Commission considered the SRJ framework crucial because it builds on human rights to recognize intersecting and systemic oppression, engages power dynamics responsible for the exclusion and marginalization of groups, facilitates movement building, and reinforces governmental accountability.[22]

Adolescents, especially unmarried girls, are disadvantaged compared to married women. This positioning diminishes the power of choice for girls that the individual rights paradigm presupposes everyone has in the same measure. Rather than presuming choice, the SRJ paradigm foregrounds justice to consider the social, cultural, and political factors that affect girls' sexual and reproductive decision-making.[23]

To better survive and maintain SRH and well-being in pandemic events such as COVID-19, adolescents need more than just the availability of reproductive health services, education, and information. Justice requires that society supports adolescents to develop intrinsic resilience. Resilience is possible when adolescents enhance their self-esteem shored up by a community that accepts their emerging sexual and gender identities.[24] 'From this perspective, adolescent sex is an essential developmental basis for healthy adult sexuality rather than an inherently dangerous risk to be silenced, shamed, and suppressed'.[25]

11.3 Adolescence and the emergence of sexual identities

The Committee on the Rights of the Child (CRC) describes adolescence as a life stage characterized by growing opportunities, capacities, and energies; the CRC draws attention to the emergence of the sense of self that characterizes adolescence, including emerging identities, beliefs, and sexualities.[26] The committee reiterates the need for society to support adolescents transitioning into adulthood. An essential aspect of this support is to help adolescents exercise agency progressively to take care of and protect themselves.[27]

Adolescence is a critical period to appreciate. Suleiman and others shed light on the physiological events from puberty that shape adolescents' affective and social behaviours, such as their interest in sex, love, and romantic relationships.[28] Indeed, the YFHS evaluation study found that young adolescents between the ages of 10 and 14 have such interests because, by these ages, they engage in sex talk.[29] The Global Early Adolescent Study (GEAS), a component of which was implemented in Malawi, corroborates the YFHS evaluation study. It found that adolescents aged between 10 and 14 engage in romantic relationships.[30] The society also recognizes this interest, which is why society's deliberate effort starts to shape adolescent sexual behaviour towards that expected of the genders.[31] Sulieman and others confirm that it is developmentally normal for adolescents to behave this way. Those early crushes and beginnings of romance are normative. Through these, adolescents negotiate their sexual identities, create social relationships, and learn the skills for adult relationships. In developing their personal and social identities, adolescents learn to balance autonomy and social connectedness, forming the basis for their evolving journey towards the full development of personality and adult decision-making.[32]

When adults adopt negative attitudes towards adolescent sexual behaviour because it does not conform to cultural norms, they go against nature. When adults maintain repressive attitudes towards adolescents, for instance, by criminalizing normative adolescent sexual conduct, it drives adolescent behaviours underground so that adolescents get disconnected from the guidance and support they need from parents and caregivers.[33]

11.4 Home

The concept of home is central to this chapter. In this section, we describe the notion of home. Governments' confinement measures to curb the COVID-19 pandemic forced adolescents to stay home. Home became the focal place where adolescents had to deal with adversity from the pandemic while trying to maintain sexual health and well-being.

The broadest understanding of home is a place of belonging.[34] Home is represented in many ways, most times as a physical structure, but it can also be a feeling, a metaphor, or a symbol.[35] Home is not just a physical structure or dwelling; it is that emotional place associated with the most influential and ambivalent early psychological experiences that continue to influence the person's life.[36] This ambivalence or mixed feelings about home are understood to be central to relationships that make the home, such as the family, because moral entailments, expectations, and obligations characterize kin relationships.[37]

Another perspective of the home is that it is a place of centring, where one 'finds oneself' physically and emotionally, constituting a meaning system indispensable to one's identity.[38] It is where a person is at peace because they are comfortable with who they are, with their identity. It also presumes significant others' acceptance of one's identity, including family members.

On the other hand, Monica Goldrick provides a spiritual and aspirational definition of home:

> *'Home' is about much more than where we live physically. It is not just where we sleep, and it is not just the nostalgic home of our childhood or our wished-for childhood. It is a spiritual and psychological place of liberation. Home is a space, where we could all belong – with each other – strengthened by what we take from those who have come before us, creating a safe haven for those who will come after us.*[39]

Goldrick suggests that the spiritual definition of home is an ideal or an aspiration mainly because the home may not be a secure and safe place for most people. While for some home may be that place of belonging, for others, constraints such as class, race, and social-cultural norms about gender and sexuality shape the experience of home.[40] Furthermore, adverse conditions such as poverty and violence also shape the experiences of home. Therefore, home is an aspiration or an ideal, a continuous search and yearning for safety, belonging, and acceptance.

Our chapter's idea of bringing adolescents home draws on this existential and psychological notion of home as that place, albeit ambivalent, for which people long and search, which they may already have found or are in the continuous process of creating. Making or creating a home is, therefore, creating that space or place in which children and adolescents thrive not only because they have material support but also because of the emotional quality of home life.[41] An essential aspect of this emotional quality is a healthy bond between parents or parent figures and adolescents. Such a bond cannot develop if parents deny, suppress, or oppress the sexual identity of the adolescent.[42]

11.5 Family

The family has many definitions from the various perspectives of sociology, psychology, anthropology, etc.[43] Family means different things to different people in diverse contexts.[44] For instance, in Africa, family includes extended relationships that in the Western context are not considered family. On the other hand, a lesbian couple and their child may be recognized as a family in Europe, but that would not be the case in most parts of Africa. Nevertheless, in whatever way people experience or practise family, it fundamentally is an indispensable 'organ of the society that gives birth to and socialises the new members of the society'.[45]

In this chapter, we do not attempt to define family. It suffices to adopt the description of family in Africa's human rights treaties. The African Charter on Human and Peoples' Rights (African Charter) and the African Charter on the Rights and Welfare of the Child (ACRWC) consider the family 'the natural unit and basis of society'. The ACRWC's preamble says that[46]

> *the child occupies a unique and privileged position in the African society and that for the full and harmonious development of his (sic) personality, the child should grow up in a family environment in an atmosphere of happiness, love and understanding.*[47]

This understanding of family reflects consensus about what the family should mean, at least for the child. The notion of the family links to the idea of home as a place to meet the child's and adolescent's emotional needs. An experience of happiness, love, and understanding presupposes the acceptance of the child's emerging sexual and gender identities.

Love, happiness, and understanding are qualities of home, where one has a sense of belonging, security, emotional connection, and acceptance. The African Charter recognizes that states must protect the family's physical and moral health and support it to carry out its functions as the custodian of morals and values.[48] The African Charter also recognizes that within the family context, the state should eliminate discrimination against women, children, persons with disabilities, and the elderly. The state should ensure that the family protects the rights of the children.[49] In other words, the family should provide a home for the child.

Home and family are, therefore, distinct but related concepts. Home is where people belong and feel accepted. In contrast, the family constitutes the relationships and practices that involve raising the next generation of human beings. The link between family and home materializes because raising the next generation of humans implies that the family should provide for a stable home.[50]

The notion of family has a political clout under international law because the law recognizes children's rights to a family. However, the concept of family necessarily conjures up the notion of home in the sense of both a physical place and a metaphorical or spiritual place, as described by McGoldrick. A concept of family that does not include home would be empty of the content that gives the family its worth. The obligation of states to ensure that the family contributes to the child's development means that the state should support families to provide physical and emotional security for the child. The family should be sensitive to the needs of children when they transition to adulthood during adolescence, including their sexual needs, for instance, sexual safety and security.[51]

The African Committee of Experts on the Rights and Welfare of the Child (ACERWC) explains that the family is

> *a place of personal (including informal, spontaneous and sometimes, frivolous) relations or interactions, as well as a place of safety, security, stability and affirmation to a person's sense of self-worth and human dignity. This is particularly important for children because the existence of a suitable family environment is fundamental to the realisation of their rights as contained in the African Children's Charter.*[52]

The family plays a critical role in providing for and satisfying both the psychological and emotional needs and the child's and adolescent's physical and material needs.[53] The family should, therefore, create a suitable environment to meet these needs for the child or adolescent, to create a home that is a place of belonging and acceptance of the multiple identities of the developing adolescent.[54]

Adolescents face challenges concerning SRH and sexual well-being when their families and communities do not accept them as sexual beings. Even more problematic is when parents repress developmentally normal adolescent sexual behaviours. States are complicit, for instance, when they criminalize consensual sexual conduct between adolescents as these negatively impact the sexual well-being of adolescents.[55]

The notion of 'bringing adolescents home' draws on the psychological concept that home is where people long to be, return, and create for the next generation. The search for a perfect home is a never-ending process, partly because the home, as an existential condition, is always an imperfect place. However, as that might be the case, human beings survive by creating homes for the next generation, and the next generation survives in homes created by the past generation. Creating 'home', therefore, means merging the past with the future. As McGoldrick has put it, 'The process of finding home involves each of us, as a fundamental part of the existential search, identifying and claiming disavowed parts of ourselves that we have to make peace with as part of the journey'.[56] Indeed, for adolescents, making peace with their emerging sexualities is vital to being at home or finding a home with the family.

Yet, people can face serious challenges at home. As McGoldrick has pointed out, albeit in the context of the US,

> *home in our society has not been a safe place for most people in our country – not for women, children, people of color, or gays and lesbians, given the pervasiveness of corporal punishment, child sexual abuse, the mistreatment and devaluing of women, and the appalling racism and homophobia of our society.*[57]

The reality described by McGoldrick is true not only for the US but also for Africa that some children grow up experiencing domestic violence, including sexual and gender-based violence.[58] Indeed, the COVID-19 pandemic demonstrated that home is not a cosy, safe, and secure place for everyone.[59] Society does violence to adolescents when instead of accepting their sexuality, it represses and oppresses them for exhibiting developmentally normal sexual behaviour.[60] Evidence from Kenya, for instance, reveals that the lockdown coincided with a new trend where victims of sexual violation were increasingly children of a young age, and the perpetrators were someone from home or a neighbour.[61] There is also evidence of queer youth facing challenges of staying at home with parents or guardians who do not tolerate their sexual and gender diversity.[62] The lockdown cut off queer youth from the emotional support of friends and significant others who accept their sexual identity.[63]

11.6 The school: a second home

For most children, school is the next place they spend most of their time, apart from their family. They meet friends and forge friendships, including potential romantic relationships. The family and the school may be the two most significant places for many African adolescents. If the family makes the first home, then the school is a second home; indeed, the teacher is like a second mom (or dad).[64]

Apart from providing education, the school serves an essential function as an extension of the family, as a second home. When the COVID-19 pandemic disrupted schooling, the fallback place was the family. School closures had the effect of exerting unprecedented pressure on families. When adolescents returned home, pregnancies and sexual violence increased, revealing that something was wrong at and within the home. The challenges adolescents faced at home during the lockdown are undoubtedly due to complex factors, including economic stress.[65] However, this chapter asserts that families have challenges recognizing adolescents as sexual beings and are unprepared to support them on matters relating to sex and sexuality. For instance, parents fail to communicate with their children about safe sex.[66]

Now, getting back to education, according to Article 29 of the UNCRC, education aims to develop the full potential of the child's identity and personality. The first general comment of the CRC explained the significance of Article 29 that education should consider the child's unique developmental needs and diverse evolving capacities.[67] These developmental needs necessarily include sexuality.

Article 11 of the ACRWC recognizes the right to education. The ACERWC agreed with the CRC that education should empower children to take up positive values and responsibilities. The ACERWC has said, 'Well educated children are better able to value respect for human rights, develop to their fullest potential, and appreciate responsibilities as a positive means of giving back'.[68] In other words, education prepares the child for citizenship roles, including respecting the rights of others.

However, education in school has continuities with education at home. The link is social values. A family is a place of learning about such values. The ACERWC has said that,

> *The family is therefore considered to be an ideal environment for teaching and learning positive values such as respect for adults, respect for the rights of others, and learning to handle responsibilities including actively taking part in the care of younger siblings.*[69]

The school is not the exclusive environment for educating the child. Education begins at home, in the family.[70] Children learn responsibilities to the community through a properly functioning family, that is, relations and practices. The ACERWC reiterates the CRC's position that education fosters respect for human rights and fundamental freedoms.[71] Children are expected to 'maintain good and healthy relations with their peers and play with other children in a spirit of respect, tolerance and equality with one another'.[72] Thus, the ACERWC conceives a link between the family and the educational institution. It recognizes that the school's positive impact on children depends on positive role-modelling and examples in the school environment taught by example in the family.[73]

Therefore, the family and school are a continuous education ecosystem that shapes the adolescent's life, career, and vocation.[74] Adolescents learn about relationships at home, family, and school, formally or informally. Ideally, the school, just like the family, must meet the emotional needs of the adolescent. The adolescent must also find nurturance in the second home. Sometimes, however, adolescents may find more acceptance among peers at school than in the family. The discrepancy may not seem consequential, at least not until something like the COVID-19 pandemic forces the adolescent to stay home with family. When schools closed during the COVID-19 pandemic, learners who found the school more accepting of their sexual identity than their family found life more challenging at home, for instance, queer youth.[75]

11.7 Sexual and reproductive health services

In a report that sparked some controversy, the UN Special Rapporteur on the right to education, Vernor Muñoz (2004–2010), sought to explain the right to sexual education from a gender and diversity perspective. In the report, the Rapporteur highlighted the interdependence of sexuality, health, and education.[76] The Rapporteur said that achieving sexual health and well-being requires that people receive comprehensive sexual education in school and outside school.[77] The Rapporteur believed that the state and the family play complementary roles in providing sexual education and shaping children's identities, both in and out of school.

Some governments have taken measures to assist adults in parenting adolescents. For instance, the US government published a booklet to support parents in helping their children through early adolescence.[78] In Kenya, the Department of Health also issued guidance on adolescence.[79] These publications fall into a different category from the usual public policy documents because policy aims to frame or address a particular problem or issue recognized in the political or public arena as requiring government attention.[80] In contrast, the two publications from the US and Kenya referenced above are guides on parenting adolescents. In any case, the point is that these two governments, Kenya and the US, recognize the family as the primary institution to nurture adolescents and that parents play an essential role.

Special Rapporteur Muñoz recognized the essential linkages between education, sexual health, and well-being, but also the roles of society, especially the family, as a fundamental unit of society. The three institutions, therefore, family, education, and health, should provide integrated support to adolescents.

11.8 Integrated support during pandemics like COVID-19

The three institutions, family, education, and health, presumably worked relatively well to various extents in pre-pandemic times, depending on the context. However, the measures to contain the COVID-19 pandemic disrupted educational and health institutions, and the family had to keep adolescents at home. Families could not handle the functions ordinarily shared with the education and health sectors, for instance, children's needs for friends and SRH services. The restrictions on movement and separation from friends negatively impacted the evolving identities of adolescents, including increased vulnerability to gender-based violence, early marriages, unintended pregnancies, and female genital mutilation.[81]

Meherali and others report that in Ethiopia, 'Even daughters in their early adolescence were forced to get married because of the limited presence of local authority officials and schoolteachers, who otherwise would cause hindrances in early marriages'.[82] The report attested that schools positively affect the prevention of early marriages. However, one could also read that the report suggests family dysfunction because when children left school and went back home, they married. The family somehow enabled or failed to prevent children from getting married. The problem had to do with the home where the children stayed. One crucial lesson from the pandemic is that families need support to handle adolescents during lockdown times. A critical aspect of this support is understanding adolescents and accepting their emerging sexualities and related behaviours as a normative aspect of their sexual development.

Indeed, why were some adolescents exposed to a high risk of intra-household and intimate partner violence at home?[83] The factors, arguably, are complex and intertwined, including the anxieties and stresses of adults to provide for and support their families in uncertain economic times. However, in that mix is the fact that parents failed to recognize the sexual needs of adolescents.

UNFPA observed that a significant challenge for young people is that the family or home may not accept them as sexual beings:

> *adolescents' sexual thoughts, feelings and needs do not go away in the context of a pandemic. Furthermore, the discomfort, reticence and biases about acknowledging adolescents as sexual beings may be even stronger in times of crisis.*[84]

The UNFPA points to a foundational issue: the 'discomfort, reticence and biases about acknowledging adolescents as sexual beings'. When families are not at home with the emerging sexuality and gender identities associated with adolescence, they may be inadequately prepared to support adolescents at any time, especially in times of adversity. For instance, the inability to talk openly with adolescents about sex and consent may disadvantage adolescents because they might not recognize a situation of sexual abuse. Adolescents should have the necessary knowledge and information to make choices about sex grounded in accepting adolescents as sexual and gendered beings by the family. Families, however, may not spontaneously understand adolescents as requiring such support. As mentioned earlier, the US and Kenya have supported parenting families with guidance on raising adolescents. Positive parenting on sexuality is critical to ensuring that adolescents are at home with their sexuality.[85] When adolescents are at home in the family because they feel accepted, it is easier for them to be at home with themselves even as they venture out into the broader environment, including the school. They are also likely to use sexual health services, such as contraceptives, without fearing their parents.

11.9 Challenges for adolescents: acceptance of sexual identities

Generally, there has been more emphasis on the school as the main ground for dealing with sexuality issues than the family. For instance, in the joint general comment on ending child marriage, the African Commission on Human and Peoples' Rights (ACHPR) and the ACERWC encourage states to provide comprehensive sexuality education and information in schools, including consent to sex, consent to marriage, and gender, sexuality, and social norms.[86] However, the treaty monitoring bodies have said little about accepting adolescent sexual identity in the family. Indeed, even in educational institutions, the effectiveness of sexuality education is based on, among other things, whether the adolescent student is at the same time accepted or positioned as sexual.

11.9.1 The learner of sexuality education as a sexual subject

Louisa Allen engages the position of the learner as sexual (or not) in several of her works. In 'Denying the sexual subject', as the title suggests, she points out that although schools might teach sexuality education, they may still promote a cultural understanding that denies the student as a sexual being or, in other words, fails to accept the student as a sexual being. This discrepancy has implications for the agency of the adolescent as it may encourage the adolescent to deny their being sexual and thus make it harder for them to exercise sexual autonomy.[87] In Malawi, for instance, there has been such a long-standing contradictory discourse when, on the one hand, the Ministry of Health promotes access to contraceptives, including condoms, for everyone. On the other, the Ministry of Education prohibits the distribution of condoms in schools or the vicinity.[88] One of the challenges with adolescents accessing contraceptives is that health providers refuse to provide condoms to unmarried adolescents. The underlying problem here is that adolescents are not permitted to be sexual, so even if they require condoms and contraceptives, adults make access difficult.[89]

It would appear, therefore, that a significant challenge is the fundamental attitude of adults towards adolescent sexual identity. What Allen says about education applies to the health system: 'The production of contradictory sexual identities not only can be disempowering for the student but ultimately may not serve what has been an underpinning philosophy of sexuality education's effectiveness – the production of sexually responsible citizens'.[90]

Although most countries have embraced the idea of comprehensive sex education, and there is evidence of a positive impact of its implementation, they are not delivering it impactfully to adolescents and young people.[91] Sexuality education still faces several challenges in Africa, including curriculum delivery, engaging sexuality issues too late when students have an earlier sexual debut, and a shallow curriculum content.[92]

Therefore, the pandemic's negative impact on the SRH of adolescents is also about the pre-pandemic attitudes of parents and adults towards adolescents as sexual beings. Families should not send children to school with the hope that the education system would be for the adolescent what the family has failed, that is, to be that place that accepts the sexual and gender identity of the adolescent. Achieving a better environment for adolescents requires a collective change of attitude towards adolescents. The COVID-19 pandemic has enabled stakeholders to think about such old challenges in new ways, such as transformative education of girls because of the observation that, currently, girls who come out of the education system believe that they are subordinate to boys.[93] We believe there is a need for no less than a cultural transformation.

11.9.2 Culture and adolescent sexuality

Culture is a complex phenomenon, and introducing sexuality makes it even more complicated. Cultural relativity complexifies any talk about sexuality because each culture will justify its approach to sexuality. However, evidence shows that a culture that promotes acceptance of the adolescent as a sexual being makes it easier for adolescents to pursue sexual well-being.

This part of the chapter draws mainly on the work of Schalet, who compared the acceptance of adolescent sexuality in two cultures: the United States of America (US) and the Netherlands. The two countries have comparable wealth and technological advancement but have widely varying demographics on teen pregnancy.[94] The US has a high rate of teen pregnancies, while the Netherlands has one of the lowest teenage pregnancy rates in the world. Schalet observed that adolescent sexuality is treated like a problem in American culture. It is denied and moralized. Consensual sex between adolescents is considered abnormal and discouraged under moral or penal law. In contrast, in Dutch culture, adolescent sexuality is accepted as normal. Dutch parents do not try to prohibit sex. Instead, they aim to enable adolescents to make positive decisions and take responsibility for their sex lives. Dutch culture emphasizes talking about sex openly and honestly.[95]

According to Schalet, resources and services do not explain the vast differences in teenage pregnancy rates between the two countries. Rather, a plausible explanation for the difference in the rates of teenage pregnancies is the cultural approaches to adolescent sexuality. In the US, adolescents are treated with scepticism that they cannot handle sexuality maturely unless under strict control. In contrast, in the Netherlands, adolescents are accepted as sexual. Parents' attitudes in the Netherlands are that adolescents will eventually find their way around sexual relationships if society guides them appropriately.[96]

What Schalet says about culture as an essential contributor to the welfare and sexual well-being of adolescents in the Netherlands compared to the US is true about Africa. Cultures that accept adolescents as sexual beings are better adapted to supporting adolescents to navigate sexuality. When adolescents are not accepted as sexual, parents treat them with scepticism or are overly anxious about their sexual behaviours. In that case, it is difficult for adolescents to be at home with their evolving sexuality. Also, it is less likely that adults would provide the necessary support to help the adolescent cultivate resilience to face an adult sexual life.

11.10 Cultural norms as a causative factor for disparities before, during, and after the pandemic

The COVID-19 pandemic's effects on African teenagers were related to services and resources as well as societal perceptions of adolescents as sexual beings. Much of the evidence generated around the impact of COVID-19 on adolescent SRH in Africa focuses on resource limitations and the failure of services. Resources and services were critical but are only part of the picture.

In their article, Ssebunya and others discuss how existing gender, cultural, and socio-economic factors fuel inequalities in accessing sexual and reproductive health and rights (SRHR) services among adolescents and young people in low- and middle-income countries.[97] One of their observations was the lack of data that tracked the impact of such factors before the pandemic. However, they point out that existing social and cultural practices negatively impacted health outcomes for adolescents during the pandemic. For instance, the lack of acceptance of pre-marital sex caused girls to be shy in accessing SRHR services and made healthcare workers reluctant to provide services to adolescents.[98] If these social and cultural factors are not addressed, they will not only affect post-pandemic recovery efforts, but it will also mean that in the wake of another pandemic, Africa will not have taken the necessary strides to strengthen resilience for adolescents. Therefore, Africa should address economic factors and create enabling social and cultural conditions for young people to benefit maximally from any economic interventions. This would take no less than transforming culture, including the attitudes towards adolescent sexuality.

11.11 Transforming culture

To achieve a fundamental reorientation of norms towards adolescent sexualities, Schalet proposes an *ABC* and *D* conceptual model.[99] The *A* stands for *autonomy*, *B* for *building* good romantic relationships, *C* for *connectedness* with parents and caregivers, and *D* for recognizing *diversities* and removing *disparities*.

Autonomy is about having control over and managing one's life. At the emergence of sexual identity, adolescents need to acquire the skills to manage their bodies, emotions, and relationships with others. Adolescents should then gradually gain sexual autonomy, navigate sexual desire and pleasure, understand their sexual wishes, recognize their boundaries, and learn to anticipate and prepare for sexual acts.[100] Recognizing the child's evolving capacities and providing age-appropriate education and information to facilitate skills development is also essential.

Skills building in romantic relationships is a critical aspect of adolescent development. Indeed, as Suleiman and others have said, 'One of the most important transitions occurring during puberty is the motivation and desire to engage in romantic love'.[101] It is a universal biological phenomenon that, at puberty, adolescents become primed to learn about love and sex.[102] Societies should acknowledge that children and adolescents want to know about love and sex and seek to build new relationships, even if they may not be in love yet or are not yet having sex.[103] When research on the impact of COVID-19 on adolescent SRH focuses primarily on resources and services, inevitably, the recommendations are limited to calling attention to more resources and services, and there is relatively little engagement with social and cultural factors.

No matter the challenging environments in which people find themselves, such as a pandemic or humanitarian crisis, the drive to learn about love and sex is an existential condition for adolescents. It will shape adolescents to seek and eventually find the sex they desire, with or without the support of adults.[104] However, if they have the full support and guidance of adults, they are likely to make positive choices about their love and sexual lives, including deciding whether to have sex or not.[105]

The C in the ABC and D model represents adolescents' connectedness with significant persons. The research findings by Suleiman and others corroborate Schalet's that the relationship with parents plays an influential role in adolescents' romantic and sex lives. They reference behavioural research that demonstrates that positive relationships between adolescents and parents are associated with a delayed sexual debut. Youth with positive and open communication with their parents have less sexual experience, increased condom use, fewer unintended pregnancies, and fewer sexual partners.[106] Such research should encourage parents to confidently offer constant and unwavering support to the adolescent on sexuality matters. The failure of parents to undertake this responsibility would not be cured by more effort and resources spent on education and health institutions to provide services to adolescents.

Lokot and Avyakan discuss the challenges adolescent girls face under imposed constraints. Apart from material challenges such as lack of resources, structural challenges like social norms about sexuality and their intersection with sex and age prevent vital information on SRH from reaching girls. The decreased mobility of girls because of their sex and age also results in low access to critical health services.[107] Power relationships and systematic inequalities, including gender norms, shape adolescents' experiences and emerging sexualities.[108] Accepting an adolescent's emerging sexual and gender identities entails addressing the power relations that shape early romantic relationships and the systemic inequalities entrenched in societal value systems, such as gender norms that negatively impact adolescents.[109] Bringing adolescents home would not materialise without addressing these social influences on the adolescent.

The idea that school closure meant more girls' exposure to sexual activities, resulting in sexual health problems, for instance, needs further interrogation.[110] The underlying assumption is that schools function to keep girls away from sexual relations. This may be true in some circumstances but not in others. For instance, colleges that bring girls and boys together for extended periods create greater opportunities for sexual conduct than at home. The issue should not be whether girls (or adolescents) are exposed to opportunities for sex. The question should be how adolescents handle the reality that love, and sex are always possible, whether at home, in the community, or at school. Therefore, the problem should not be conceived as being about sex opportunities for adolescents, and the solution the restricting of those opportunities. Rather, families should empower adolescents to practise safe sex if they choose to have sex, and help adolescents recognize and avoid sexual coercion, abuse, or violence. The closure of schools certainly impacted adolescents' sexual health and well-being, but the social and cultural context also made a crucial difference. 'Efforts to support adolescents and young adults must also attend to broader impacts on their sexual and reproductive lives, including their ability to form and maintain romantic relationships and experience their sexuality in positive ways'.[111]

Finally, Schalet's D in the ABC and D model stands for Diversity and Disparities. Adolescents are not a homogenous group. Their identities reflect the difference, among others, in gender, ability, and sexual orientation. Cultures should not be selective about which adolescents to support because justice requires that all adolescents be treated equally and fairly. A justice approach also addresses disparities because, for instance, adolescents with a disability may face unique challenges that put them at a disadvantage compared to adolescents without a disability.[112] States should ensure that all adolescents have a fair chance at getting the support needed to maintain optimum sexual health and well-being.

11.12 Bringing adolescents home

Adolescents are resilient to challenges in their sexual and reproductive lives if their sexual agency is supported. When parents fail to recognize and accept adolescents as sexual, they fail to provide adolescents with the support they need about sexuality. Parents must ensure that the family is, first and foremost, a home for the adolescent, where they are loved and accepted to develop a sense of belonging. This includes recognizing adolescents in their diversity as sexual and gendered and supporting them to meet their sexual and relationship needs. In some cultures, for instance, parents buy their children condoms.[113] Such a practice is an example of acceptance of the adolescent as sexual. In other cultures, this would be abhorrent. Yet, it is those cultures that accept adolescents as sexual that fare better at promoting the sexual health and well-being of their adolescents, as Schalet's study demonstrated.

In this chapter, 'bringing adolescents home' is a metaphor for acknowledging adolescent sexual and gender identities and supporting them to navigate sexual and intimate relationships. Adolescents should be most at home in the family as the fundamental unit of society.

11.13 Future pandemics and the way forward

Governments should facilitate creating the conditions in which every child and adolescent realizes SRHR to the extent of their evolving capacities. However, SRHR cannot be realized only by making economic and social resources and services available. The attitudes of parents and families towards child and adolescent sexuality, as explained in this chapter, are a critical factor. Failure to accept children and adolescents as sexual creates challenges for them, for instance, to report abuse or sexual violation because the child may not have the confidence to initiate such a discussion.[114]

Africa does not only need economic resources and interventions to achieve better SRH for adolescents, but it must also address cultural and gender norms about adolescent sexuality to ensure that adolescents enjoy equitable access to SRH services and care at any time, including during pandemic times. COVID-19 made the cracks visible and exacerbated adolescent SRH problems, which means that ongoing SRJ labour is needed in relation to adolescents. If adolescents are 'at home', they are less likely to feel adrift and suffer negative consequences in future pandemics. It is important that this labour of justice, of bringing adolescents home, is effected *before* crises hit.

Governments should, therefore, raise awareness among parents about accepting the transformation the child undergoes at puberty, leading to the emergence of sexuality and gender identities. This also entails decriminalizing consensual and non-exploitative sex between adolescents because such state-sanctioned punitive approaches reinforce stigma and negative attitudes towards normative adolescent sexualities. Governments should support the institutional environments of the family, school, and health facilities to enable adolescents to build the necessary skills to navigate sexual relationships. This would include, for instance, teaching comprehensive sexuality education in schools and training providers such as healthcare workers and educators to address stigma around adolescent sex and sexuality.

11.14 Conclusion

The COVID-19 pandemic caused severe life disruptions that impacted adolescents' SRHR. However, adolescents already faced challenges around access to SRH services, which was exacerbated during the pandemic. The quality of relationships in the family, especially in cases where adolescent sexuality is repressed or oppressed, contributed to the weakened resilience of adolescents to withstand the disruptions caused by the pandemic.

The family is a fundamental unit of society and the basis for ensuring the respect of children's SRHR. When families and communities accept adolescents as sexual beings, the foundations for respecting their sexual and reproductive rights are created. This acceptance is crucial to building adolescents' resilience to adversity. Only when society is at home with adolescents will adolescents better survive challenges impacting their SRH, such as the disruptions of social, educational, and health services caused by the COVID-19 pandemic.

Notes

1 L Gittings et al "Now my life is stuck!': Experiences of adolescents and young people during COVID-19 lockdown in South Africa' (2021) 16 *Global Public Health* 951–952; C Groenewald et al 'Adolescent sexual and reproductive health during the COVID-19 pandemic: A mini review' (2022) 4 *Frontiers in Reproductive Health*.

2 G Murewanhema 'Adolescent girls, a forgotten population in resource-limited settings in the COVID-19 pandemic: Implications for sexual and reproductive health outcomes' (2020) 37 *The Pan African Medical Journal*; S Meherali et al 'Impact of the COVID-19 pandemic on adolescents' sexual and reproductive health in low- and middle-income countries' (2021) 18 *International Journal of Environmental Research and Public Health*.

3 R Eghtessadi et al 'Safeguarding gains in the sexual and reproductive health and AIDS response amidst COVID-19: The role of African civil society' (2020) 100 *International Journal of Infectious Diseases*.

4 P International Living under lockdown: Girls and COVID-19 (2020).

5 FC Mukumbang et al 'Unspoken inequality: How COVID-19 has exacerbated existing vulnerabilities of asylum-seekers, refugees, and undocumented migrants in South Africa' (2020) 19 *International Journal for Equity in Health*; N Kantamneni

'The impact of the COVID-19 pandemic on marginalized populations in the United States: A research agenda' (2020) 119 *Journal of Vocational Behavior*.
6 C Groenewald et al (n 1 above) 5–6; Z Duby et al 'Navigating education in the context of COVID-19 lockdowns and school closures: Challenges and resilience among adolescent girls and young women in South Africa' (paper presented at the Frontiers in Education, 2022).
7 BO Ahinkorah et al 'COVID-19 pandemic worsening gender inequalities for women and girls in sub-Saharan Africa' (2021) 2 *Frontiers in Global Women's Health*.
8 As above, 3.
9 Evidence to Action Project Evaluation of youth-friendly health services in Malawi (2014) 162.
10 As above, 163.
11 As above, 167.
12 Institute for Reproductive Health, Georgetown University, Exploring social norms around reproductive health affecting unmarried adolescent girls and young women in Burundi (2021) 21.
13 Evidence to Action Project (n 9 above) 185.
14 Population Council et al 'Advancing girls' education in light of COVID-19 in East Africa: A synthesis report' (2021).
15 LS Ho et al 'Health system resilience during COVID-19 understanding SRH service adaptation in North Kivu' (2022) 19 *Reproductive Health*; Z Duby et al 'Adaptation and resilience: Lessons learned from implementing a combination health and education intervention for adolescent girls and young women in South Africa during the COVID-19 pandemic' (2022) 2 *Frontiers in Health Services*.
16 KS Hall et al 'Centring sexual and reproductive health and justice in the global COVID-19 response' (2020) 395 *Lancet*.
17 AM Starrs et al 'Accelerate progress-sexual and reproductive health and rights for all: Report of the Guttmacher–Lancet Commission' (2018) 391 *Lancet* 2646.
18 T Morison 'Reproductive justice: A radical framework for researching sexual and reproductive issues in psychology' (2021) 15 *Social and Personality Psychology Compass*.
19 L Ross & R Solinger *Reproductive justice: An introduction* (2017).
20 See T Morison et al *Sexual and reproductive justice: From the margins to the centre* (2022).
21 CI Macleod et al 'Articulating reproductive justice through reparative justice: Case studies of abortion in Great Britain and South Africa' (2017) 19 *Culture, Health & Sexuality* 610.
22 High Level Commission on the Nairobi Summit on ICPD25 Follow-up 'Sexual and reproductive justice as the vehicle to deliver the Nairobi Summit commitments' (2022).
23 TS Bakhru 'Thinking transnationally: Reproductive justice in a globalized era' in TS Bakhru (ed) *Reproductive justice and sexual rights: Transnational perspectives* (2019).
24 V Enejoh et al 'Impact of self esteem on risky sexual behaviors among Nigerian adolescents' (2016) 28 *AIDS Care*.
25 JD Fortenberry 'Sexual learning, sexual experience, and healthy adolescent sex' (2014) 2014 *New Directions for Child and Adolescent Development* 40.
26 Committee on the Rights of the Child (CRoC) 'General comment no. 20 (2016) on the implementation of the rights of the child during adolescence' 6 December 2016 CRC/C/GC/20 para 16.
27 As above, CRC/C/GC/20 para 19.

28 AB Suleiman et al 'Becoming a sexual being: The 'elephant in the room' of adolescent brain development' (2017) 25 *Developmental Cognitive Neuroscience* 210.
29 Evidence to Action Project (n 9 above) 51.
30 AD Smith et al 'Why do young people engage in dating relationships during early adolescence? An inter-generational qualitative analysis from Blantyre, Malawi' (2022) 24 *Culture, Health & Sexuality*.
31 RW Blum et al 'It begins at 10: How gender expectations shape early adolescence around the world' (2017) 61 *Journal of Adolescent Health*.
32 JH Pfeifer & ET Berkman 'The development of self and identity in adolescence: Neural evidence and implications for a value-based choice perspective on motivated behavior' (2018) 12 *Child Development Perspectives* 162.
33 In the court case judgement of *Teddy Bear Clinic for Abused Children and Another v. Minister of Justice and Constitutional Development and Another* 2014 (2) SA 168 (CC) at para 89, Justice Sisi Kampepe expressed the view that "Rather than deterring early sexual intimacy, the provisions (criminalising consensual adolescent sexual conduct) merely drive it underground, far from the guidance that might otherwise be provided by parents, guardians and other members of society".
34 MC Marchetti-Mercer 'New meanings of "home" in South Africa' (2006) 38 *Acta Academica* 192.
35 IN Magat 'Israeli and Japanese immigrants to Canada: Home, belonging, and the territorialization of identity' (1999) 27 *Ethos* 120.
36 R Rubenstein *Home matters: Longing and belonging, nostalgia and mourning in women's fiction* (2001) 1–2.
37 M Palmberger 'Relational ambivalence: Exploring the social and discursive dimensions of ambivalence–the case of Turkish aging labor migrants' (2019) 60 *International Journal of Comparative Sociology* 75.
38 As above.
39 M McGoldrick 'Homelessness and the spiritual meaning of home' in M McGoldrick & KV Hardy (eds) *Re-visioning family therapy: Addressing diversity in clinical practice* (2019) 97–98.
40 As above, 98.
41 GN Wambua et al 'The role of attachment relationship in adolescents' problem behavior development: A cross-sectional study of Kenyan adolescents in Nairobi city' (2018) 12 *Child and Adolescent Psychiatry and Mental Health*; S Demuth & SL Brown 'Family structure, family processes, and adolescent delinquency: The significance of parental absence versus parental gender' (2004) 41 *Journal of Research in Crime and Delinquency* 61.
42 MM Moretti & M Peled 'Adolescent–parent attachment: Bonds that support healthy development' (2004) 9 *Paediatrics and Child Health*.
43 S Maharramova 'Increased awareness about "a definition of family" ' *InterConf* (2022).
44 R Mafumbate 'The undiluted African community: Values, the family, orphanage and wellness in traditional Africa' (2019) 9 *Information and Knowledge Management*.
45 A Pathak 'Discussing the indispensability of family as a social institution' (2017) 7 *International Journal of Humanities and Social Sciences* 91–92.
46 The African Charter on Human and Peoples' Rights Article 18; the African Charter on the Rights and Welfare of the Child Article 18.
47 Organization of African Unity (OAU) *African charter on the rights and welfare of the child* 11 July 1990 CAB/LEG/24.9/49 (1990), preamble.
48 As above, Article 18 (1) and (2).

49 As above, Article 18
50 This resonates with the thinking of the ACRWC that family constitutes 'common sense of responsibility for one another's wellbeing, based on individual roles, functions and practices to maintain the family cohesion within a larger societal collective'. ACERWC Gen Com on Article 31 para 29.
51 KR Mitchell et al 'What is sexual wellbeing and why does it matter for public health?' (2021) 6 *The Lancet Public Health*.
52 African Committee of Experts on the Rights and Welfare of the Child *General comment on article 31 of the African charter on the rights and welfare of the child on the responsibilities of the child* (2017) para 30.
53 E Okon 'Towards defining the 'right to a family' for the African child' (2012) 12 *African Human Rights Law Journal* 384.
54 M McGoldrick 'Preface' in M McGoldrick & KV Hardy (eds) *Re-visioning family therapy: Addressing diversity in clinical practice* (2019) xiii.
55 R Tallarico et al 'Age of consent: A case for harmonizing laws and policies to advance, promote and protect adolescents' sexual and reproductive health rights' (2021) 25 *African Journal of Reproductive Health*.
56 McGoldrick (n 54 above) xiii.
57 As above, 98.
58 NJ Dlamini 'Gender-based violence, twin pandemic to COVID-19' (2021) 47 *Critical Sociology*.
59 H Cowie & C-A Myers 'The impact of the COVID-19 pandemic on the mental health and well-being of children and young people' (2021) 35 *Children & Society* 68; Amnesty International 'Southern Africa: Homes become dangerous place for women and girls during COVID-19 lockdown' available at www.amnesty.org/en/latest/press-release/2021/02/southern-africa-homes-become-dangerous-place-for-women-and-girls-during-covid19-lockdown/.
60 AB Suleiman et al (n 28 above).
61 LM Stevens et al 'Children's vulnerability to sexual violence during COVID-19 in Kenya: Recommendations for the future' (2021) 2 *Frontiers in Global Women's Health*.
62 Centre for Human Rights University of Pretoria 'Understanding the disproportionate impact of COVID-19 on LGBTIQ+ persons in Africa' (2020).
63 N Nyagah 'COVID-19 pandemic: A perfect storm for LGBTI youth' Web blog article *Labour Research Intensive* 27 May 2020 available at www.lrs.org.za/2020/05/27/covid-19-pandemic-a-perfect-storm-for-lgbti-youth/.
64 Y Morales-Alexander '"School is the child's second home": Family engagement from a Latino sociocultural perspective' (2021) 42 *Journal of Early Childhood Teacher Education* 465.
65 P Mahlangu et al 'Impact of COVID-19 lockdown and link to women and children's experiences of violence in the home in South Africa' (2022) 22 *BMC Public Health*; Population Council et al (n 14 above).
66 BW Maina et al 'Parent–child sexual and reproductive health communication among very young adolescents in Korogocho informal settlement in Nairobi, Kenya' (2020) 17 *Reproductive Health*.
67 UN Committee on the Rights of the Child (CRC) 'General comment no. 1 (2001), article 29 (1), the aims of education' 17 April 2001 CRC/GC/2001/1 para 1.
68 African Committee (n 52 above).
69 As above, para 28.
70 Organization of African Unity (OAU) (n 47 above) art.18.
71 African Committee (n 52 above) para 35.
72 As above.

73 African Committee (n 52 above) para 36.
74 A Barton et al 'Understanding the connection between family-school engagement and education system transformation' (2021).
75 N Nyagah (n 63 above).
76 United Nations General Assembly 'Report of the United Nations special rapporteur on the right to education' 23 July 2010 A/65/162.
77 As above, paras 11–12.
78 United States Department of Education Office of Communications & Outreach Helping your child through early adolescence: For parents of children from 10 through 14 (2005).
79 Ministry of Health (Kenya) 'Understanding adolescence: A guide for adolescents' (2021).
80 A Hassel 'Public policy' in JD Wright (ed) *International encyclopedia of the social & behavioral sciences* (Second Edition) (2015).
81 S Meherali et al (n 2 above).
82 As above.
83 P Banati et al 'Intersecting vulnerabilities: The impacts of COVID-19 on the psycho-emotional lives of young people in low- and middle-income countries' (2020) 32 *European Journal of Development Research* 1627.
84 UNFPA 'Not on pause: Responding to the sexual and reproductive health needs of adolescents in the context of the COVID-19 crisis' *Technical Brief* (2020).
85 L Widman et al 'Parent–adolescent sexual communication and adolescent safer sex behavior: A meta-analysis' (2016) 170 *JAMA Pediatrics*.
86 Joint General Comment of the African Commission on Human and Peoples' *Rights and the African committee of experts on the rights and welfare of the child on ending child marriage* (2017) para 36.
87 L Allen 'Denying the sexual subject: Schools' regulation of student sexuality' (2007) 33 *British Educational Research Journal* 222.
88 K Nash et al ' "Our girls need to see a path to the future"–perspectives on sexual and reproductive health information among adolescent girls, guardians, and initiation counselors in Mulanje district, Malawi' (2019) 16 *Reproductive Health*.
89 V Chandra-Mouli et al 'Contraception for adolescents in low and middle income countries: Needs, barriers, and access' (2014) 11 *Reproductive Health*.
90 Allen (n 87 above) 222.
91 P Machawira et al 'Progress and challenges with comprehensive sexuality education: What does this mean for HIV prevention in the ESA region?' in *Preventing HIV among young people in Southern and Eastern Africa* (2020).
92 AJ Mturi & AL Bechuke 'Challenges of including sex education in the life orientation programme offered by schools: The case of Mahikeng, North West province, South Africa' (2019) 23 *African Journal of Reproductive Health*; BE Ocran 'Teacher approaches, attitudes, and challenges to sexuality education: A case study of three junior high schools in Ghana' (2021) 25 *African Journal of Reproductive Health*.
93 Population Council et al (n 14 above).
94 AT Schalet *Not under my roof* (2011) 205.
95 AT Schalet 'Must we fear adolescent sexuality?' (2004) 6 *Medscape General Medicine*.
96 Schalet (n 94 above) 205.
97 RN Ssebunya et al 'Disparities in accessing sexual and reproductive health services and rights among adolescents and young people during COVID-19 pandemic: Culture, economic, and gender perspectives' (2022) 9 *Current Tropical Medicine Reports*.
98 As above, 237.

99 AT Schalet 'Beyond abstinence and risk: A new paradigm for adolescent sexual health' (2011) 21 *Womens Health Issues*.
100 As above, S6.
101 AB Suleiman et al (n 28 above).
102 As above, 218.
103 C Odimegwu et al 'Regional differences in positive sexual behaviour among youth in sub-Saharan Africa' (2019) 51 *Journal of Biosocial Science*.
104 D Bhana 'Love, sex and gender: Missing in African child and youth studies' (2017) 42 *Africa Development*.
105 H de Graaf et al 'Parental support and knowledge and adolescents' sexual health: Testing two mediational models in a national Dutch sample' (2010) 39 *Journal of Youth and Adolescence*.
106 AB Suleiman et al (n 28 above) 214.
107 M Lokot & Y Avakyan 'Intersectionality as a lens to the COVID-19 pandemic: Implications for sexual and reproductive health in development and humanitarian contexts' (2020) 28 *Sexual and Reproductive Health Matters* 41.
108 As above, 42.
109 C Moreau et al 'Measuring gender norms about relationships in early adolescence: Results from the global early adolescent study' (2019) 7 *SSM Population Health*; A Kågesten et al 'Understanding factors that shape gender attitudes in early adolescence globally: A mixed-methods systematic review' (2016) 11 *PLoS One*.
110 G Murewanhema (n 2 above).
111 LD Lindberg et al 'The sexual and reproductive health of adolescents and young adults during the COVID-19 pandemic' (2020) 52 *Perspectives on Sexual and Reproductive Health* 78.
112 CG Ngwena 'Reproductive autonomy of women and girls under the convention on the rights of persons with disabilities' (2018) 140 *International Journal of Gynecology & Obstetrics*.
113 D Borison 'Parents and sex education: Teaching about condoms' available at https://yourteenmag.com/health/teen-sexuality/parents-teaching-sexual-responsibility.
114 S Angelides 'Feminism, child sexual abuse, and the erasure of child sexuality' (2004) 10 *GlQ: A Journal of Lesbian and Gay Studies*.

12

IMPACT OF COVID-19 ON HEALTHCARE PROVIDERS IN AFRICA

Adetoun T. Adebanjo

12.1 Introduction

The COVID-19 pandemic has had a huge negative effect on global health care. Naturally, the focus was on those infected by the virus and the impact on communities and economies. Even though healthcare workers were on the frontline of the outbreak, their welfare was put on the backburner. However, as the real heroes of the COVID-19 pandemic, it is important to shine the light on the impact of COVID-19 on healthcare workers. Their mental health and well-being must be made top priority. Based on previous pandemics like the H1N1 influenza (bird flu) and SARS, issues that healthcare workers typically face in such situations have been identified to include stress, anxiety, depression, and post-traumatic stress disorder (PTSD).[1] Similarly, with respect to the COVID-19 pandemic, issues that healthcare workers face have been identified as including anxiety, hyperarousal, hypervigilance, sleep disturbance, depression and grief, and survival guilt,[2] as well as uncertainty, difficulties achieving a balance in their roles, and stigmatization.[3] All healthcare workers have been categorized as needing support irrespective of their role or level of exposure.[4] The many challenges associated with the COVID-19 pandemic that medical workers face have been identified as heightening their anxiety levels and fears for their personal safety to a level reminiscent of war conditions.[5] These conditions can undermine their decision-making ability and affect the quality of their interaction with patients.[6]

WHO has been vocal on how the pandemic has impacted frontline workers globally. WHO estimates that between January 2020 and May 2021, as many as between 80,000 and 180,000 healthcare workers could have died from COVID-19, with a median of 115,500 deaths.[7] As of July 2020,

DOI: 10.4324/9781032671437-15

more than 10,000 healthcare workers had been infected with COVID-19 in Africa.[8] These figures underscore the need for better protection. The words of WHO's regional director for Africa shed light on this issue:[9]

> The growth we are seeing in covid-19 cases in Africa is placing an ever-greater strain on health services across the nation. This has very real consequences for the individuals who work in them, and there is no more sobering example of this than the rising number of health worker infections.

The director stated that 'one infection among health workers is one too many' as medical staff work to save lives endangered by the virus.[10] Priority must therefore be given to the health and well-being of these workers who risk their lives under harsh conditions to manage the pandemic and its effects, more so in Africa where many of the healthcare systems are stretched beyond capacity and groaning under the pressure.

This chapter will identify the many challenges faced in the African health sector with the onslaught of COVID-19 and the impact of the pandemic on healthcare workers, with a focus on two African countries, namely Nigeria and South Africa. As aptly captured by Quadri et al, understanding the issues affecting the healthcare community in Africa will enable identification of potential targets for the purpose of preventing and mitigating burnout.[11] The chapter will also include a brief discussion on the impact felt by frontline workers in other countries. It will then conclude by making recommendations on how African countries can better improve their healthcare systems and responses to national health emergencies, and better support their healthcare workers through COVID-19 and future health emergencies.

At the start of the COVID-19 pandemic, 69 healthcare workers (including doctors, nurses, and residents) were surveyed on the impact of the pandemic on them.[12] Three key concerns were explored, namely what healthcare workers were most concerned about, the messaging and behaviours needed from leaders, and other useful sources of support.[13] Recurring sources of anxiety identified included lack of access to PPE, being exposed to COVID-19 at work and then taking it home to family members, lack of rapid access to testing should they develop symptoms, and uncertainty about whether the workplace will support them and their families should they become infected.[14] These sources of anxiety were then consolidated into five requests from these healthcare workers, namely hear me, protect me, prepare me, support me, and care for me.[15] It is necessary to have early psychosocial support from employers addressing these requests and focusing on creating a psychologically safe environment, consistent communication, and reliable team support.[16]

The vantage position that healthcare workers occupy during a public health emergency like the COVID-19 pandemic has earned them the designation of 'witnesses and victims'.[17] They are first-hand witnesses of the devastation caused by COVID-19 and are usually victims themselves, either through losses encountered at work or in their own personal lives. Their physical, mental, and general health and well-being must therefore receive priority.

12.2 Legal framework for protecting healthcare workers during public emergencies

Conflicts often arise on the rights and obligations of healthcare workers in their capacity as essential workers during public health emergencies, and it can be tricky to balance their rights and welfare against the greater good. For instance, due to extreme pressure on the healthcare system, the priority will be to stretch available resources to ensure provision of the best available healthcare services under the circumstances. In this situation, healthcare workers, while navigating uncharted waters, also have to contend with the possibility of incurring liability while doing their jobs. As Oliva et al bluntly put it, as the pandemic ends (or wanes), there is a high possibility that the grief for lives lost will morph into anger, or greed, resulting in criminal and civil proceedings against healthcare providers.[18] It is therefore imperative that countries provide some form of protection for their health workforce.

For instance, the US provided this under emergency laws, namely the Public Readiness and Emergency Preparedness Act (Prep Act) Declaration and the Coronavirus Aid, Relief, and Economic Security Act (the CARES Act). These were in addition to state laws (known as Good Samaritan Laws) and executive orders which shield 'good Samaritans' or 'bystanders', in this case, health workers, from liability when they provide care in emergency situations.[19] The basis of these laws is that bystanders, for fear of litigation or getting into trouble, do not refuse to come to the aid of those needing help.[20] The protection under these Good Samaritan Laws were then extended to cover care provided during the pandemic. Limitations to this would include gross negligence and criminal conduct. In spite of these protections, it has been suggested that some adventurous patients and their attorneys may look for loopholes and institute suits challenging these health worker protections.[21] Such suits would however be deemed unlikely to succeed.

The Prep Act Declaration provides immunity from liability for healthcare professionals and other qualified persons who administer COVID-19 countermeasures. They are protected from liability regarding claims for loss arising from the use of a COVID-19 'countermeasure', for example an approved COVID-19 vaccine that is, except in the case of wilful misconduct. These exceptions act as a necessary check on the powers of healthcare workers while also safeguarding the interests of patients.

Furthermore, healthcare workers themselves are unfortunately an at-risk group in the context of COVID-19.[22] Antecedents of public health emergencies such as SARS and Ebola support this assertion. For instance, in Vietnam, all but one of the people who died from SARS were doctors and nurses,[23] while in Nigeria, healthcare workers in the facility that treated patient zero during the Ebola crisis in 2014 paid the ultimate price.[24] It is therefore of paramount importance that their health and well-being are given the attention it deserves.

Public health emergencies including pandemics present conflicting obligations on the government. On the one hand, it is the obligation of the government to protect public health while relying on healthcare workers, and on the other hand, it is its obligation to also protect and respect the rights of the healthcare workers involved. Regrettably, the Forced Labour Convention of 1930 – which prohibits the use of forced labour – is silent on work during public emergency, thereby potentially leaving room for such situations. Many countries used their sweeping powers under their emergency declarations to suspend rights such as the rights of essential workers to go on strike. This may be because strikes are seen as creating conflicts between job duty, obligations to patients, labour rights, public health, and public interest.[25]

The obligation to protect healthcare workers derives from Occupational Health and Safety laws,[26] as well as the duty of care owed to healthcare workers by their employer.[27] These laws may have different names and fine prints in different countries. However, the effect would be the same, that is that healthcare settings implement control measures to eliminate or minimize risks to workers.[28] Unfortunately, the standards to which employers in healthcare settings would be held is unclear, given that pandemic response, available resources, and information on transmission and treatment continue to evolve.[29] Notwithstanding, certain measures must be taken to protect healthcare workers, including the provision of good personal protective equipment (PPE) like N95 masks over regular surgical masks, offering the option of telehealth consultations where possible, moving vulnerable healthcare workers to non-patient-facing roles, and offering opportunity to work from home where feasible.[30]

Healthcare workers have faced ethical and moral dilemmas in the provision of care during previous public health emergencies like SARS, Ebola, and HIV/AIDS, where the consensus had been that healthcare workers had the duty to treat patients, given the availability of adequate safety measures resulting in low risks of infection.[31] Discussions at the height of the HIV/AIDS crisis reaffirmed that what distinguished healthcare workers from others was their devotion to caring for the sick. To this end, it has been said:[32]

This moral ideal defines the core element of being a medical professional. The obligation is not chosen. It is inseparable from the choice to become a doctor. To reject this ethical ideal is to reject the profession.

However, it must be stressed that affirming the healthcare worker's ethical duty to care for the sick imposes a correlative duty on administrators and others to quickly develop and deploy procedures to maximize the safety of frontline physicians and nurses.[33] It is submitted that a moral obligation to protect healthcare workers and prioritize their welfare must be taken to exist by all and sundry as a healthy healthcare worker is a productive one.

It is also helpful to view healthcare workers as first and foremost members of the society who must also be protected like every other individual. They do not deserve less attention and care just because they are frontline workers.

During the COVID-19 pandemic, healthcare workers have been faced with preventable risks to their safety, such as exposure to patients without PPE, PPE shortage, and the use of substandard ones. Healthcare workers were infamously gagged and threatened to prevent them speaking out on these system failures.[34] Doctors in some countries instituted legal proceedings against the authorities for breach of duty in the procurement of PPE. A group of doctors in Spain got judgement against their regional government for compensation ranging from 5,000 to 49,000 euros to 153 doctors working in the province of Alicante.[35] Some of their complaints included being given one face mask per week, having to reuse gowns while hospitals kept protective gears locked up, and having to improvise, making their own PPE.[36] The situation lasted for 3 months, by which time thousands of healthcare workers had been infected.[37] Needless to say, this is putting valuable lives at risk. Given the nature of their job, made even more dangerous by the pandemic, priority ought to be given to the protection and well-being of healthcare workers. Highlighting the lack of care for their welfare, a US doctor said:[38]

> After examining a hypoxic woman . . . who likely has COVID, I had to clean my single-use face shield that I've worn the past three days with disinfectant used to clean hospital beds since we ran out of sanitizing wipes **#GetMePPE**

The above scenarios are harmful not only to the physical health of healthcare workers but also to their mental health, and many felt uncertain about their fate.[39]

Protecting the health and well-being of healthcare workers should be seen as a priority. After all, in the words of the WHO director-general, 'no country, hospital or clinic can keep its patients safe unless it keeps its health workers safe'.[40] Prioritizing the welfare of healthcare workers is key to ensuring a functioning healthcare system and society.[41]

12.3 Healthcare providers in Africa pre-COVID

Africa continues to play catch-up with other continents in every sphere including politics, health, economic growth, infrastructural development, and social services. The health sector receives little to no attention in many African countries. Run-down facilities that are inadequately staffed, outdated equipment, non-availability of diagnostic tools, insufficient supply of medication, shortage of healthcare workers, and underpaid and overworked staff are typical problems with healthcare delivery in these countries.[42] Thus, being a healthcare provider in Africa already came with a lot of unique challenges. The COVID-19 crisis has only added to these challenges.

Africa has not done enough to train, secure, and protect its most valuable assets in the health sector – its health workforce, and the fallout from this continues. As aptly stated, increasing hospital supplies and bed spaces will be of no consequence without the availability of healthcare workers.[43] The ability of each healthcare worker to care for a high volume of patients must be maximized.[44]

The continent also has a track record of healthcare worker shortage. Several factors account for this. Firstly, there are not enough health workers being trained within the system. Many African countries have only one medical school (e.g. Namibia and Lesotho) Unfortunately, as has been emphasized at a high-level forum meeting on the Millennium Development Goal (MDG) on Health held in the Nigerian capital of Abuja in December 2005, addressing the shortage of human resources was crucial to strengthening health systems and achieving the MDG on health.[45] A 2004 report put the number of healthcare workers in Africa at 750,000 for the total population of 682 million people, meaning the ratio was 0.8 healthcare worker per 1,000 people.[46] Even though there has been an improvement, with the ratio growing up to 2.3 healthcare workers per 1000 people,[47] this still falls short. For a better perspective, the Americas have a ratio of 24.8 healthcare workers per 1000 people.[48] This shows that Africa needs to improve on its healthcare provider-to-patient ratio.

Poor remuneration of healthcare workers has also been a long-standing problem on the continent, resulting in healthcare workers seeking greener pastures in systems with better remuneration and welfare packages. This has been the singular most common reason for the brain drain in Africa's health sector. The meagre sums that they are paid as allowances reflect the low premium placed on Africa's medical personnel. A good example is the issue of hazard allowance, which has been found in many cases to be inadequate; for example until the explosion of the COVID-19 pandemic in Nigeria, the hazard allowance for medical doctors in Nigeria was N2,000 (US$4.70) per month. Following the outcry, it was reviewed to N5,000 (US$11.74) per month. This was further reviewed upwards in December 2021 to between N34,000 and N40,000 (US$79.83–US$93.92) for medical doctors[49] and was met with protests and calls for further review.[50] Meanwhile, Nigerian senators were paid a whopping N1.2 million (US$2,817.57) as 'hardship allowance'[51] and N1.24 million (US$2911.49) for the 'purchase of newspapers' monthly.[52] This disparity shows the little premium placed on healthcare workers and health care generally in Nigeria.

Migration of African health workers to more prosperous economies in search of the proverbial 'greener pasture' and further training is also a major contributor to the continent's depleted health workforce. Every year, thousands of health workers leave the continent to pursue careers elsewhere. The development of bilateral agreements to check this practice does not appear to have put a dent in this phenomenon. It has been alleged that there are more Malawian doctors practising in Manchester, England, than in the whole of Malawi.[53] Unfortunately, African governments have largely been unable to address this problem. Some, like the Nigerian government, have chosen to ignore the glaring problems in the sector, resorting instead to bullying tactics, with Nigeria's minister of labour and employment infamously stating that Nigeria had more than enough doctors and that it could afford to let go of whomever was inclined to leave.[54] These statements attracted huge backlash as it was deemed reckless and untrue.[55] National representatives of Nigerian healthcare workers blamed the mass exodus on poor working conditions and harsh economic realities.[56] In place of these brash tactics, African governments should formulate plans to address brain drain by revamping their healthcare systems and providing adequate training and support for healthcare workers.

12.4 Impact of COVID-19 on the fundamental rights of healthcare providers in Africa

The negative impact of the pandemic on frontline workers globally has been well-documented. It is agreed that interventions are urgently needed to forestall negative effects like stress, burnout, and secondary traumatization on healthcare workers.[57] Maintaining the health and mental well-being of healthcare workers is crucial to sustaining safe and quality care of the general population during the pandemic.[58] Unfortunately, while there have been discussions on the impact of COVID-19 on the mental health and well-being of healthcare workers on an international scale, little, if any, attention is being paid to this issue in Africa.

The scenario in Africa was made worse by widespread misinformation and untruths relating to the genesis of the virus, modes of transmission, treatments, and cure. Drugs such as hydroxychloroquine, chloroquine (commonly used to treat malaria in Africa), ivermectin, and azithromycin (an antibiotic) and vitamins had been touted as cures for COVID-19. A group of healthcare workers had notoriously gone on air to proclaim hydroxychloroquine as the 'cure' for COVID-19, causing further confusion.[59] There were reports of these drugs flying off the shelves thereafter,[60] and some of the healthcare workers in the above survey, particularly from Tanzania, Egypt, and Ethiopia, admitted treating COVID-19 patients with these drugs.[61] Conspiracy theories were also common, creating a tense and distrustful environment, ultimately affecting healthcare workers.

The negative impacts of the pandemic transcended the realm of health and well-being of health workers. It extended to other spheres, affecting their income, transportation and access to the workplace, family, and social lives, all of which traverse various fundamental rights. Apart from rights like freedom of movement, freedom of assembly, and freedom of association which were commonly taken away in several jurisdictions at different times during the pandemic, other fundamental rights that healthcare workers in Africa have been deprived of include the following.

12.4.1 Right to health

The right to health is guaranteed in international and regional human rights instruments such as under Articles 12 and 16 of the International Covenant on Economic, Social, and Cultural Rights (ICESCR) and the Banjul Charter respectively. Unfortunately, this right has been one of the most threatened for healthcare workers in the face of the COVID-19 pandemic. By the very nature of their work, they are among the demographics considered most exposed to COVID-19. Unfortunately, the risk of exposure also extends to their immediate family members. A staggering 89% of those surveyed by Quadri et al expressed worry about exposing their immediate families to COVID-19.[62]

The effect of the pandemic on healthcare workers can be seen as two-fold: As carers for the sick and as patients themselves. This is because the nature of their jobs exposes them to the risk of infection. Working in healthcare settings generally increases their risk of exposure. For those healthcare workers such as ophthalmologists and dentists who have to work in very close proximity with patients, the risk becomes higher.[63] Also, as noted by Chersich et al, many healthcare workers in Africa would be considered high-risk individuals for COVID-19 given the high rates of non-communicable diseases among them.[64]

As noted by WHO, at a point, 16% of COVID-19 infections in Sierra Leone were among healthcare workers, while they accounted for 6.1% of infections in Cote d'Ivoire.[65] Unfortunately, these estimates were for a point in time early in the pandemic, and the infection rate for health workers was expected to increase. Thus, healthcare workers found themselves weighed down not only by the demands of working to prevent infections and treating the infected but also by a higher risk of exposure than most.

COVID-19 has had a huge impact on the mental health of millions of people. The number of people needing access to mental health services increased significantly during the pandemic. However, substantially less attention has been focused on preserving the psychological well-being of healthcare workers.[66] Several healthcare workers found themselves playing the roles of psychiatrists to patients needing reassurance, or a listening ear, and many struggled to find a balance in the midst of the chaos. For many, especially those in high-risk wards or settings, the very nature of their work put them at serious risk of developing PTSD and post-traumatic stress syndrome (PTSS).[67] Factors that come into play include their level of exposure, age, gender, marital status, and previous mental health issues.[68] Factors that could help prevent or alleviate the effects of PTSD include family and social support, the support of colleagues and supervisors, and training.[69]

In their study, Quadri et al found that there was an increase in the number of healthcare workers who had experienced daily depressive symptoms.[70] Shanafelt et al have opined that it is necessary to understand the specific sources of the anxiety and fear felt by healthcare workers before an effective approach to support them can be developed, as addressing these concerns should take precedence over the teaching of 'generic approaches' to stress reduction or resilience.[71]

12.4.2 Right to dignity

Article 1 of the Universal Declaration guarantees the right to dignity. Since the start of the pandemic, there has been a rise in health worker abuse in the hands of patients and their families. This abuse is fuelled by factors including fear and ignorance surrounding the disease and mistrust of the healthcare system. In Nigeria for example, the conspiracy theories included that the pandemic was a hoax; that covid-19 was linked to 5G; and entering into the realm of the even more bizarre, that COVID-19 vaccines were designed to alter human DNA as a prelude to global domination.[72]

12.4.3 Right to just and favourable conditions of work

Article 7 of the ICESCR guarantees the right to favourable conditions of work which not only protects remuneration but also advocates safe and healthy working conditions, as well as reasonable limitations of working hours. The conditions under which healthcare workers in Africa have had to work since the COVID-19 pandemic began have been anything but safe and healthy. The average healthcare worker is overworked, with many experiencing burnout, as it has already been pointed out. Challenges to safe and healthy work environments in Africa's health sector include lack of access or limited access to basic medical resources such as PPE, masks, and gloves; overpopulation, high-density living conditions, which affect social distancing; and lack of access to basic sanitary items such as soap, water, hand sanitizers, and wipes.[73] In April 2020, two doctors – a husband and wife who had been exposed to COVID-19 on the job – launched legal proceedings against the UK government for its failure to adequately provide PPE, as well as for the lack of adequate guidance on proper use.[74] The Doctors' Association UK (DAUK), the Good Law Project, and the Hourglass charity initiated judicial review proceedings following the UK government's refusal to open an inquiry into the failure to provide PPE for healthcare workers, which is believed to have contributed to the illnesses and deaths of many.[75]

A major review by the British Medical Association (BMA) found that the UK government failed in its duty of care to protect healthcare workers during the COVID-19 pandemic.[76]

12.4.4 Right to social services

The rights of healthcare workers to access social services has also been affected by COVID-19 restrictions. Article 25 of the Universal Declaration protects this right. Availability of social services was scaled down significantly following the imposition of lockdowns, curfews, and work-from-home orders. Unfortunately, even though many countries had imposed movement restriction measures, health workers as essential workers were exempted from these orders. Hence, they had to navigate their way to work in uncertain terrains. There were reports of several healthcare workers being harassed and attacked by law enforcement officers on their way to work.[77]

Also, commuting to work became more difficult for those relying on public transport, cab services, and carpooling. The above survey noted a reduction in the number of health workers going to work by bus and an increase in those who had resorted to walking. Reasons for this could vary; however, the fact that walking is at no cost cannot be overlooked.

12.4.5 Right to work/survival

The right to work is guaranteed under Article 23 of the Universal Declaration, Article 7 of the ICESCR, and Article 15 of the Banjul Charter. For instance, a study conducted in April and May of 2020 on the impact of COVID-19 on health workers[78] in 13 African countries reported that as many as 49% of those surveyed had experienced a reduction in income.[79] This would naturally put further strain on their finances and family life, especially for those in settings where healthcare worker remuneration was already poor.

12.4.6 Right to health of health providers to health-related goods and services

Healthcare providers have the right to health-related goods and services. However, long before COVID-19, non-availability of basic medical supplies had been an ongoing issue in Africa. Shortage of ventilators and intensive care capabilities has always been a huge limitation to saving critically ill patients in Africa.[80]

Shortages of PPE, oxygen cylinders, and ventilators became a general cause for concern worldwide during the COVID-19 pandemic, with a disproportionate shortage found in Africa.[81] As aptly captured, the 'global jostling' for supplies meant that supplies to Africa was limited.[82] To ease these shortages, countries and organizations with access to supplies of PPE sent supplies to those needing them.[83] It is noteworthy that even where PPE was available, healthcare workers often had to contend with the weight of full protective gear with no option of going without if they were to continue treating patients.[84] Unfortunately, as it has been noted, other problems that arose were epileptic power supply which threatened the use of certain equipment, for example ventilators, and the lack of adequately trained personnel to use them.[85] To circumvent the problem of ventilator shortage in Africa, Madzimbamuto has proposed that African healthcare systems focus instead on using other more available and less costly equipment and manoeuvres to obtain the much-needed oxygen supply.[86]

As COVID-19 became more widespread, most countries also experienced immense pressure on space. As beds in isolation wards filled up, it became a norm to build emergency/makeshift structures for isolating and treating COVID-19 patients. In places like Nigeria, it was challenging to get workers or volunteers to work in COVID isolation wards and centres. To get workers on board, the government had to offer small incentives. Unfortunately, as is common in Nigeria, the government did not fulfil its promises. In most cases, payments stopped after the first month or two. It is unclear how these issues were resolved, if they were ever resolved.

The toll of COVID-19 on healthcare workers in select countries in Africa

As aptly put, the COVID-19 pandemic generated a 'parallel pandemic' of deteriorating mental health for existing mental health patients and those needing or seeking mental health support for the very first time.[87] COVID-19 would seem to have opened the door wide. Although the availability of vaccines eased some of the fears associated with the pandemic, by giving 'physical immunity', they did not cover 'psychological immunity' for the healthcare workers on the frontline.[88] Access to COVID-19 vaccines has been deemed to create a 'pandemic paradox' where, on the one hand, the world experiences hope brought on by the availability of vaccines and, on the other hand, despair brought on by the increased risks due to an ever-mutating virus manifesting in tougher variants and sub-variants.[89] The situation causes tension, fatigue, and confusion, to name a few.[90]

As it will be virtually impossible for this chapter to have an in-depth discussion on all African countries, the chapter will focus on two countries in Africa, namely South Africa and Nigeria. South Africa is recognized as one of the countries that were worst-hit by COVID-19, with high rates of infection and deadly variants and sub-variants. Although not on the same trajectory with South Africa, Nigeria has experienced different waves of the COVID-19 pandemic. The country with its large population size and troubled healthcare sector can also be used to highlight the implication of COVID-19 on the health and well-being of healthcare providers in Africa.

Nigeria

Prior to COVID-19, most fundamental rights of Nigeria's healthcare workers were already greatly eroded. This has only gotten worse since the pandemic began. Constitutionally guaranteed rights including the right to health, the right to dignity, the right to work, and the right to just and favourable working conditions are regularly eroded not only in the health sector but also across different sectors in Nigeria. In addition to international human rights instruments, the Nigerian Constitution also guarantees rights including the right to health, dignity, and favourable conditions of work.[91]

As of 24 October 2023, Nigeria had 266,675 official COVID-19 cases and 3,155 deaths.[92] The numbers are generally believed to be much higher however, due to reasons like the country's poor surveillance system[93] and the reluctance to present for testing due to stigmatization.

Nigeria's health sector can easily be summarized as being 'in shambles'. The myriad of problems berating the country's health sector predate the COVID-19 pandemic. Africa's most populous nation has one of the highest maternal (with 20% of global maternal deaths)[94] and infant mortality rates in the world (with 110.8 deaths per 1,000 live birth rate)[95]; one of the highest HIV cases in the world, with 1.9 million people living with HIV[96]; and a high rate of non-communicable diseases (NCDs), even though life expectancy rose from 54.6 (1998) to 64.3 (2019).[97] This indicates massive failure to preserve the right to health as guaranteed under various international human rights instruments and section 17(3)(d) of the Nigerian Constitution.

Meanwhile, public healthcare facilities are underfunded and not well-maintained. Equipment is often outdated or barely working. Medicines are not readily available, including the most basic ones such as paracetamol, for pain relief. Add to these the incessant strike actions embarked on by healthcare workers in Nigeria, many of which have occurred during the COVID-19 pandemic.[98] These strike actions hinder the delivery of good healthcare services in Nigeria. Unfortunately, they are common across different sectors in Nigeria and are indicative of the government's failure to guarantee the right to just and humane conditions of work under section 17(3)(b) of the Constitution. These are some of the reasons that public health facilities in Nigeria have been loosely referred to as 'death traps'.[99] Nigeria's political class are notorious for shunning the country's healthcare facilities, and instead engaging in medical tourism in countries with better health care.[100] Nigerian presidents have themselves been at the forefront of medical tourism, with President Muhammadu Buhari having spent almost 200 days – as of April 2021 – outside Nigeria on medical treatment.[101]

It is against this backdrop that healthcare workers in Nigeria have to work. Some have died in the course of performing their duties due to associated risks. Nigeria has experienced a number of public health emergencies in recent years. Apart from the Ebola crisis which took the lives of some healthcare workers, others have died from infections picked up at work during the country's Lassa fever epidemic. Nigeria's healthcare workers believe that not much value is placed on their lives and the work that they do.

When COVID-19 spread to Nigeria in 2020, the country's health sector was ill-prepared, and the odds were stacked against the country considering challenges like its huge population size, widespread poverty, healthcare worker shortage, and poor infrastructure.[102] Immediate problems included non-availability of materials for protection and prevention such as masks, lack of adequate facilities for isolation, and stigmatization of suspected cases leading to many people hiding symptoms or infections. Many people later diagnosed with COVID-19 often presented to hospitals – in some cases private hospitals and clinics – without disclosing symptoms. Hence, COVID-19 cases were being diagnosed in facilities ill equipped to do so. Even though it was standard requirement to disclose information such as coughing or symptoms of flu, recent travel to or through places with known COVID-19 cases, and contact with someone who has been ill before entering healthcare settings and other places, these requirements were hardly complied with. These factors contributed to the vulnerability of healthcare workers to COVID-19. By September 2020, as many as 2,175 healthcare workers had been diagnosed with COVID-19 in Nigeria.[103]

Nigeria's persistent dependence on external aid to tackle public health emergencies remains a challenge to its handling of these emergencies. This dependence minimizes the important role of healthcare workers, as no matter the dedication or availability of the healthcare worker, lack of training and non-availability of necessary equipment in handling such emergencies put them at risk and leave them helpless to act. For instance, until the timely intervention of WHO and some other countries, PPE supply challenges and healthcare worker training remained a problem. With WHO-led Infection and Prevention control (IPC) training of healthcare workers across the country, there was a drop in the number of healthcare worker infections.[104] Similarly, when COVID-19 vaccines became available, more developed countries had access before countries like Nigeria did. Some of the initial worries about the vaccines centred around the availability of 24-hour power supply to keep the vaccines viable, given the country's well-known power supply problem. Fortunately, the country appears to have managed its COVID-19 vaccine supplies, although there have been rumours of big batches of vaccines going bad. Fortunately for Nigeria, able countries have stepped forward to support others less fortunate. Hence, Nigeria has hugely benefitted from vaccine donations from external sources such as the US and the Africa Union (AU), with both estimated to have provided about 18 million vaccine doses to Nigeria.[105] The position of perpetual receiver of aid, even in the face of a pandemic, can be seen as one which will negatively affect the morale of healthcare workers. Uncertainty about if or when vital supplies like PPE and later vaccines would be available could cause problems like stress, anxiety, and sleeplessness.

Not much acknowledgement is accorded to those who lose their lives in service during public health emergencies. This knowledge can lead to negative emotions such as dejection, depression, nonchalance, or loss of interest in their work for those who are left behind. For example there was no recognition of healthcare workers who had lost their lives after being infected during the Ebola crisis of 2014. One of such was Dr Stella Ameyo Adadevoh, an accomplished medical doctor, who died after being infected while treating Nigeria's patient zero during the Ebola outbreak in 2014.[106] Due to Dr Adadevoh's quick thinking and proactive measures, the country was saved from an outbreak. Patrick Sawyer, Nigeria's Ebola patient zero, was a high-ranking Liberian national who was in Nigeria to attend a conference and had presented at the hospital after falling ill on arrival in Lagos, Nigeria.[107] Despite protests from the patient and immense pressure from the Liberian government, Dr. Adadevoh stuck to her guns about quarantining the patient and testing him for Ebola, which he later tested positive for, thereby saving the country from a potential outbreak of the deadly disease.[108] She fell ill soon after and passed away on 19 August 2014.

On 20 October 2014, WHO declared Nigeria Ebola-free, having had a total of 19 positive cases with 11 survivors.[109] Four of the casualties were those who had initial contact with patient zero, namely Dr Adadevoh, Dr Amos Abaniwo, Justina Ejelonu (a nurse), and Evelyn Uko (a nurse aide).[110] Sadly, the Nigerian government made no efforts to celebrate Dr Adadevoh's legacy and her contribution to the society, neither was any meaningful support offered to her family and loved ones who were left to pick up the pieces.[111] Any efforts by Nigeria to recognize Dr Adadevoh only came after a public outcry, and such effort felt contrived and insincere. Meanwhile, recognition poured in from other sources but not the government of her country. She received the 2018 ECOWAS prize for Excellence among others,[112] and Google honoured her with a doodle on her 62nd posthumous birthday.[113] Shockingly, her name and those of other heroic healthcare workers who served at the centre of the country's Ebola outbreak were missing from the 2014 National Honours award list of over 300 honourees, most of whom were observed to be serving government officials being recognized simply because of the public office they held.[114] The government's excuse that the awards were not given posthumously was a weak one at best. As has been pointed out, the rules governing the awards were silent on this issue. Besides, the federal government had in 2018 conferred the same honours posthumously on other citizens.[115] Also, an argument can also be made for Dr Adadevoh's colleagues who were similarly infected but survived. Nigeria's Lassa fever outbreaks have also recorded their fair share of healthcare worker infections and deaths, with 71 healthcare worker deaths recorded between 1969 and 2021. Of the 211 reported cases in January 2022, five were healthcare worker infections.[116] At least four healthcare workers were reported to have died in the first quarter of 2022 (one medical doctor with WHO in Benue state in January, one doctor in February 2022, and two medical doctors in Oyo state in March 2022).[117] As of September 2023, the official number of healthcare workers infected by Lassa fever was 49.[118] In December 2021, following the infection and deaths of two consultant gynaecologists after treating an infected pregnant woman in Lafia, Nassarawa state, the Nigerian Medical Association observed that the N5,000 hazard allowance was far from commensurate with the risks involved and called on government to increase this allowance.[119] As observed by the Nassarawa state NMA chairman: 'Medical doctors face great risks on a daily basis while carrying their duties. We are doing this job because we love it, especially because it concerns humanity'.

Unfortunately, witnessing these events and the seeming disregard for their welfare will expectedly result in waning enthusiasm and disillusionment of many healthcare workers. To undo the damage in its health sector, Nigeria needs to begin to respect and uphold the fundamental rights of its health workforce.

South Africa

South Africa is one of the countries most affected by COVID-19. It experienced several waves of COVID, with increasingly deadly variants and sub-variants. As of October 2023, South Africa had recorded 4,092,483 COVID-19 cases in total and 102,595 deaths.[120] The number of deaths was high at 102,595.[121]

The country's health sector, already under strain pre-COVID, had been stretched to the limit during the pandemic. Once considered a top destination for employment within the continent for healthcare workers, South Africa's healthcare system has faced imminent collapse in recent years.[122] This is attributable to a combination of factors, which include healthcare worker shortages, healthcare worker concentration in the private sector, unequal distribution of public healthcare workers among the provinces, public sector underfunding, and an unequal system in which most cannot afford exorbitant rates of private health care.[123] The shortage of healthcare workers has been given as a reason for physical and mental exhaustion among South African healthcare workers.[124] South African public health facilities have been found to be especially riddled with problems such as poor hygiene and infection control measures, overcrowding, high patient-to-staff ratios, turning away patients sometimes with dire consequences for the persons turned away, medical negligence and ensuing litigation, and shortage of medicine and equipment.[125] This situation had already created an unhealthy environment for healthcare workers in the country. All these factors interfere with the enjoyment of the right to health by not only healthcare workers but also the general population.

Unfortunately, South Africa had been faced with a 'multiple burden of disease' prior to the COVID-19 outbreak, what with its long-drawn battle with HIV/AIDS, tuberculosis, and a growing burden of non-communicable diseases.[126] The COVID-19 pandemic placed further burden on the system and compounded the problems of South Africa's healthcare workers. In an online survey involving 7,607 South African healthcare workers conducted between April and May 2020, 23.7% of those surveyed displayed poor general health.[127] The study observed a difference in the levels of general health among the different categories of healthcare workers surveyed, with nurses faring the worst with respect to health, well-being, and psychological distress. For instance, 44.4% of nurses reported poor general health and well-being, as against medical practitioners at 31.1% and other health professionals at 24.5%.[128] Nurses also fared the worst with regard to psychological distress, with 24.7% reporting severe psychological distress, compared to 14.3% of medical practitioners reporting the same.[129] These findings tallied with those from two other surveys from New York, USA,[130] and China,[131] which also found the highest levels of distress among nurses. As has been pointed out, these survey findings in South Africa show that indicators of distress were already heightened among South African healthcare workers at the start of the pandemic.[132]

Another survey of doctors and nurses in the KwaZulu-Natal Province showed that 51.5% presented with depression, 47.2% with anxiety, and 44.3% with stress, with significantly high percentages in the severe to extremely severe range.[133] This is not surprising, as South Africa is acknowledged as one of the countries that were worst hit by COVID-19 with astronomically high infection rates and case numbers.[134] This in turn increased the likelihood of healthcare worker infections, given their position as COVID-19 frontline workers. In the first year of the pandemic, almost 16,000 healthcare worker infections were recorded in KwaZulu-Natal's public sector alone, with 335 deaths.[135]

Dawood et al acknowledge the high likelihood of a collision of 'professional grief' and 'personal grief' for healthcare workers,[136] which could have a negative effect on the mental health and well-being of the healthcare worker. Professional grief is grief experienced by healthcare workers due to the loss of patients, while personal grief is grief due to the loss of loved ones.[137]

The high number of healthcare worker deaths recorded in South Africa has further deepened the country's healthcare worker shortage. By August 2020, 181 healthcare workers had died in South Africa, and just over a year later, the numbers had exploded to more than 1,300.[138] Sadly, the actual figures were believed to be much higher, possibly double the quoted figure.[139] To put things in proper perspective, the September 2021 death tally was given to be the equivalent of the staff strength of the Chris Hani Baragwanath Hospital, the largest hospital in South Africa.[140] As has been observed, there seemed to be no tangible plan to fill the void created by the losses.[141] Illustrating the impact of the loss, Dr Maggie Mojapelo-Mokotedi, the founder of the Healthcare Workers Heroes Memorial referred to the deaths as a 'professorial apocalypse'.[142]

An innovation of the KwaZulu-Natal health department can offer guidance to others on providing support for healthcare workers during pandemics. The KwaZulu-Natal Department of Health developed a 'mental health toolkit' for health workers and the general public to help them deal with the psychological impact of COVID-19 on them.[143] This mental health toolkit, which was available on the department's webpage, covered issues and contained resources on coping with stress, well-being of healthcare workers, moral injury, and regular emotional check-ins, among many others.[144] These efforts support the protection of the right to health.

Of note is the Healthcare Workers Heroes Memorial mentioned earlier, which celebrates the lives of the hero South African healthcare workers who died in active service to humanity during the COVID-19 pandemic.[145] The memorial was founded by Dr Mojapelo-Mokotedi, herself a healthcare worker, following her COVID-19 battle and survival, and the passing of her sister from COVID-19.[146] The memorial was not only to honour the memories of those who had died but also to support their families and advocate for those who were left.[147] The website collates names of the 'fallen heroes' and displays their images on a wall.[148] The memorial is a great initiative, as it helps celebrate those who have paid the ultimate sacrifice during the pandemic but have seemingly not been given the recognition that they deserve given the circumstances. A wall of remembrance erected by the South African Nursing Council (SANC) was unveiled in March 2023 in honour of nurses who lost their lives to COVID-19.[149] These initiatives could have a two-pronged effect, in that they not only celebrates those who are gone, but it could also help in giving their colleagues who are left behind some form of closure and reassurance that they are not alone. This could provide some much-needed psychological boost, contributing positively to their overall health and well-being.

12.5 Recommendations for mitigating the impact of the pandemic on healthcare providers in Africa

One obvious fact that emerged as COVID-19 spread on the African continent was the lack of preparedness on the parts of African governments to handle a national emergency on the scale of COVID. Even though the virus did not arrive on the continent until well after others, buying Africa a little time to prepare, Africa was still ill-prepared for COVID-19. It is therefore important for Africa to learn from its mistakes and the consequences of a lack of preparedness. Doing so will help its preparation for future public health emergencies, as better preparedness is expected to affect/impact things like case numbers, rate of spread, fatalities, and management. It could also allow early formulation of plans for support for frontline workers.

This section will consider a number of interventions for reducing the negative impact of the pandemic on healthcare workers. Some of them are general and operational in nature, as they are not targeted specifically at the health and well-being of healthcare workers but at ultimately reducing the burden of the pandemic on them. These include maintaining strong and functional emergency response plans, encouraging telehealth consultations, and deploying more healthcare workers in mobile testing units. On the other hand, tailor-made interventions for preserving the health and well-being of healthcare workers include the provision of psychological care for them, adapting the 'battle buddy' programme, and holistically harnessing all-round support from a robust network (including family and colleagues) for health workers. These will be discussed in further detail below.

It is usual for countries to have a disaster management plan in anticipation of events including public health emergencies. It is therefore concerning that in spite of this, African countries struggled to implement sound COVID-19 emergency responses. Many did not even have stock of basic protective equipment. To address the burden of health emergencies like COVID-19 on healthcare workers, African countries would do well to develop and maintain very strong emergency response plans. It is also suggested that in addition to having the plans in place, healthcare workers would benefit from having preparatory exercises (drills) where public health emergency situations are simulated. This would aid healthcare workers to be better prepared should the situation arise; and it could help recognize an emergency and curtail the spread of any contagion, instil more confidence in them, and generally ease some of their fears of 'the unknown'. Tessema et al. note the low number of healthcare workers who had received COVID-19 training and updated guidelines for the provision of care during COVID-19.[150] This prevents healthcare workers from performing at their optimum.

Avoiding unnecessary traffic at/attendance of healthcare facilities will reduce the risk of infection and spread. Adopting telehealth or telemedicine as an alternative method of consultation is an efficient way of achieving reduction in in-person consultations and scaling back on outpatient clinics. This would especially be a timely intervention in African health settings where physical distancing between patients and staff would be deemed challenging due to the history of overcrowding in healthcare facilities.[151] As COVID-19 spread, many countries provided for medical personnel to have consultations via telehealth.[152] Telehealth could be through different means of communication including telephone, email, video call, or conference (which involves using Internet-supported and government-approved applications like Skype,

Microsoft Teams, and Zoom).[153] Telehealth through video calls could be more reassuring to patients because of the possibility of being able to see and speak with their healthcare provider in real time and getting feedback. The availability of visual aid with video telehealth consultations could also give reassurance to patients, carers, and family, with the added advantage of being able to show things like scars and growths to their healthcare provider and being more reliable in ascertaining a patient's identity. Unfortunately, this option might not be readily available in many healthcare settings in Africa, which struggles with poor Internet and electricity supply, which are important for telehealth consultations.[154] The situation would be worse in rural and remote areas where Internet and power supply are poor or non-existent.[155]

Another limitation of a general nature to the option of telehealth would be the kind of healthcare services needed. For example, patients would need to be physically present for services like surgery, blood work, and imaging.[156] For example, healthcare systems had to at different times postpone elective surgeries when systems were being stretched due to the pandemic and resume them when there was respite.[157]

Deployment of healthcare workers in mobile testing units to remote or COVID-19 infection cluster areas could also be key to stemming the tide of the virus. The role played by these mobile testing units during the Ebola crisis in West Africa of 2014 has been emphasized, wherein testing units went around villages, detecting infection clusters and building temporary treatment centres.[158] The overall effect was that already stretched resources were focused on where they were mostly needed while some semblance of life could continue in unaffected areas.[159] It is believed that adequate training, preparation, and kitting up would be vital to the successful operation of these mobile testing units, as it would give reassurance to healthcare workers deployed to service these testing units. To also encourage healthcare workers to sign up, appropriate incentives could be offered in the form of bonuses and days off.

To help healthcare workers in dealing with the impact of the COVID-19 pandemic on their health and well-being, it is necessary to first understand their experiences. As has been pointed out, the best way to understand their concerns is to ask them.[160] Healthcare workers on the continent feel that their voices are not being heard. Creating a dedicated platform through which their voices are heard and their worries are taken into consideration will go a long way towards healing for many.

Chersich et al emphasize the importance of providing psychological care for frontline workers. They recognize the challenges to formal or structured interventions and raise the possibility of informal interventions.[161] Examples of informal interventions are counsellors or retired colleagues visiting healthcare workers' rest areas/break rooms to lend a listening ear. Healthcare workers can themselves take advantage of the availability of social media platforms to seek support from and offer support to colleagues. The advent of social media platforms has seen people with common interests interacting and forming alliances. It is common to see these families, colleagues, church members, and alumni of schools forming 'groups' on Meta (formerly Facebook) and WhatsApp. Of note is the South African Vula Mobile platform, which is an online medical referral application in South Africa through which healthcare workers get advice from one another and refer patients.[162] The application connects healthcare workers 'by providing a safe and secure platform to share advice'.[163]

Consciously providing support for healthcare workers can help mitigate the impact of the pandemic on them. Carmassi et al highlighted the importance of support from different sources, including family, society, colleagues, and supervisors, in combating stress and other negative effects of previous public health emergencies like SARS and MERS.[164] This can be adapted for the COVID-19 pandemic. Many healthcare workers relied on the support of family members during COVID-19. Social support, where available, gave healthcare workers the renewed energy to face the pandemic. For instance, in countries like the UK, the US, and Australia, healthcare workers were celebrated and given special treatment in accessing certain services. This was a welcome development, as previously, many had missed out on things like groceries due to the rampant panic buying that became the hallmark of the pandemic.[165] By the time healthcare workers were able to get to the shops, they had been emptied of essentials. In March 2020, a video of a UK nurse who had broken down following futile efforts to get groceries went viral.[166] This video resonated with many frontline workers and could have been instrumental in measures later introduced to curtail panic buying and cater for the needs of frontline workers. The public later made conscious efforts to appreciate the good work of healthcare workers, with kind gestures such as deliberate applause and providing free coffee or food for healthcare workers being rampant. In Australia for example, they were given exclusive early morning access to shop for groceries by major retailers on certain days of the week.[167]

Harnessing the power of positive coping strategies has also been identified as a means of preventing PTSD.[168] Positive coping strategies include the use of humour and planning, the acceptance of work-related risks, the ability to speak about and share their experiences, having strong religious beliefs, and having the motivation to learn different skills.[169] Negative coping skills or maladaptive coping skills such as avoidance, hostile confrontation, and self-blame, on the other hand, were more likely to have negative effects on mental health and well-being.[170]

The possibility of using a digital support package (e-package) to support the psychological well-being of healthcare workers during and after COVID-19 has also been explored. Blake et al developed this package using Agile methodology and trialled it on a diverse group of healthcare workers from the UK.[171] Participants, among other things, suggested that materials available online needed to go beyond the usual rhetoric of promoting health and should rather address specific issues facing healthcare workers during COVID and those that were relevant to the workplace environment.[172] The authors observed that this package generated interest quickly, having been accessed 17,633 times and gaining more than 50,000 exposures within the first seven days of its release.[173] On the whole, healthcare workers reacted positively to the digital support package.

Also, the Psychological Resilience Intervention developed by Albott et al could be adapted for healthcare workers in Africa. Modelled after the US Army Battle Buddy system (which assigns a 'battle buddy' to every soldier to assist them in and out of combat throughout their military career), the Psychological Resilience Intervention aims to help equip healthcare workers with the ability to cope with COVID-19 and the stresses it creates for them.[174] This intervention aims to use the personal resilience-promoting principles on focused attention to self-care, self-efficacy, and social connection and to provide quick access to mental health consultation and support as necessary.[175]

It is essential that the rights and welfare of healthcare workers are given priority, in order to harness the best that this group has to offer. Improving the overall health and well-being of healthcare workers in Africa during the COVID-19 pandemic will have a ripple effect of improving patient care and overall healthcare delivery.

12.5.1 Future pandemics and the way forward

The 2014 Ebola outbreak in West Africa has been described as exposing weaknesses in the global capacity for timely outbreak detection and containment in resource-poor settings.[176] In particular, COVID-19 can be said to have further exposed, just like previous public health issues before it, the weaknesses in Africa's health systems and brought the inadequate protection of healthcare workers to the fore. As public health emergencies are a constant challenge to global health systems, it is expedient that appropriate mechanisms be put in place to meet these emergencies should they occur. Countries with more advanced healthcare systems are known to have contingency plans in place for dealing with public health emergencies. Unfortunately, many were found wanting when COVID-19 struck. For instance, despite its touted 'pandemic preparedness' and despite boasting renown infectious disease and public health establishments such as the Centres for Disease Control and Prevention (CDC) and the Department of State Biosecurity Engagement Program, the US has been described as 'unprepared, overconfident and inept at pandemic control'.[177] Africa generally has a history of inadequate preparedness for public health emergencies. A study on African states' influenza preparedness revealed that while majority (74%) had a plan, most were inadequate and lacking in operational clarity.[178] Vital issues such as case management, triage procedures and identification of treatment facilities, and the maintenance of essential services were poorly outlined or absent.[179] The reasons for these are not far-fetched: As pointed out by Daszak et al, epidemics do not occur in a vacuum. Rather, they exploit society's connectivity and are impacted by issues such as social divides, economic disparities, and injustices, which invariably lead to inequities in the provision of healthcare services.[180]

Going forward, it is essential for states to build and improve on their health systems. Most African countries would need to start with the provision of basic health care and amenities, which were mostly lacking during the COVID-19 and previous pandemics. It is also necessary to have clear and practical infectious disease preparedness plans, which should be adapted specifically to suit each country's healthcare system. Another measure that can significantly halt the spread of infectious diseases could be drastically limiting cross-border travels. Unfortunately, this may be deemed non-feasible. There have also been calls for the revision of the International Health Regulations of 2005 to include states' obligations to report public health events to WHO as they are detected and to revise the classification system to allow international response to growing outbreaks before the declaration of a public health emergency of international concern.[181]

12.6 Conclusion

The chapter discussed the effect of COVID-19 on healthcare providers on the African continent. It examined the many problems beleaguering healthcare systems in Africa before the COVID-19 pandemic to show that health care in Africa was already troubled, with profound negative effects on the continent's healthcare workers. The pandemic further exacerbated an already dire situation, with large percentages of healthcare workers experiencing challenges to their physical, professional, and mental health and well-being, including stress, anxiety, insomnia, burnout, depression, and PTSD. Unfortunately, even though the physical and mental health of healthcare workers has begun receiving attention globally, not much has been done to help them in Africa. The chapter has therefore stressed the importance of providing support for healthcare workers in Africa to enable them cope with the impact of COVID-19 on them. The chapter shows the need to prioritize the rights and welfare of healthcare workers, given the high-risk nature of their work, and highlights the importance of allowing them to provide health care without the added pressure of frivolous lawsuits, all the while recognizing applicable limitations.

Through a discussion of the healthcare systems in two focus African countries (Nigeria and South Africa), the chapter has highlighted the challenges peculiar to the rights and welfare of healthcare workers in Nigeria, drawing comparisons from countries with more established healthcare systems. The chapter then concludes by suggesting ideas and interventions for the long-term to mitigate the impact of the pandemic on healthcare workers that goes beyond mere formalities to practical, healthcare worker-focused solutions.

Notes

1 Blake et al 'Mitigating the psychological impact of COVID-19 on healthcare workers: A digital learning package' (2020) 17 *International Journal of Environmental Research and Public Health* 2997.
2 CS Albott et al 'Battle buddies: Rapid deployment of a psychological resilience intervention for healthcare workers during the coronavirus disease 2019 pandemic' (2020) 131(1) *Anesthesia & Analgesia* at 2 available at www.anesthesia-analgesia.org (accessed 4 June 2022).
3 R Buselli et al 'Professional quality of life and mental health outcomes among health care workers exposed to SARS-CoV-2 (COVID-19)' (2020) 17 *International Journal of Environmental Research and Public Health* 6180.
4 Blake et al (n 5 above).
5 Albott et al (n 6 above)
6 MF Chersich et al 'COVID-19 in Africa: Care and protection for frontline healthcare workers' (2020) 16 *Globalization and Health* 46.
7 WHO (n 3 above).
8 WHO African Region 'Over 10,000 health workers in Africa infected with COVID-19' 23 July 2020 available at www.afro.who.int/news/over-10-000-health-workers-africa-infected-covid-19 (accessed 24 October 2023).
9 As above.
10 As above.
11 NS Quadri et al 'COVID-19 in Africa: Survey analysis of impact on health-care workers' (2021) 104(6) *American Journal of Tropical Medicine and Hygiene* at 2169.
12 T Shanafelt et al 'Understanding and addressing sources of anxiety among healthcare professionals during the COVID-19 pandemic' (2020) 323 *Journal of the American Medical Association* at 2133–2134.
13 Shanafelt et al (n 16 above).
14 As above.
15 As above.
16 Blake et al (n 5 above).
17 MW Rabow et al 'Witnesses and victims both: Healthcare workers and grief in the time of COVID-19' (2021) 62(3) *Journal of Pain and Symptom Management* 647.
18 A Oliva et al 'Liability of healthcare professionals and institutions during COVID-19 pandemic in Italy: Symposium proceedings and position statement' (2020) 16 *Journal of Patient Safety* e299–e302, at e301.
19 H.R.8330 – Good Samaritan Act (94th Congress 1975–1976); West & Varacallo 'Good Samaritan Laws' 20 September 2021 available at www.ncbi.nlm.nih.gov/books/NBK542176 (accessed 24 October 2023).
20 West & Vacarallo (n 23 above).
21 Kolbert 'Legal protections for New York healthcare providers during COVID-19 – and what's next' available at www.thedoctors.com/articles/legal-protections-for-new-york-healthcare-providers-during-covid-19and-whats-next/ (accessed 15 August 2022).
22 JM Dean et al 'Obligations of Australian health services as employers during COVID-19' (2021) 45 *Australian Health Review* 622–626, at 622.

23 EJ Emmanuel 'The lesson of SARS' (2003) 139(7) *Annals of Internal Medicine* 589–591.
24 This is discussed in further detail under 12.4.6 below.
25 YT Li & J Ng 'Moral dilemma of striking: A medical worker's response to job duty, public health protection and the politicization of strikes' (2021) 1–10 *Work, Employment and Society* at 3.
26 For example, in Australia, the corresponding federal law is the Work Health and Safety Act of 2011.
27 Dean et al (n 26 above) at 623.
28 As above.
29 As above.
30 As above.
31 Emmanuel (n 27 above).
32 As above.
33 As above.
34 Carville et al Bloomberg 'Hospitals tell doctors they'll be fired if they speak out about lack of gear' 31 March 2020 available at www.bloomberg.com/news/articles/hospitals-tell-doctors-they-ll-be-fired-if-they-talk-to-press#xj4y7vzkg (accessed 23 October 2023).
35 Raphael Minder, *New York Times*, 12 Jan 2022 'Spanish doctors who lacked protective gear early in the pandemic win compensation' available at www.nytimes.com/2022/01/12world/spanish-doctors-ppe-settlement.html (accessed 24 October 2023).
36 Minder (n 39 above).
37 As above.
38 Carville et al (n 38 above).
39 As above.
40 WHO 'Keep health workers safe to keep patients safe: WHO' 17 September 2020 available at www.who.int/news/item/17-09-2020-keep-health-workers-safe-to-keep-patients-safe-who (accessed 23 October 2023).
41 As above.
42 Jiyao Chen et al 'Mental health during the COVID-19 crisis in Africa: A systematic review and meta-analysis' (2021) 18 *International Journal of Environmental Research and Public Health* 10604.
43 Shanafelt et al (n 16 above).
44 As above.
45 Nullis-Kapp 'Health worker shortage could derail development goals' (January 2005) 83(1) *Bulletin of the WHO*.
46 As above.
47 S Naicker et al 'Shortage of healthcare workers in developing countries – Africa' (Spring 2009) (Suppl 1) *Ethnicity & Disease*: S1–60–4.
48 Quadri et al (n 15 above) 2169–2175.
49 This was done via circular No. SWC/S/04/S.218/11/406 of 22 December 2021
50 Deborah Tolu-Kolawole Punch Newspapers 25 December 2021 'FG increases hazard allowance from N5,000 to N4,000 for doctors, N34,000 for others' available at https://punchng.com/fg-increases-hazard-allowance-from-n5000-to-n40000-n34000-for-others (accessed 24 October 2023).
51 Kenneth Odoeme Nigeria Info FM 5 August 2021 'Health workers receive N5,000 hazard allowance' available at www.nigeriainfo.fm/news/hardfacts/health-workers-receive-n5000-hazard-allowance-nard/ (accessed 23 October 2023).
52 Samuel Akpan The Cable Newspapers (Nigeria) 7 April 2021 'MATTERS ARISING: Striking doctors on N5,000 hazard allowance but senators get N1.2millionfornewspapers'availableatwww.thecable.ng/matters-arising-striking-

doctors-receive-n5000-hazard-allowance-but-senators-get-n1-2m-for-news papers (accessed 23 October 2023)

53 Nullis-Kapp (n 49 above).

54 Chukwuma Muanya & Eniola Daniel Guardian Newspapers 29 April 2019 'Doctors can leave, Nigeria has enough, says Ngige' available at https://guardian.ng/news/doctors-can-leave-nigeria-has-enough-says-ngige/ (accessed 23 October 2023).

55 As above.

56 As above

57 Buselli et al (n 7 above).

58 Chersich et al (n 10 above)

59 SH Spencer & A Fichera 28 July 2020 'In viral video, doctor falsely touts hydroxylchloroquine as COVID-19 cure' available at www.factcheck.org/2020/07/in-viral-video-doctor-falsely-touts-hydroxylcholoroquine-as-covid-19-cure/ (accessed 24 October 2023).

60 Christine Farr CNBC 7 April 2020 'Patients with autoimmune diseases are running out of hydroxylchloroquine' available at https://wwwcnbc.com/2020/04/07/patients-with-autoimmune-diseases-running-out-of-hydroxychloroquine.html (accessed 24 October 2023); I Murray Sun Herald Newspapers 25 August 2021 'Ivermectin is flying off Coast store shelves despite warnings the new hydroxylchloroquine' available at www.sunherald.com/news/coronavirus/article253694393.html (accessed 24 October 2023).

61 At 2172.

62 At 2170.

63 Chersich et al (n 10 above).

64 As above.

65 WHO (n 12 above).

66 Albott et al (n 6 above).

67 C Carmassi et al 'PTSD symptoms in healthcare workers facing the three coronavirus outbreaks: What can we expect after the COVID-19 Pandemic' (2020) 292 *Psychiatry Research* 113312.

68 As above.

69 As above.

70 Quadri et al (n 15 above).

71 Shanafelt et al (n 16 above).

72 N Nwosu-Igbo UNICEF Nigeria 17 February 2022 'Vaccine equity: US donated COVID-19 vaccines benefit Nigerians – the United States Government helps strengthen global vaccine equity' available at www.unicef.org/nigeria/stories/vaccine-equity-us-donated-covid-19-vaccines-benefit-nigerians (accessed 24 October 2023).

73 GA Tessema et al 'The COVID-19 pandemic and healthcare systems in Africa: A scoping review of preparedness, impact and response' (2021) 6 *BMJ Global Health* e007179.

74 Reuters 24 April 2020 'Doctors launch legal challenge to UK government over protective kit' available at www.reuters.com/article/us-health-coronavirus-britain-legal-idUSKCN22533P (accessed 24 October 2023).

75 A Rimmer 'COVID-19: Doctors launch judicial review over PPE failures' (2020) 369 *BMJ* m2301.

76 BMA Press release 19 May 2022 'The UK government "failed in its duty of care" to doctors and the healthcare workforce in its handling of the pandemic, says BMA' available at www.bma.org.uk/bma-media-centre/the-uk-government-failed-in-its-duty-of-care-to-doctors-and-the-health-workforce-in-its-handling-of-the-pandemic-says-bma (accessed 24 October 2023).

77 Reuters 20 May 2020 'Nigerian doctors to strike over treatment by police during lockdown' available at www.reuters.com/article/us-health-coronavirus-nigeria-healthcare-idUSKBN22W22R (accessed 24 October 2023).
78 These were made up of physicians, nurses, pharmacists, students, and medical officers.
79 Quadri et al (n 15 above) at 2172.
80 FD Madzimbamuto 'Ventilators are not the answer in Africa' (2020) 12(1) *African Journal of Primary Health Care and Family Medicine* at 2517
81 Quadri et al's survey confirmed 'relative scarcity of ventilators in African facilities' (n 15 above) at 2174); Madzimbamuto (n 84 above) at 2517.
82 Chersich et al (n 10 above).
83 African Union 'Africa CDC receives third donation of medical supplies from Jack Ma Foundation, co-hosts global MediXChange webinar on COVID-19' available at https://africacdc.org/news-item/africa-cdc-receives-third-donation-of-medical-supplies-from-jack-ma-foundation-co-hosts-global-medixchange-webinar-on-covid-19/ (accessed 23 October 2023); Welsh Government 26 August 2021 'Press release: 7.2 million of PPE equipment sent from Wales to Namibia' available at https://gov.wales/£7-2m-ppe-equipment-sent-wales-namibia (accessed 23 October 2023).
84 CY Liu et al 'The prevalence and influencing factors in anxiety in medical workers fighting COVID-19 in China: A cross-sectional survey' (2020) 148 *Epidemiology and Infection* e98, 1–7 at 2.
85 Quadri et al (n 15 above) at 2174,
86 Madzimbamuto (n 84 above) at 2517–2518.
87 United Nations (UN) 28 January 2021 'COVID-19: Mental illness, a 'parallel pandemic' available at https://unric.org/en/covid-19-mental-illness-a-parallel-pandemic/ (accessed 24 October 2023).
88 B Dawood et al '"Unheard", "uncared for" and "unsupported": The mental health impact of COVID-19 on healthcare workers in KwaZulu-Natal Province, South Africa' (2022) 17(5) *PLoS One*.
89 UN (n 91 above).
90 As above.
91 Sections 17(3)(d), 17(2)(b) and 17(3)(b)&(c) of the Constitution of the Federal Republic of Nigeria, 1999.
92 Nigeria Centre for Disease Control (NCDC) 'COVID-19 NIGERIA' available at https://covid19.ncdc.gov.19/report (accessed 24 October 2023).
93 C Ohia et al 'COVID-19 and Nigeria: Putting the realities in context' (2020) 95 *International Journal of Infectious Diseases* 279–281.
94 ID Sule et al Daily Trust 9 January 2021 'Nigeria: Why Nigeria's maternal mortality amongst highest in the world' available at http://dailytrust.com/why-nigerias-maternal-mortality-amongst-highest-in-the-world/ (accessed 24 October 2023).
95 UNICEF 'Country profiles – Nigeria: Key demographic indicators' available at https://data.unicef.org/country/nga (accessed 24 October 2023).
96 National Agency for the Control of AIDS (NACA) 'Nigeria prevalence rate' available at https://naca.gov.ng/nigeria-prevalence-rate (accessed 24 October 2023).
97 B Angell et al 'Population health outcomes in Nigeria compared with other West African countries, 1998–2019: A systematic analysis for the global burden of disease study' (2022) 399 *Lancet* 1117–1129.
98 Akpan The Cable Newspapers (n 56 above).
99 M Ahmadu-Suka, Daily Trust Newspapers 12 October 2017 'Nigerian hospitals are death traps, group alleges' available at https://dailytrust.com/nigerian-hospitals-are-death-traps-group-alleges (accessed 24 October 2023); E Mekwunye, Bella Naija 7 June 2016 'The death camps called government hospitals in

Nigeria! Read the story of how Ekene lost his dad' available at www.bellanaija.com/2016/06/the-death-camps-called-government-hospitals-in-nigeria-read-the-story-of-how-ekene-lost-his-dad/ (accessed 24 October 2023).

100 Odoeme (n 55 above).

101 Akpan The Cable Newspapers (n 56 above).

102 N Nwosu-Igbo UNICEF Nigeria 7 April 2020 'In the frontline of Nigeria's struggle with COVID-19: Healthcare workers such as doctors and nurses are in the frontline of the COVID-19 response in Nigeria' available at www.unicef.org/nigeria/stories/frontline-nigerias-struggle-covid-19 (accessed 24 October 2023).

103 WHO, Nigeria 10 September 2020 'Combatting healthcare worker infection in Nigeria' available at www.afro.who.int/news/combatting-health-worker-infections-nigeria (accessed 24 October 2023).

104 As above.

105 Nwosu-Igbo UNICEF (n 106 above)

106 T Ogunlesi, Guardian Newspapers 21 Oct 2014 'Dr Stella Ameyo Adadevoh: Ebola victim and everyday hero' available at www.the.guardian.com/lifeandstyle/womens-blog/2014/oct/20/dr-stella-ameyo-adadevoh-ebola-doctor-nigeria-hero (accessed 24 October 2023)

107 Ogunlesi (n 110 above).

108 As above.

109 WHO Nigeria 20 October 2014 'WHO declares Nigeria Ebola-free' available at www.afro.who.int/news/who-declares-nigeria-ebola-free (accessed 24 October 2023).

110 E Onyeji, Premium Times Newspapers 19 August 2020 'Stella Adadevoh: Six years after, Nigeria yet to honour medic who saved country from Ebola' available at www.premiumtimesng.com/news/headlines/409760-stella-adadevoh–six-years-after-nigeria-yet-to-honour-medic-who-saved-country-from-ebola.html (accessed 24 October 2023).

111 Ogunlesi (n 110 above).

112 Dr Ameyo Stella Adadevoh Health Trust 30 June 2019 'ECOWAS honors Dr. Ameyo Stella Adadevoh' available at www.drasatrust.org/ecowas-honors-dr-ameyo-stella-adadevoh/ (accessed 24 October 2023).

113 Available at www.google.com/doodles/stella-adadevohs-62nd-birthday (accessed 24 October 2023).

114 Ogunlesi (n 110 above).

115 Onyeji (n 114 above).

116 WHO 14 February 2022 'Lassa fever – Nigeria' available at www.who.int/emergencies/disease-outbreak-news/item/lassa-fever–nigeria (accessed 24 October 2023).

117 Deborah Tolu-Kolawole Punch Newspapers 6 March 2022 'Lassa Fever kills four doctors, infects 38 health workers' available at https://punchng.com/lassa-fever-kills-four-doctors-infects-38-health-workers/ (accessed 24 October 2023).

118 NCDC 'Lassa fever situation report, Epi week 37: 11th-17th September 2023' available at https://ncdc.gov.ng/diseases/sitreps/lassa-fever (accessed 24 October 2023).

119 Collins Sunday Punch Newspapers 21 December 2021 'N5,000 hazard allowance not enough, Nassarawa doctors beg Sule' available at https://punchng.com/n5000-hazard-allowance-not-enough-nassarawa-doctors-beg-sule/?utm_source=auto-read-also&utm_medium=web (accessed 24 October 2023).

120 Dept of Health, Republic of South Africa 'COVID-19 daily updates and cases' available at https://sacoronavirus.co.zacovid-19-daily-cases/ (accessed 24 October 2023).

121 As above.
122 WT Maphumulo & BR Bhengu 'Challenges of quality improvement in the healthcare of South Africa post-apartheid: A critical review' (2019) 42(1) *Curationis* a1901.
123 R Rensburg 7 July 2021 'Healthcare in South Africa: How inequity is contributing to inefficiency' available at www.wits.ac.za/news/latest-news/opinion/2021/2021-07/healthcare-in-south-africa-how-inequity-is-contributing-to-inefficiency.html# (accessed 24 October 2023).
124 Maphumulo & Bhengu (n 126 above).
125 As above.
126 As above.
127 I Naidoo et al 'South African health professionals' state of wellbeing during the emergence of COVID-19' (2020) 110(10) *South African Medical Journal* 956.
128 As above.
129 As above.
130 Ari Shecter et al 'Psychological distress, coping behaviours, and preferences for support among New York healthcare workers during the COVID-19 pandemic' (2020) 66 *General Hospital Psychiatry* 1–8.
131 J Lai et al 'Factors associated with mental health outcomes among health care workers exposed to coronavirus disease 2019' (2020) 3(3) *JAMA Network Open* e203976.
132 Naidoo et al (n 131 above).
133 Dawood et al (n 92 above)
134 W Fengler et al 'South Africa after COVID-19 – light at the end of a very long tunnel' available at www.brookings.edu/articles/south-africa-after-covid-19-light-at-the-end-of-a-very-long-tunnel/ (accessed 24 October 2023).
135 Dawood et al (n 92 above).
136 As above.
137 Rabow et al (n 21 above).
138 M Heywood, Daily Maverick 7 September 2021 'More than 1,300 healthcare workers in South Africa have died of COVID-19' available at www.dailymaverick.co.za/article/2021-09-07-more-than-1300-healthcare-workers-in-south-africa-have-died-of-covid-19/ (accessed 24 October 2023).
139 As above.
140 As above.
141 As above.
142 As above.
143 KwaZulu-Natal (KZN) Province, Republic of South Africa 'COVID-19 mental health toolkit' available at www.kznhealth.gov.za/mental/covid19.htm (accessed 24 October 2023).
144 As above.
145 M Heywood, Daily Maverick, 13 August 2020 'Healthcare heroes: Memorial to hospital workers unveiled' available at www.dailymaverick.co.za/article/20-08-13-healthcare-heroes-memorial-to-hospital-workers-unveiled/ (accessed 24 October 2023); www.facebook.com/healthcareheroesmemorial/ (accessed 24 October 2023).
146 Heywood (n 142 above).
147 Heywood (n 149 above).
148 As above.
149 K Masweneng Times Live, 30 March 2023 'Memorial wall unveiled to honour nurses who died during COVID-19' available at www.timeslive.co.za/news/

south-africa/2023-03-30-memorial-wall-unveiled-to-honour-nurses-who-died-during-covid-19/ (accessed 24 October 2023)
150 Spencer & Fichera (n 63 above) at 6.
151 Chersich et al (n 10 above).
152 SN Gajarawala & JN Pelkowski 'Telehealth benefits and barriers' (2021) 17 *The Journal for Nurse Practitioners* 218–221 at 218.
153 As above, at 221.
154 KH Moahi 'Health information networks for telehealth in Africa – challenges and prospects: A review of the literature' (1999) 49 *Libri* 43–50, at 44–45.
155 RE Scott & M Mars 'Telehealth in the developing world: Current status and future prospects' (2015) *Smart Homecare Technology and Telehealth* 25–37, at 31.
156 S Watson, Harvard Health Publishing 'Telehealth: The advantages and disadvantages' 12 October 2020 available at www.health.harvard.edu/staying-healthy/telehealth-the-advantages-and-disadvantages (accessed 24 October 2023).
157 COVIDSurg Collaborative 'Elective surgery cancellations due to the COVID-19 pandemic: Global predictive modelling to inform surgical recovery plans' (2020) 107 *British Journal of Surgery* 1440–1449, at 1440.
158 Chersich et al (n 10 above).
159 As above.
160 Shanafelt et al (n 16 above).
161 Chersich et al (n 10 above).
162 Vula Mobile 'About us' available at www.vula-mobile.com/about-us (accessed 24 October 2023).
163 Vula Mobile 'How it works' available at www.vula-mobile.com/how-it-works (accessed 24 October 2023.
164 Carmassi et al (n 71 above).
165 N Slawson & L Bachelor, Guardian Newspapers 22 March 2020 'Coronavirus: UK panic-buyers urged to think of frontline workers' available at www.theguardian.com/world/2020/mar/21/coronavirus-uk-panic-buyers-urged-to-think-of-frontline-workers (accessed 24 October 2023).
166 Guardian Newspapers 20 March 2020 'Nurse in tears after coronavirus panic buying leaves shelves empty of food – video' available at www.theguardian.com/world/video/2020/mar/20/nurse-in-tears-coronavirus-panic-buying-leaves-shelves-empty-food-video (accessed 24 October 2023).
167 E Knopf 9News Australia 29 March 2020 'Woolworths extends 'community hour' shopping to frontline workers during coronavirus crisis' available at www.9news.con.au/national/coronavirus-woolworths-community-shopping-hours-times-health-care-workers-emergency-services-coles (accessed 24 October 2023).
168 Carmassi et al (n 71 above).
169 As above.
170 As above.
171 Blake et al (n 5 above).
172 As above.
173 As above.
174 Albott (n 6 above) at 2.
175 As above, at 5–6.
176 P Daszak et al 'Commentary – infectious disease threats: A rebound to resilience' (2021) 40(2) *Health Affairs* 204 available at www.healthaffairs.org/doi/pdf/10.1377/hlthaff.2020.01544 (accessed 31 July 2023).
177 As above, at 204.

178 EZ Sambala et al 'Pandemic influenza preparedness in the WHO African region: Are we ready yet?' (2018) 18 *BMC Infectious Diseases* 567, at 10; G Ortu et al 'Pandemic influenza preparedness in Africa is a profound challenge for an already distressed region: Analysis of national preparedness plans' (2008) 23(3) *Health Policy Plan* 161–169.
179 Ortu et al (n 182 above) at 161.
180 Daszak et al (n 180 above) at 206.
181 As above, at 207.

13

IMPACT OF COVID-19 ON THE ENJOYMENT OF RIGHTS TO ABORTION CARE AND THE ROLE OF TRANSPARENCY

Benson Chakaya Atonga

13.1 Introduction

The COVID-19 pandemic significantly impacted access to reproductive health services, including abortion health care. States across the globe implemented various containment measures to slow the spread of the virus, including lock-downs, travel restrictions, and social distancing guidelines. While these measures were necessary to protect public health, they resulted in unintended consequences for reproductive health services, in particular access to abortion care.[1]

The pandemic demonstrated the critical role that transparency can play in public health crises and emergencies, specifically in ensuring continued access to vital health services and adherence to government response measures. Access to abortion care is an emotive issue in most African countries, with laws and regulations varying widely.[2] In some countries, abortion is illegal, while in others, it is legal but heavily restricted.[3] In countries where abortion is legal, access to safe and affordable abortion services can be limited due to a lack of transparency in the healthcare system. Transparency is essential in ensuring that individuals have access to accurate information about their reproductive health options, including abortion.

African countries have a duty to ensure transparent communication about their disaster or pandemic management and response plan, including vital health services that are affected and measures that are taken to maintain access to critical health services. However, with the uncertainty created by the COVID-19 pandemic, clear communication would have reduced confusion and mistrust, enabling women and girls to continue accessing appropriate and safe reproductive health services without fear. Healthcare providers, too,

DOI: 10.4324/9781032671437-16

had the responsibility to embody transparency in their care delivery strategy by providing clear information about the conditions for safe abortion and supporting patients' make informed choices. This way transparency helps build trust between the patient and the healthcare provider, ensuring that the patient has access to safe, legal, and timely abortion care.

A key aspect of transparency is guaranteeing availability of information, and in the context of abortion care, this information should be about the legal status of abortion, the availability of abortion services, and the risks and benefits of different abortion methods in pandemic times. Most countries in Africa, either by design or by omission, lack accurate and comprehensive information about abortion. This situation was worsened by the COVID-19 pandemic when information was not forthcoming at the onset where confusion and misinformation were a daily norm.

13.2 Impact of COVID-19 containment measures

The rapid spread of the virus across the globe prompted the World Health Organization (WHO) to declare the state of pandemic for the virus in March 2020.[4] While various African countries were swift in deploying emergency public health responses to contain the spread of the virus, the responses were generic and ad hoc and did not acknowledge intersectional health needs, particularly women's and girls' access to abortion care services.[5] Limitation of mobility and closure of primary healthcare facilities and market days, which would ordinarily provide an opportunity for most women to discretely access services, left many with no vital sexual and reproductive health (SRH) services. The effect is an exacerbation of pre-existing gender inequalities where women cannot access vital health and support services.[6]

While most African countries have restrictive abortion laws, which limit women's and girls' access to abortion care even in normal circumstances, the outbreak of the novel coronavirus (COVID-19) towards the end of 2019 further limited access to abortion and post-abortion care services by disrupting the health system, with most governments opting to suspend SRH services.[7] COVID-19-related social and economic challenges experienced by many families made it difficult for women and girls to afford abortion and post-abortion care services in few private clinics that maintained operation.[8] Most countries classify abortion care as either 'elective' or 'non-essential', effectively banning the service.[9]

According to reported data, there was 'an increase in demand for abortion and post abortion care, reductions in provision, and increases in barriers to accessing these services during the pandemic'.[10] The restrictions placed on mobility due to lockdowns and curfews limited the ability of women and girls to access abortion care services.[11] For instance, in Zimbabwe and Kenya, the respective governments banned public transport, restricting mobility, thus making it difficult for women and girls living in rural areas to travel to urban centres to receive abortion services.[12] According to Marie Stopes International, travel restrictions prevented women from obtaining maternity and post-abortion care or contraceptive services in Madagascar.[13]

The disrupted global manufacturing and supply chains as well as overwhelmed health facilities had a direct impact on the availability of reproductive health commodities, especially contraceptives and abortion pills, on the continent.[14] Most African countries do not manufacture pharmaceutical products and rely on global pharmaceutical manufacturers. The closure of boarders and trade restrictions worsened the disruption, leading to shortages and high cost of contraceptives.[15] The resultant effect was that women and girls found it challenging to use contraceptives, leading to an increase in unwanted pregnancies and resorting to unsafe abortions.[16]

The United Nations Population Fund (UNFPA) estimated that the pandemic interfered with contraceptive use for about 12 million women, resulting in as many as 2.7 million unintended pregnancies in its first year.[17] Evidence indicates that most women and girls with unwanted pregnancies would choose to terminate them safely.[18] However, in a pandemic situation where access to abortion services was withdrawn, most ended up in unsafe abortions.[19] Marie Stopes International estimated that 1.2 million unsafe abortions were procured in the first 6 months of the pandemic.

COVID-19 disproportionately affected minor and adolescent girls who had to spend long periods confined to their homes with no access to contraceptives and abortion care for those who became pregnant. According to a UNFPA global survey, mothers of adolescents are hesitant to speak about sexual and reproductive health and rights (SRHR) with their adolescent girls.[20] It was reported that some parents denied their adolescent girls permission to seek SRH services at health facilities.

The situation was worsened by the unavailability of youth-friendly services following closure and, in some cases, conversion of centres offering youth-friendly services into COVID-19 quarantine and recovery centres.[21] Furthermore, cases of pregnancy resulting from sexual abuse and violence increased, leading to high demand for abortion care and child marriages. In most African countries criminalizing access to abortion care even during pregnancy because of sexual violence or incest, many resorted to unsafe abortion.[22]

Moreover, the limitation of mobility through curfews and lockdowns made it difficult for adolescents and young women, including victims of sexual violence and abuse, to access emergency contraceptives. The rights of adolescents to manage their sexual and reproductive needs as well as any sexually related complications were also compromised.[23] In addition, laws and policies that require third-party authorization for adolescents to access contraceptives were listed as contributing factors to an increase in unwanted pregnancies and consequently resorting to unsafe abortion.[24],[25]

COVID-19 prevention measures adopted by governments increase the cost of seeking and accessing SRH services, making them unaffordable to many. The requirement for undertaking an expensive COVID-19 test and the prospect of being quarantined at your own cost discouraged women and girls from accessing safe abortion care in health facilities. Healthcare providers were forced to innovatively provide access to SRH services, particularly contraceptives and abortion care, through digital technologies that facilitate telemedicine.

Healthcare providers utilized online platforms to give information and deliver drugs to their clients. 'Telemedicine was encouraged as an intervention to provide services for safe and easy access to medical abortions, counselling, and screening to adolescents'.[26] Moreover, adolescent-friendly telephone conversation lines were created to provide additional information to adolescents on contraceptive availability and how to self-medicate and manage side effects.

At the onset of COVID-19, most governments either scaled down or totally withdrew SRH services, including abortion and post-abortion care, and considered them nonessential services.[27] The justification for withdrawal of services was to free up resources to manage the COVID-19 pandemic. Healthcare providers were also affected, with many being reassigned to COVID-19-related responses.[28] This decision was worsened by rising numbers of healthcare providers contracting and dying of COVID-19. The decision affected the availability of commodities as well as abortion and post-abortion services in primary health facilities. In Kenya, a report indicated that the lack of supplies, for instance, pregnancy test kits, delayed women and girls from identifying pregnancies, thus impacting their timely access to abortion services.[29]

The existence of COVID-19-related stigma, misinformation about what constitutes an essential health service, ended up amplifying the stigma that already surrounds abortion service, making it difficult for women and girls to access the service. A lack of information on the pandemic created uncertainty, making women and girls fear travelling to health facilities for SRH services. This was evident in Ethiopia, where reports indicated that most of the women who obtained abortion never visited health facilities due to the perception that abortion and post-abortion care were not included as essential health services.[30]

A further report indicated that due to inaccessibility of abortion and post-abortion care services, some women resorted to using medication abortion from pharmacies and chemist. In some cases, others self-managed the abortion at home and lacked follow-up care, while others resorted to abortions using local products or went to informal providers, had unsafe abortions, and experienced delays in getting help.[31]

The restriction of movement confined most people at home, which could have led to increased demand for sex among partners which might have increased disagreements and hence the risk of sexual coercion or unwanted sex.[32] There were also reports of women and girls being overburdened by household chores, including caring of children, the sick, and the elderly members of the society, that increased levels of stress and conflict with partners.[33] Sex-related violence against women was also reported as widespread in most countries, including rape, incest, and intimate partner violence, including marital rape and first sexual experiences that occur through coercion.[34] Acts of sexual violence generate unwanted pregnancies and the use, by victims, of unsafe abortion with its consequences such as psychological trauma.[35]

13.3 Transparency in COVID-19 pandemic

The COVID-19 pandemic undoubtedly brought to light the critical importance of transparency in managing and addressing major emergencies and crises. Transparency refers to the quality of being open, clear, and honest in communication, decision-making, and action. Whenever, the public is faced with an uncertain emergency or crises of the magnitude of the COVID-19 pandemic, they look up to their governments for guidance and assurance. During the COVID-19 pandemic, there was uncertainty that made the public to want to know what is happening, how it was to affect them, and what steps were being taken to control it. Without openness, it is impossible to provide this information, and the public is likely to be thrown into confusion or even panic.

Transparency is a concept that attracts a near universal acceptance as a norm, a principle, and a measure of conduct in society.[36] It has been linked to the right to access information, legalisation, legality, and good governance or effectiveness.[37] As a public health concept, transparency denotes the ability of stakeholders and the public to obtain accurate, timely, and relevant information about health issues. This definition can be expanded to encompass the need for openness and accountability of healthcare providers and policy-makers in providing information and services related to health care.

Transparency is critical in understanding and managing public health crises and pandemics such as COVID-19. It facilitates trust between governments, healthcare organizations, and the public during pandemics. By publishing and sharing accurate, understandable information about the virus' spread, severity, and management strategies, governments and healthcare organizations instil trust and confidence among the public. The trust, dispelling conspiracy theories and speculation, hence encourages individuals to adhere to preventive measures such as wearing masks, social distancing, and getting vaccinated.

At the start of the COVID-19 pandemic, most countries operated in an opaque manner, with little or no information being shared on containment measures and how essential healthcare services were to be accessed, resulting in misinformation, panic, confusion, and mistrust as most people resisted containment measures. However, as COVID-19 intensified, and following the publication of information guidelines by WHO on which services were essential, availability of treatment, distribution of protective equipment, and severity of the disease, government ministries of health begun to provide daily updates on COVID-19, numbers of those infected, hospitalizations, and fatalities.

With the lessons learnt from the COVID-19 pandemic, embracing transparency where authorities share accurate information about the virus, its spread, and the measures taken to control it, the public is more likely to comply with regulations and guidelines. Moreover, transparency ensures that people can make informed decisions about their health, such as seeking medical treatment or taking preventive measures to reduce their risk of contracting the virus. This includes having access to information about symptoms, testing, and vaccines.

Finally, transparency significantly reduces misinformation, rumours, and conspiracy theories that can harm public health efforts. Availing accurate and timely information ensures that people are less likely to believe false claims and more probable to follow guidelines to protect themselves and others. Transparent communication promotes equality and non-discriminatory access to information about the virus and public health measures. This is important for marginalized communities who may be disproportionately affected by the pandemic. Transparency holds governments and health authorities accountable for their actions and decisions during the pandemic and allows the public to monitor and evaluate government responses to the crisis and advocates for better policies.

13.4 Normative frameworks for transparency

In the context of human rights and access to abortion laws and policies, transparency is a pivotal tool in guaranteeing legal certainty that ensures laws are 'knowable and stable so that people can adjust their behaviour accordingly', more so when dealing with criminal laws regulating certain conduct without stating explicitly and definitely what conduct is punishable. Transparency can be equated to a process that ensures that effects of a legal instrument are readily understandable, and the scope of its derivative rights and obligations is easy to assess for the addressee and rights-holders.[38]

Moreover, transformative transparency can be interpreted as a concept or principle that promotes fundamental freedoms and human rights. Drawing on the concept of reproductive justice, transparency can be argued as a tool that promotes women's decisional security in accessing reproductive health rights, including abortion service and realization of gender equality and non-discrimination. Transparency can be applied to secure abortion as a fundamental right and to vindicate women accessing the service as well as the healthcare provider offering abortion care.

While acknowledging the importance of transparency in African states affairs, the African Commission updated the declaration on freedom of expression in 2019,[39] which had been adopted through a 2002 resolution, recognizing the right to access information held by public entities.[40] Furthermore, the Maputo Protocol, in General Comment 2, calls on states to ensure the provision of correct information, education, and awareness on SRH, namely contraception and abortion treatment. This appeal is carried out through the Maputo Plan of Action for the operationalization of the Sexual and Reproductive Health and Rights Continental Policy Framework initiative. The Plan of Action urges African states to take steps to enact abortion laws in the most expansive ways and to create awareness among healthcare practitioners and communities about the situations under which abortion is legal.[41]

Similarly, the Universal Declaration of Human Rights emphasizes the significance of transparency and accountability in public governance, including healthcare service delivery.[42] Article 19 acknowledges the right to freedom of expression, which includes the right to seek, receive, and share information and views about health and healthcare services. Furthermore, the UN Human Rights Committee published General Comment 26 on Article 19 of the International Covenant on Civil and Political Rights (ICCPR) in 2011, which specifically affirms that Article 19 encompasses a general right of access to information held by public institutions.[43]

The International Covenant on Economic, Social, and Cultural Rights (ICESCR)[44] is an important normative framework that recognizes everyone's right to the best health possible. Article 12 of the ICESCR emphasizes the need of transparency in the provision of healthcare services, including the availability of necessary information and education to guarantee that individuals may make the best healthcare choices. For example in General Comment 22 of the CESCR, the suggestion on access to accurate information emphasizes the importance of access to accurate information in the realization of economic, social, and cultural rights. It also establishes a framework for nations to implement policies that promote and defend access to information.

Article 16 of the International Convention on Elimination of All Forms of Discrimination Against Women (CEDAW)[45] guarantees women equal rights in deciding 'freely and responsibly on the number and spacing of their children and to have access to the information, education and means to enable them to exercise these rights'.

The UN Special Rapporteur on the right of everyone to the enjoyment of the highest attainable standard of physical and mental health has called on states to ensure accurate, evidence-based information regarding abortion and its legal availability.[46] Furthermore, the Special Rapporteur has reiterated that all individuals and groups have the right to access to evidence-based information on SRH, including safe abortion and post-abortion care.[47]

Furthermore, the information should be provided in accessible formats,[48] and states have a duty to ensure that information is available in a timely manner, in a form that is accessible to all, including those with disabilities, and in a language that is understood by the public. Finally, states have an obligation to allow health information, including abortion information, to flow freely without state interference on moral or other grounds.[49]

13.5 COVID-19-related and reproductive health injustice

While COVID-19 pandemic had a significant impact on reproductive health services, including access to abortion care, most governments exploited the pandemic to pass new anti-abortion laws or enforce existing laws more stringently.[50] Most countries imposed far-reaching restrictions on access to abortion services during the pandemic. These restrictions violate the right to reproductive health and placed women's lives at risk.

For instance, in Kenya, the government suspended all SRH services except those deemed emergencies. This move led to a significant decline in the number of women accessing abortion services.[51] In Nigeria, some states used the pandemic as an excuse to restrict access to abortion services. These restrictions extend to circumstances where pregnancy poses a danger to the woman's life, health, or, in cases of rape or incest, foetal anomaly.[52]

Furthermore, in most countries, abortion was deemed a non-essential service, and as a result, many clinics and hospitals that provide abortion care closed or reduced their services. This resulted in serious difficulty for women and girls accessing contraceptives and SRH information and education, including access to safe and legal abortion care for those with unwanted pregnancies. This is particular in areas where there are already legal restrictions and limited resources for reproductive health services.

In addition to limiting access to abortion care, governments' COVID-19 response and containment measures have also perpetuated reproductive health injustice by exacerbating existing inequalities. For example, individuals who are already marginalized, such as women with disability, adolescent girls, and women living in rural and remote areas, may face additional barriers to accessing abortion care during the pandemic. These women and girls live in areas where abortion services are limited or areas that have limited access to transportation.

Moreover, the pandemic also led to a decrease in funding for reproductive health services, including abortion care. Most African governments redirected resources to address the pandemic, which resulted in less or no funding for other health services, including reproductive health services. This made it even more difficult for individuals to access the care they needed, particularly in areas where resources were already limited.

13.6 African regional human rights norms

Similar to the international human rights law, African human rights legal instruments place a duty on states to mitigate any discriminatory impacts of their emergency responses. While states may justify their actions when faced with extraordinary public health crises such as COVID-19, certain fundamental rights, such as access to health, cannot be derogated from. According to the Human Rights Council and the Siracusa Principles, states are under an obligation to ensure that any public health measures taken that limit individuals' rights and freedoms must be lawful, necessary, and proportionate and cannot have a discriminatory impact on specific persons or marginalized groups.[53],[54] According to WHO, 'the right to the highest attainable standard of health' implies a clear set of legal obligations on states to ensure appropriate conditions for the enjoyment of health for all people without discrimination.[55]

Access to health is provided for under various human rights instruments at the continental level. The African Charter on Human and Peoples' Rights (the Charter)[56] affirms the right to health, including reproductive health, as an integral component of the right to life, dignity, and well-being.[57] The Charter recognizes women's right to health, which extends to reproductive healthcare services, including safe and legal access to abortion.[58]

The Charter prohibits any form of discrimination based on sex, gender, and any other status or medical condition, in the enjoyment of the right to health.[59] This includes ensuring that women have equal access to reproductive health services, including abortion care of high quality. The Charter requires that states take measures to safeguard the reproductive health rights of women, including through funding and implementing comprehensive reproductive health policies that promote safe and legal abortions.

Moreover, Article 16 of the Charter protects women against harmful medical practices, particularly female genital mutilation, early and forced marriages, and, in general, any form of exploitation or coercion that deprives women of their human rights. The protection against harmful medical practices explicitly includes abortion when it is not conducted according to medical standards, including when it is done in unsafe conditions, which can lead to severe health consequences.

The African Commission is a regional body established under the African Charter with a mandate to promote and protect human rights across the African continent.[60] The African Commission receives and investigates complaints of violations and abuses committed by state parties to the Charter.[61] In case of a violation of the Charter, the Commission may issue recommendations to the state parties, urging them to take corrective measures, provide reparations to the victims, and implement the provisions of the Charter fully. The Commission plays a crucial role in advancing the sexual and reproductive rights of women on the continent. It has adopted important resolutions and general comments relating to the SRHR of women in the region.

With regard to the COVID-19 pandemic, the African Commission issued a statement in June 2020, calling on African states to ensure that SRH services, including abortion care, are considered essential services and access to them is protected even during the pandemic.[62] The Commission urged states to eliminate legal barriers that impede access to abortion care and ensure that health facilities providing these services are adequately resourced, with trained health personnel, to provide safe and quality abortion care.[63] The Commission also urged states to ensure access to relevant information and access to safe SRH care services; protect adolescents, particularly girls, from domestic and sexual violence; and ensure that their access to SRH services is not disrupted.[64]

The African Charter on the Rights and Welfare of a Child[65] is another important instrument protecting children's rights to health, including reproductive health. The Children's Charter is a legally binding instrument that protects the rights of children and adolescents in Africa. The Children's Charter recognizes the right of children and adolescents to access contraceptives and abortion care.[66]

Furthermore, Article 14 obligates states to 'take all appropriate measures to ensure that children and adolescents have access to appropriate information and services in order to protect them from unwanted pregnancies and sexually transmitted infections'. Moreover, states have a duty to take 'all appropriate measures to ensure that children and adolescents have access to safe and effective methods of contraception'.

Similarly, Article 16 of the Children's Charter protects children against abuse and torture and includes adolescents' rights to access contraceptive and legal abortion services, especially children who are victims of sexual violence and abuse. Moreover, state parties to the Charter have a duty to ensure adolescents are provided with appropriate information and counselling on the risks and consequences of unsafe abortion.

In the context of the COVID-19 pandemic, adolescent girls faced the challenge of a legal requirement for parental consent or third-party authorization. The African Commission has elaborated that 'article 14 of the Maputo Protocol requires that states formulate precise standards and guidelines for health providers, stating that the consent of parents and their authorisation is not required for the minor to access contraceptive or abortion care'.[67]

In 2021, the African Committee of Experts on the Rights and Welfare of the Child (ACERWC) published General Comment 7, in which it elaborates that the age of consent should not hinder adolescents' access to SRH services.[68] During the COVID-19 pandemic, it was reported that parents avoided providing sexuality information and education to their adolescent girls and barred them from seeking SRH services; existence of laws and policies on third-party authorization can be an impediment to adolescent access to abortion care.

While many countries do not provide child- and adolescent-friendly services, including abortion care to minors who are survivors of sexual abuse and violence, ACERWC calls on states to provide emergency contraception and safe termination of pregnancies for minors and adolescents.[69] The reason is that girls in child marriages are at a high risk of pregnancy-related health complications, and medical abortion in the instances contemplated by Article 14 (2) (c) must be provided.[70]

A more specific regional human rights instrument protecting the rights of women is the Protocol to the African Charter on Human and Peoples' Rights on the Rights of Women in Africa (Maputo Protocol).[71] Article 14 of the Maputo Protocol guarantees women the right to health, including SRH. The protocol identifies women's rights to SRH to include 'the right to control their fertility, the right to decide the number of children and the spacing of children, the right to choose any method of contraception, and the right to have family planning education'.[72]

Significantly, Article 14 (2) (c) of the Maputo Protocol provides for medical abortion in cases of sexual assault, rape, incest, and where the continued pregnancy endangers the mental and physical health of the mother or the life of the mother or the foetus.[73] The article is a critical tool that facilitates protection and promotion of women's and girls' rights to access abortion and post-abortion services during a public health emergency such as COVID-19. The provisions underscore the importance of ensuring that women can access critical medical services and that governments should take proactive action to guarantee access even in times of pandemics such as COVID-19.

Unlike the clawback on access to abortion that was witnessed in many states in the US, Africa countries like Sierra Leone enacted legislation that domesticated provisions of the Maputo Protocol on abortion. Moreover, various countries have domesticated the Maputo Protocol which played a vital role in ensuring that women and girls accessed abortion care, particularly those who were victims of sexual violence and abuse during the COVID-19 pandemic.

Moreover, the Maputo Protocol addresses stigma and discrimination in relation to access to abortion care and post-abortion care where state parties are required to remove impediments to health services reserved for women, including ideology- or belief-based barriers. States must ensure that 'administrative laws, policies and procedures of health systems and structures cannot restrict access to contraceptives and abortion care based on religious beliefs. Stigma and discrimination are significant barriers to access to abortion care, as evidenced during COVID-19, where services such as abortion care required only by women were non-essentialized.[74]

13.6.1 General comment 2

To provide more transparency on Article 14(2)(c) of the Maputo Protocol, the African Commission adopted General Comment 2, which provides interpretive guidance to state parties on the overall and specific obligations towards effective implementation of rights to abortion as envisaged in the Protocol.[75] The General Comment emphasizes the importance of state parties ensuring that women and girls have access to information and education on contraceptives and abortion care, particularly adolescent girls. In addition, state parties must ensure that educational institutions at primary, secondary, and tertiary levels include SRH education in their school programmes.[76]

13.6.2 General states' obligations

Under the obligation to respect, state parties are required to refrain from hindering, directly or indirectly, women's rights and to ensure that women are duly informed about abortion services. State parties are to ensure availability, accessibility, acceptability, and good-quality reproductive health care, including safe and legal abortion care for women. Moreover, state parties have a duty to ensure services that are comprehensive, integrated, rights-based, sensitive to the reality of women in all contexts, and adapted to women with disabilities and youth, free from any coercion, discrimination, and violence.[77]

Therefore, state parties have a duty to recognize that access to abortion care is an essential healthcare service and, hence, ensure that these services are available even in times of public health emergencies such as the COVID-19 pandemic. This means allocating adequate resources, including human resources, medical supplies, and equipment, to ensure that service provision is not interrupted, particularly during a public health emergency.

Closely related to the COVID-19 pandemic is the requirement for the state parties to take necessary measures to prevent third parties from interfering with the enjoyment of women's sexual and reproductive rights. This is specific to the rights of vulnerable groups such as adolescent girls, women with disabilities, those with HIV/AIDS, and women in situations of conflict. The obligation entails the formulation of standards and guidelines clearly highlighting that the consent and involvement of third parties, including, but not limited to, parents, guardians, spouses, and partners, should not be invoked where adolescents and adult women are seeking contraception and safe abortion services in the cases provided for in the Protocol.[78]

With regard to the promotion obligation, state parties are 'to create legal, economic, and social conditions that enable women to exercise their sexual and reproductive rights in relation to contraception and safe abortion, as well as to enjoy them'. This is an essential step towards eliminating stigma and discrimination related to reproductive health, which includes, but is not limited to, supporting women's empowerment, sensitizing, and educating communities, religious leaders, traditional chiefs, and political leaders on women's sexual and reproductive rights including abortion, as well as training healthcare workers.[79]

Furthermore, the obligation to fulfil rights requires that state parties adopt relevant laws, policies, and programmes that ensure the fulfilment de jure and de facto of women's sexual and reproductive rights, including the allocation of sufficient and available resources for the full realization of those rights.[80] Therefore, policies must be established that ensure women can access safe and legal abortion care without being exposed to additional risks of infection with COVID-19. This can be realized by availing additional resources for telehealth services to allow women to consult with healthcare providers and receive medication abortion care in a safe and convenient manner. The supply chain and manufacturing sector was severely affected by the COVID-19 pandemic. Thus, the general comment is very relevant as it emphasizes the availability of supplies through procurement systems that function properly to guarantee access to SRH commodities to all women, especially rural women.

Likewise, the general comment elaborates on the duty of state parties to ensure availability, accessibility, and acceptability of procedures, technologies, and comprehensive and good-quality services, using technologies based on clinical findings. This guide is useful in the context of the COVID-19 pandemic where healthcare organizations and their clients capitalized on technology to continue providing services despite disruptions, for instance, the use of telemedicine and self-medication for abortion care. Telemedicine can be a useful tool for providing abortion care during a pandemic, and governments need to explore ways of expanding access to telemedicine for abortion care, including through the adoption of telemedicine regulations and guidelines.

Furthermore, the general comment elaborates that abortion care services should include the methods recommended by WHO-updated guidelines and be based on clinical findings, including procedures. Moreover, the equipment and medicines recommended by WHO should be included in the lists of national essential products and medicines. With the new WHO abortion care guidelines of 2022 recommending self-medication through medical abortion, states have a duty to ensure availability of misoprostol and mifepristone, provide accurate information on its use, and train healthcare providers to ensure that women who choose this method can terminate pregnancy safely.[81]

Finally, the general comment calls on state parties' duty to avoid all unnecessary or irrelevant restrictions on the profile of the healthcare providers authorized to practise safe abortion and the requirements of multiple signatures or approval of committees in the cases provided for in the Protocol. The call on state parties is most relevant to the COVID-19 pandemic context which experienced an accurate shortage of healthcare providers due to the overstretched health system under the COVID-19 patient load. Most women and girls opted to use midwives and traditional healers. Equipping these cadres of healthcare providers with training and competencies to offer abortion care in an environment that is conducive is vital to ensuring the availability of safe abortion care services to women and girls.

Finally, the African Union adopted a comprehensive framework for the promotion of women's rights and gender equality in Africa. The Maputo Plan of Action 2016–2030 is a Sexual and Reproductive Health and Rights Continental Policy Framework that seeks to take the continent forward towards the goal of universal access to comprehensive sexual and reproductive health services in Africa beyond 2015. The framework was adopted by the African Union in 2016 and is named after the city of Maputo, Mozambique, where it was signed.[82] One key area of focus in the framework is the protection of women's reproductive rights, including their right to access safe and legal abortion care and services. The plan recognizes unsafe abortion as a major public health issue in Africa and that women and girls who are denied access to safe and legal abortion services are at risk of serious health complications and even death.

13.7 United Nations Human Rights mechanism

Abortion care is a fundamental human right that is recognized by several regional and international human rights normative frameworks. The COVID-19 pandemic, on the other hand, posed significant difficulties to the right to health, including access to abortion care. Although not explicitly recognized, international human rights frameworks such as the ICCPR,[83] CEDAW,[84] and ICESCR[85] recognize the right to abortion services. Most African countries have ratified these international human rights treaties and incorporated them into their national legal systems.

Although the ICESCR outlines various rights, including the right to health,[86] it does not directly include the right to abortion. However, the committee charged with the mandate of implementing the ICESCR, through General Comment 22, has stated that 'states have a core obligation to ensure, at the very least, minimum essential levels of satisfaction of the right to sexual and reproductive health, including measures to prevent unsafe abortion'.[87] The general comment is relevant to the right to abortion care because it defines governments' duty to guarantee that women have access to abortion services that are safe, legal, and affordable, as well as comprehensive information about the procedure and post-abortion care.[88] The Human Rights Committee issued a statement on the right to access abortion services in the context of the pandemic. Through the statement, they reaffirmed that 'states must ensure that women and girls have access to safe and legal abortion services, including in the context of the COVID-19 pandemic'.

The Committee on the Rights of the Child has recommended that 'states ensure access to safe abortion and post-abortion care services, irrespective of whether abortion itself is legal'.[89] Similarly, the Committee on the Rights of the Child has emphasized the right of the child, in accordance with evolving capacities, to confidential counselling and to access to information without parental or guardian consent.[90] It has also recommended that 'states should review and consider allowing children to consent to certain medical treatments and interventions without the permission of a parent, caregiver, or guardian, such as HIV testing and sexual and reproductive health services, including education and guidance on sexual health, contraception and safe abortion'.[91]

13.8 Self-management and medical abortion care

It is predicted that the world shall experience a shortage of up to 18 million health workers by the year 2030, with low- and middle-income countries shouldering most of the shortage.[92] The COVID-19 pandemic made this projection almost certain when routine health services were disrupted and existing health systems were overwhelmed. Telemedicine and self-medication played a key role in ensuring continuation of access to health services despite COVID-19-related limitation on mobility coupled with the fear of contracting the virus. Most healthcare organizations embraced telemedicine and self-medication to reach clients, especially with medical abortion care services.

Medical abortion care involves taking two pills, mifepristone and misoprostol, to terminate a pregnancy. Mifepristone blocks the hormone progesterone that is essential for sustaining a pregnancy, while misoprostol induces contractions to expel the embryo or foetus. The medication has a success rate of 95–98%, thus a viable option for women who are in their first 10 weeks of pregnancy.[93] Adopting medical abortion through self-management has the potential to significantly improve access to safe, timely, affordable, and person-centred abortion care. Mifepristone and misoprostol regimens have enormous potential for reproductive health care, including in addressing geographic disparities in abortion services.

WHO abortion care guidelines recommend that in the first 12 weeks of pregnancy, a medical abortion can be safely self-managed by the pregnant person outside of a healthcare facility in whole or in part.[94] The guide recommends that the woman, girl, or other pregnant person have access to accurate information, quality medicine, and support from a trained health worker (just in case they need or want it during the process).[95]

Self-management approaches are empowering for women because of their non-invasive nature and because they safeguard women's right to privacy and autonomy. This cannot be said of the surgical abortion because medication abortion does not require any medical instruments or anaesthesia. The pills are taken orally or vaginally at home, and the process of termination occurs naturally. This reduces the stress and stigma associated with a clinic visit and allows women to maintain their privacy and control over their bodies.[96]

In addition, medication abortion presents low risk of complications. Evidence indicates that although rare, serious complications, such as infection or haemorrhage, occur in less than 0.3% of cases. In contrast, surgical abortion carries a higher risk of injury to the cervix or uterus, and, in rare cases, requires hospitalization. Medication abortion is also associated with less pain and a shorter recovery time compared to surgical abortion.

To guarantee women and girls even safer self-management of medical abortion, it is imperative that African countries adopt health policy reforms that ensures greater transparency on legal position bearing in mind that WHO already approved and recommended medical abortion as a safe pregnancy termination method. Firstly, improving access will mean decriminalizing and destigmatizing abortion and registering medicines involved and dispensing at a reasonable price. Secondly, providers should be trained to offer medication abortion support as part of comprehensive abortion care and provide accurate information and counselling to patients.[97]

13.9 Conclusion

Africa has an enabling legal and policy framework that protects access to the best attainable standards of health that includes reproductive health and access to abortion. The African Charter on Human and People's Rights guarantees that women have safe and legal access to abortion as part of their right to health. This is critical to realizing the reproductive rights of women and girls, promoting gender equality, and advancing their overall health and well-being. State parties to the Charter must, therefore, take measures to ensure that women have access to safe and legal abortion services, and provide comprehensive reproductive health services that meet international human rights standards.

African governments should embrace telemedicine and self-managed medication abortion through health policy reforms, particularly for women living in rural or remote areas, who face transportation barriers or have limited access to clinics. Telemedicine, where patients receive medical advice and support via a telephone or video link, has been proven to be as safe and effective as clinic-based care. Self-managed medication abortion, where women can obtain and use pills without direct medical supervision, is also feasible and safe when provided with comprehensive instructions and follow-up care. Telemedicine surmounts many of the barriers created by the COVID-19 pandemic. However, the success of medical abortion lies with governments' acceptance of registration and inclusion of mifepristone and misoprostol on their national essential medicine lists and work towards procurement of these medications.

The concept of transparency as applied to access to health, including abortion rights, is crucial during public health emergencies like COVID-19 as it supports openness and accountability, especially in protecting fundamental rights that cannot be derogated by a crisis or pandemic. Preparedness for a crisis or a pandemic is key to sustaining access to health, particularly SRH. African countries should not continue being unprepared and unresponsive to public health emergencies and resort to limiting fundamental human rights such as access to safe and legal abortion, and governments must pick up important lessons.

Notes

1 K Tang 'SRH: A key issue in the emergency response to the coronavirus disease (COVID-19) outbreak' (2020) 17(1) *Reproductive Health* 59.
2 A Bankole et al 'From unsafe to safe abortion in sub-Saharan Africa: Slow but steady progress' *Guttmacher Institute* (2020).
3 As above.
4 World Health Organization 'WHO Director-General's opening remarks at the mission briefing on COVID-19' available at www.who.int/dg/speeches/detail/who-director-general-s-opening-remarks-at-the-mission- briefing-on-COVID-19 (accessed 12 March 2023).
5 L Lopez et al 'Racial and ethnic health disparities related to COVID-19' (2021) 325 *JAMA* 719–20.
6 VK Chattu & S Yaya 'Emerging infectious diseases and outbreaks: Implications for women's reproductive health and rights in resource-poor settings' (2020) 17(1) *Reproductive Health*.
7 Brooks SK et al 'The psychological impact of quarantine and how to reduce it: Rapid review of the evidence' (2020) 395 *Lancet*.
8 M Lokot & Y Avakyan 'Intersectionality as a lens to the COVID-19 pandemic: Implications for SRH in development and humanitarian context' (2020) 28(1) *SRH Matters*.
9 E Igonya et al 'Impact of the COVID-19 Pandemic on SRH Services in Burkina Faso, Ethiopia, Kenya, Malawi, and Uganda' *African Population Health and Research Centre* (2021) available at https://aphrc.org/wp-content/uploads/2022/05/APHRC-COVID-Report-PRINT.pdf
10 A Seme et al 'Impact of the COVID-19 pandemic on adolescent SRH in Ethiopia' *New York* (2021) available at www.guttmacher.org/report/impact-COVID-19-on-adolescent-srh-ethiopia (accessed 11 February 2023).
11 CB Polis et al 'Impacts of COVID-19 on contraceptive and abortion services in low- and middle-income countries: A scoping review' (2022) 30(1) *Sexual and Reproductive Health Matters*.
12 SRT Chilunjika et al 'The COVID-19 pandemic and sexual reproductive health needs of women and adolescent girls in Zimbabwe' (2022) 8(1–2) *International Journal of Behavioural and Health Research* 59–73.
13 Marie Stopes International available at www.msichoices.org/covid-19/stories-from-the-frontline/ (accessed 10 December 2022).
14 L Lee 'COVID-19: World's biggest condom producer warns of global shortage' *Global News* (2020) available at https://globalnews.ca/news/6743979/condom-shortage-coronavirus/ (accessed 10 January 2023).
15 T Riley et al 'Estimates of the potential impact of the COVID-19 pandemic on sexual and reproductive health in low-and middle-income countries' (2020) 46 *International Perspectives on Sexual and Reproductive Health* 73–76.
16 V Sharma 'Why the promotion of family planning makes more sense now than ever before? (2020) 22(2) *Journal of Health Management* 206–214.
17 UNFPA 'Impact of COVID-19 on family planning: What we know one year into the pandemic' *Technical Not Information* as of 11 March 2021.

18 MH Asratie 'Unintended pregnancy during COVID-19 pandemic among women attending antenatal care in Northwest Ethiopia: Magnitude and associated factors' (2021) 13 *International Journal of Women's Health* 461.
19 As above.
20 United Nations Population Fund (UNFPA) 'The impact of COVID-19 on women and girls with disabilities' (2021) available at www.unfpa.org/featured-publication/impact-COVID-19-women-and-girls-disabilities (accessed 20 February 2023).
21 K Church et al 'Reproductive health under COVID-19 – challenges of responding to a global crisis' (2020) 28(1) *Sexual and Reproductive Health Matters*.
22 S Meherali et al 'Impact of the COVID-19 pandemic on adolescents' sexual and reproductive health in low- and middle-income countries' (2021) 18(24) *International Journal of Environmental Research and Public Health* 13221.
23 United Nations Children's Fund 'COVID-19: A threat to progress against child marriage' *UNICEF* (2021) available at https://data.unicef.org/resources/covid-19-a-threat-to-progress-against-child-marriage/ (accessed January 2023).
24 G Nalwadda 'Persistent high fertility in Uganda: Young people recount obstacles and enabling factors to use of contraceptives' (2010) 10 *BMC Public Health* 1–13.
25 K Wood & R Jewkes 'Blood blockages and scolding nurses: Barriers to adolescent contraceptive use in South Africa' (2006) 14 *Reproductive Health Matters* 109–118.
26 United Nations Population Funds 'Not on pause: Responding to the SRH needs of adolescents in the context of the COVID-19 crisis' available at www.unfpa.org/sites/default/files/resource-pdf/Not_on_Pause.pdf (accessed 10 February March 2023).
27 E Igonya et al 'Impact of the COVID-19 pandemic on sexual and reproductive health services in Burkina Faso, Ethiopia, Kenya, Malawi and Uganda' (2021) available at https://aphrc.org/wp-content/uploads/2022/05/APHRC-COVID-Report-PRINT.pdf (accessed February 2023).
28 M Okereke et al 'Impact of COVID-19 on access to healthcare in low- and middle-income countries: Current evidence and future recommendations' (2020) 36(1) *International Journal of Health Planning and Management* 13–17.
29 S Gichuna et al 'Access to healthcare in a time of COVID-19: Sex workers in crisis in Nairobi, Kenya' (2020) 15(10) *Global Public Health* 1430–1442.
30 K Temesgen et al 'The impact of COVID-19 infection on maternal and reproductive health care services in governmental health institutions of Dessie town, North-East Ethiopia' *G.C. medRxiv* (2020).
31 R Both et al 'I feel that things are out of my hands: How COVID-19 prevention measures have affected young people's SRH in Ghana, Indonesia, Kenya, Nepal, Uganda and Zimbabwe' *Utrecht: Rutgers* (2021).
32 A Peterman et al 'Pandemics and violence against women and children' *Center for Global Development* (2021).
33 WHO 'Addressing violence against children, women and older people during the COVID-19 pandemic: Key actions' in *COVID-19: Risk communication and community engagement* (2020).
34 J Chandra 'COVID-19 lockdown: Rise in domestic violence, police apathy: NCW' *The Hindu* available at www.thehindu.com/news/national/COVID-19-lockdown-spike-in-domestic-violence-says-ncw/article31238659.ece (accessed 12 February 2023).
35 G Barbara et al 'Characteristics of sexual violence against adolescent girls: A 10 years' retrospective study of 731 sexually abused adolescents' (2022) 14 *International Journal of Womens Health* 311–312.
36 A Bianchi & A Peters 'On power and illusion: The concept of transparency in international law' in A. Bianchi & A Peters (eds) *Transparency in international law* (2013) 2.

37 J Farrall 'United Nations sanctions and the rule of law' (2007) 40.
38 C Hood 'Transparency in historical perspective' in C Hood & D Heald (eds) *Transparency: The key to better government?* (2006) 5 and 14.
39 www.achpr.org/public/Document/file/English/Declaration%20of%20Principles%20on%20Freedom%20of%20Expression_ENG_2019.pdf (accessed 1 March 2022)
40 Art 19 *Declaration of principles on freedom of expression in Africa* 22 October 2002.
41 CG Ngwena 'Reforming African abortion laws and practice: The place of transparency' in RJ Cook et al (eds) *Abortion laws in transnational perspective: Cases and controversies* (2014).
42 UN General Assembly *Universal declaration of human rights* 10 December 1948, 217 A (III).
43 International Covenant on Civil and Political Rights CCPR/C/GC/34 General Comment No. 34 (12 September 2011).
44 UN General Assembly *International covenant on economic, social and cultural rights* 16 December 1966 United Nations, Treaty Series, vol. 993, p. 3.
45 UN General Assembly, Convention on the Elimination of All Forms of Discrimination Against Women, 18 December 1979, United Nations, Treaty Series, vol. 1249, p. 13.
46 UN Special Rapporteur on the right of everyone to the enjoyment of the highest attainable standard of physical and mental health, Interim Report to the General Assembly (2011) (UN Doc. A/66/254).
47 UN CESCR 'General comment no. 22: Article 12 of the international covenant on economic, social and cultural rights' (2016) (UN Doc. E/C/12/GC/22).
48 UN General Assembly 'Convention on the rights of persons with disabilities: Resolution/adopted by the general assembly' 24 January 2007, A/RES/61/106 Art 6; UN CRPD, General Comment No. 3 (2016) (UN Doc. CRPD/C/GC/3).
49 Report of the United Nations Working Group on the issue of discrimination against women in law and in practice (2016) (UN Doc. A/HRC/32/44).
50 Guttmacher Institute 'COVID-19 state policy update' (2021) available at www.guttmacher.org/article/2021/01/covid-19-state-policy-update (accessed 15 December 2022).
51 G Zulaika et al 'Impact of COVID-19 lockdowns on adolescent pregnancy and school dropout among secondary schoolgirls in Kenya (2022) 7 *BMJ Global Health*.
52 Ipas Nigeria 'Impact of COVID-19 Lockdown on Access to Safe Abortion in Nigeria' (2021).
53 UN Human Rights Committee 'General comment no. 29' UN Doc. CCPR/C/21/Rev.1/Add.11, 2001 available at http://ccprcentre.org/ccpr-general-comments (accessed 18 February 2023).
54 UN Commission on Human Rights 'Siracusa principles on the limitation and derogation provisions in the international covenant on civil and political rights, annex' UN Doc. E/CN.4/1985/4, 1984 available at https://undocs.org/en/E/CN.4/1985/4 (accessed 18 February 2023).
55 WHO 'Human rights' available at www.who.int/news-room/fact-sheets/detail/human-rights-and-health
56 Organisation of African Unity (OAU), African Charter on Human and Peoples' Rights ("Banjul Charter"), (African Charter) 27 June 1981, CAB/LEG/67/3 rev. 5, 21 I.L.M. 58 (1982), art 16 (accessed 17 March 2023).
57 As above.
58 As above, art 16.
59 As above, art 2 and art 18.
60 African Charter on Human and Peoples' Rights ("Banjul Charter"), 27 June 1981, OAU Doc CAB/LEG/67/3 rev. 5, 1520 UNTS 217, entered into force on October 211986.

61 Organisation of African Unity (OAU), (n 57 above) art 30 &45.
62 Special Rapporteur on the Rights of Women in Africa, Press Release of the Special Rapporteur on the Rights of Women in Africa on violation of women's rights during the COVID-19 Pandemic, African Commission on Human and People's Rights available at www.achpr.org/pressrelease/detail?id=495 (accessed 6 January 2023).
63 Resolution on Human and Peoples' Rights as the central pillar of successful response to COVID-19 and recovery from its socio-political impacts-ACHPR/Res. 449 (LXVI) 2020
64 As above.
65 Organisation of African Unity (OAU), African Charter on the Rights and Welfare of the Child, 11 July 1990, CAB/LEG/24.9/49 (1990) (accessed 17 March 2023).
66 As above.
67 African Commission on Human and Peoples' Rights. General Comment No. 2 on Article 14.1 (a), (b), (c) and (f) and Article 14. 2 (a) and (c) of the Protocol to the African Charter on Human and Peoples' Rights on the Rights of Women in Africa (2014).
68 African Committee of Experts on the Rights and Welfare of the Child (ACERWC). General Comment No. 7 on article 27 on Sexual Exploitation of the African Charter on the Rights and Welfare of the Child (2021).
69 As above
70 Ipas Nigeria Impact (n 52 above).
71 Protocol to the African Charter on Human and Peoples' Rights on the Rights of Women in Africa, adopted 11 July 2003 (Maputo Protocol).
72 Ipas Nigeria Impact (n 52 above).
73 African Commission on Human and Peoples' Rights, Protocol to the African Charter on Human and Peoples' Rights on the Rights of Women in Africa (Maputo Protocol), art 14 (2) (a) (2003).
74 As above.
75 General Comment No. 2 on art 14 (2) (a) and (c) of the Protocol to the African Charter on Human and Peoples' Rights on the Rights of Women in Africa (2014).
76 As above.
77 As above, para 42.
78 As above, para 43.
79 As above, para 44.
80 As above, para 45.
81 WHO 'WHO consolidated guidelines on self-care interventions for health: SRH and rights' (2019) available at www.who.int/reproductivehealth/publications/self-care-interventions/en/ (accessed 10 March 2023).
82 African Union Commission 'Maputo plan of action 2016–2030 for the operationalisation of the continental policy framework for SRH and rights, Addis Ababa: African Union Commission' available at https://au.int/sites/default/files/documents/30358-doc-mpoa_7-_revised_au_stc_inputs_may_se-rob-director_002.pdf (accessed 20 January 2023).
83 UN General Assembly *International covenant on civil and political rights* 16 December 1966, United Nations, Treaty Series, vol. 999, p. 171.
84 UN General Assembly (n 46 above).
85 International Covenant on Economic, Social and Cultural Rights (ICESCR), adopted 16 December 1966, art. 15 (1), G.A. Res. 2200A (XXI), U.N. GAOR, Supp. No. 16, U.N. Doc. A/6316 (1966) (entered into force on Jan. 3, 1976).
86 UN CESCR 'General comment no. 14, para 44' UN Doc. E/C.12/2000/4, 2000. Also see; www.escr-net.org/resources/general-comment-14.
87 Committee on Economic, Social and Cultural Rights 'General comment no. 22: On the right to SRH (Art. 12 of the international covenant on economic, social and cultural rights)' U.N. Doc. E/C.12/GC/22, para 49.

88 As above.
89 General Comment No. 15 (2013) on the right of the child to the enjoyment of the highest attainable standard of health, para 70. Also see, Special Rapporteur on the right of everyone to the enjoyment of the highest attainable standard of physical and mental health, A/HRC/32/32 (2016), para 113 (b).
90 Convention on the Rights of the Child General Comment No. 15 (2013) on the right of the child to the enjoyment of the highest attainable standard of health (art. 24).
91 UN Committee on the Rights of the Child (CRC) 'General comment no. 15 (2013) on the right of the child to the enjoyment of the highest attainable standard of health (art. 24)' 17 April 2013, CRC/C/GC/15, para 31
92 WHO 'Health workforce' available at www.who.int/health-topics/health-workforce#tab=tab_1 (accessed 3 March 2023).
93 P Blumenthal et al 'Providing medical abortion in low-resource settings' *Gynuity Health Projects* (2009) available at http://gynuity.org/resources/info/medical-abortion-guidebook/.
94 'Fact sheet: Self-care health interventions' available at www.who.int/news-room/fact-sheets/detail/self-care-healthinterventions.
95 As above.
96 (n 94 above).
97 As above.

Bibliography

Books and journals

A Bankole et al 'From Unsafe to Safe Abortion in Sub-Saharan Africa: Slow but Steady Progress' (2020) *Guttmacher Institute*.

A Bianchi & A Peters 'On Power and Illusion: The Concept of Transparency in International Law' in A Bianchi & A Peters (eds) *Transparency in International Law* (2013).

A Peterman et al 'Pandemics and Violence against Women and Children' (2021) *Center for Global Development*.

A Seme et al 'Impact of the COVID-19 Pandemic on Adolescent Sexual and Reproductive Health in Ethiopia' (2021) *New York*.

C Hood 'Transparency in Historical Perspective' in C Hood & D Heald (eds) *Transparency: The Key to Better Government?* (2006) 5 and14.

CB Polis et al 'Impacts of COVID-19 on Contraceptive and Abortion Services in Low- and Middle-Income Countries: A Scoping Review, Sexual and Reproductive' (2022) 30(1) *Health Matters*.

CG Ngwena 'Reforming African Abortion Laws and Practice: The Place of Transparency' in RJ Cook et al (eds) *Abortion Laws in Transnational Perspective: Cases and Controversies* (2014).

G Barbara et al 'Characteristics of Sexual Violence against Adolescent Girls: A 10 Years' Retrospective Study of 731 Sexually Abused Adolescents' (2022) 14 *International Journal of Women's Health* 311–312.

G Nalwadda 'Persistent High Fertility in Uganda: Young People Recount Obstacles and Enabling Factors to Use of Contraceptives' (2010) 10 *BMC Public Health* 1–13.

G Zulaika et al 'Impact of COVID-19 Lockdowns on Adolescent Pregnancy and School Dropout among Secondary Schoolgirls in Kenya' (2022) 7 *BMJ Glob Health*.

GD Kangaude et al 'Integrating Child Rights Standards in Contraceptive and Abortion Care for Minors in Africa' (2022) *International Journal of Gynecology & Obstetrics* 1–7.

J Chandra 'COVID-19 Lockdown: Rise in Domestic Violence, Police Apathy: NCW' *The Hindu*.

J Farrall *United Nations Sanctions and the Rule of Law* (2007) 40.

K Church et al 'Reproductive Health Under COVID-19 – Challenges of Responding to a Global Crisis' (2020) 28(1) *Sexual and Reproductive Health Matters*.

K Tang 'SRH: A Key Issue in the Emergency Response to the Coronavirus Disease (COVID-19) Outbreak' (2020) 17(1) *Reproductive Health 59*.

K Temesgen et al 'The Impact of COVID-19 Infection on Maternal and Reproductive Health Care Services in Governmental Health Institutions of Dessie Town, North-East Ethiopia' (2020) *G.C. medRxiv*. Available at https://www.medrxiv.org/content/10.1101/2020.09.20.20198259v1.full

K Wood & R Jewkes 'Blood Blockages and Scolding Nurses: Barriers to Adolescent Contraceptive Use in South Africa (2006) 14 *Reproductive Health Matters* 109–118.

L Lee 'COVID-19: World's Biggest Condom Producer Warns of Global Shortage' (2020) *Global News*.

L Lopez et al 'Racial and Ethnic Health Disparities Related to COVID-19' (2021) 325 *JAMA* 719–720.

M Lokot & Y Avakyan 'Intersectionality as a Lens to the COVID-19 Pandemic: Implications for SRH in Development and Humanitarian Context' (2020) 28(1) *Sexual and Reproductive Health Matters*.

M Okereke et al 'Impact of COVID-19 on Access to Healthcare in Low- and Middle-Income Countries: Current Evidence and Future Recommendations' (2020) 36(1) *International Journal of Health Planning and Management* 13–17.

MH Asratie 'Unintended Pregnancy during COVID-19 Pandemic among Women Attending Antenatal Care in Northwest Ethiopia: Magnitude and Associated Factors' (2021) 13 *International Journal of Women's Health* 461.

P Blumenthal et al 'Providing Medical Abortion in Low-Resource Settings' (2009) *Gynuity Health Projects*.

R Both et al 'I Feel That Things Are Out of My Hands: How COVID-19 Prevention Measures Have Affected Young People's SRH in Ghana, Indonesia, Kenya, Nepal, Uganda and Zimbabwe' (2021) *Utrecht: Rutgers*.

RJ Cook 'Transparency in the Delivery of Lawful Abortion Services' (2009) 180(3) *CMAJ* 272–273.

RJ Cook et al (eds) *Abortion Laws in Transnational Perspective: Cases and Controversies* (2014).

S Gichuna et al 'Access to Healthcare in a Time of COVID-19: Sex Workers in Crisis in Nairobi, Kenya' (2020) 15(10) *Global Public Health* 1430–1442.

S Meherali et al 'Impact of the COVID-19 Pandemic on Adolescents' Sexual and Reproductive Health in Low- and Middle-Income Countries (2021) 18(24) *International Journal of Environment Research Public Health* 13221.

SK Brooks et al 'The Psychological Impact of Quarantine and How to Reduce It: Rapid Review of the Evidence' (2020) 395 *Lancet*.

SRT Chilunjika et al 'The COVID-19 Pandemic and Sexual Reproductive Health Needs of Women and Adolescent Girls in Zimbabwe' (2022) 8(1–2) *International Journal of Behavioural and Health Research* 59–73.

T Riley et al 'Estimates of the Potential Impact of the COVID-19 Pandemic on Sexual and Reproductive Health in Low- and Middle-Income Countries' (202) 46 *International Perspective on Sex Reproductive Health* 73–76.

V Sharma et al 'Why the Promotion of Family Planning Makes More Sense Now Than Ever Before?' (2020) 22(2) *Journal of Health Management* 206–214.

VK Chattu & S Yaya 'Emerging Infectious Diseases and Outbreaks: Implications for Women's Reproductive Health and Rights in Resource-Poor Settings' (2020) 17(1) *Reproductive Health*.

International instruments

African Charter on Human and Peoples' Rights ("Banjul Charter"), 27 June 1981, OAU Doc CAB/LEG/67/3 rev. 5, 1520 UNTS 217, entered into force on 21 October 1986.

African Union Commission. Maputo Plan of Action 2016–2030 for the Operationalisation of the Continental Policy Framework for SRH and Rights, Addis Ababa: African Union Commission.

International Covenant on Economic, Social and Cultural Rights (ICESCR), adopted December 16, 1966, art. 15 (1), G.A. Res. 2200A (XXI), U.N. GAOR, Supp. No. 16, U.N. Doc. A/6316 (1966) (entered into force on 3 January 1976).

Organisation of African Unity (OAU), African Charter on Human and Peoples' Rights ("Banjul Charter"), (African Charter) 27 June 1981, CAB/LEG/67/3 rev. 5, 21 I.L.M. 58 (1982).

Organisation of African Unity (OAU), African Charter on the Rights and Welfare of the Child, 11 July 1990, CAB/LEG/24.9/49 (1990).

Protocol to the African Charter on Human and Peoples' Rights on the Rights of Women in Africa, adopted 11 July 2003 (Maputo Protocol).

Report of the United Nations Working Group on the Issue of Discrimination against Women in Law and in Practice (2016) (UN Doc. A/HRC/32/44).

Resolution on Human and Peoples' Rights as the Central Pillar of Successful Response to COVID-19 and Recovery from Its Socio-political Impacts-ACHPR/Res. 449 (LXVI) 2020.

Special Rapporteur on the Rights of Women in Africa on Violation of Women's Rights during the COVID-19 Pandemic, African Commission on Human and People's Rights.

UN Commission on Human Rights. Siracusa Principles on the Limitation and Derogation Provisions in the International Covenant on Civil and Political Rights, Annex. UN Doc. E/CN.4/1985/4, 1984.

UN General Assembly, Convention on the Elimination of All Forms of Discrimination Against Women, 18 December 1979, United Nations, Treaty Series, vol. 1249.

UN General Assembly, Convention on the Rights of Persons with Disabilities: Resolution/adopted by the General Assembly, 24 January 2007, A/RES/61/106.

UN General Assembly, International Covenant on Civil and Political Rights, 16 December 1966, United Nations, Treaty Series, vol. 999, p. 171.

UN General Assembly, International Covenant on Economic, Social and Cultural Rights, 16 December 1966, United Nations, Treaty Series, vol. 993.

UN General Assembly, Universal Declaration of Human Rights, 10 December 1948, 217 A (III).

UN Human Rights Committee. General Comment No. 29, UN Doc. CCPR/C/21/Rev.1/Add.11, 2001.

UN Special Rapporteur on the Right of Everyone to the Enjoyment of the Highest Attainable Standard of Physical and Mental Health, Interim Report to the General Assembly (2011) (UN Doc. A/66/254).

General comment

African Commission on Human and Peoples' Rights. General Comment No. 2 on Article 14.1 (a), (b), (c) and (f) and Article 14. 2 (a) and (c) of the Protocol to the African Charter on Human and Peoples' Rights on the Rights of Women in Africa (2014).

African Committee of Experts on the Rights and Welfare of the Child (ACERWC). General Comment No. 7 on article 27 on Sexual Exploitation of the African Charter on the Rights and Welfare of the Child (2021).

Committee on Economic, Social and Cultural Rights, General Comment No. 22: On the right to sexual and reproductive health.
Committee on the Elimination of Discrimination against Women, CEDAW Committee, General Recommendation No. 24: Art 12 of the Convention (Women and Health) 1999, A/54/38.
Committee on the Elimination of Discrimination against Women, General Recommendation No. 30: Women in Conflict Prevention, Conflict, and Post-conflict Situations, in Compilation of General Comments and General Committee on the Elimination of Discrimination against Women (CEDAW).
General Comment No. 15 (2013) on the right of the child to the enjoyment of the highest attainable standard of health, para. 70.
General Comment No. 2 on art 14 (2) (a) and (c) of the Protocol to the African Charter on Human and Peoples' Rights on the Rights of Women in Africa (2014).
International Covenant on Civil and Political Rights CCPR/C/GC/34 General Comment No. 34 (2011).
Special Rapporteur on the right of everyone to the enjoyment of the highest attainable standard of physical and mental health, A/HRC/32/32 (2016), para. 113 (b).
UN CESCR. General Comment No. 14, para. 44. UN Doc. E/C.12/2000/4, 2000.
UN Committee on the Rights of the Child (CRC), General Comment No. 15 (2013) on the right of the child to the enjoyment of the highest attainable standard of health (art. 24), 17 April 2013, CRC/C/GC/15.
UN CRPD, General Comment No. 3 (2016) (UN Doc. CRPD/C/GC/3).

Cases

Family Planning Association of Northern Ireland v. Minister for Health, Social Services and Public Safety, (2005) Northern Ireland Law Reports 188 (Court of Appeal).
Ministerio de la Protección Social. Resolución No. 4905 de 2006. Por la cual se adopta la Norma Técnica para la atención de la Interrupción Voluntaria del Embarazo – IVE.
PAK & Another v Attorney General & 3 Others (Constitutional Petition E009 of 2020) [2022] KEHC 262 (KLR) (24 March 2022).
Tysiac v. Poland, Application No. 5410/03, European Court of Human Rights, Judgment 20 March 2007

Legislation

Offences against the Person Act of 1861.

Guidelines and reports

'Abortion Care Guideline' (Geneva: World Health Organization, 2022).
'COVID-19: Operational Guidance for Maintaining Essential Health Services during an Outbreak' on 25 March 2020.
Fact Sheet 'Self-care Health Interventions'.
Family Health Services 'Technical Procedural Guidelines for Safe Abortion in Ethiopia' (2006).
Guttmacher Institute 'COVID-19 State Policy Update' (2021).
Guttmacher Institute 'Induced Abortion in the United States'.
Impact of the COVID-19 Pandemic on SRH Services in Burkina Faso, Ethiopia, Kenya, Malawi, and Uganda.

Ipas Nigeria 'Impact of COVID-19 Lockdown on Access to Safe Abortion in Nigeria' (2021).
Marie Stopes International 'Stories from the Frontline: In the Shadow of the COVID-19 Pandemic. COVID-19' (2021).
Pathfinder 'mHealth in Mozambique: Fulfilling Our Mission during a Global Pandemic'.
'Prevention and Management of Unsafe Abortion: Comprehensive Abortion Care Services, Standards and Protocols' (Accra: Ghana Health Service, 2006), 182–83nn61–63
The National Guideline for Implementation of the Choice on Termination of Pregnancy Act.
UNFPA 'Impact of COVID-19 on Family Planning: What We Know One Year into the Pandemic' *Technical Not Information* as of 11 March 2021.
United Nations Children's Fund 'COVID-19: A Threat to Progress against Child Marriage' (New York: UNICEF, 2021).
United Nations Population Fund (UNFPA) 'The Impact of COVID-19 on Women and Girls with Disabilities' (2021) (accessed 20 February 2023)
United Nations Population Funds 'Not on Pause: Responding to the SRH Needs of Adolescents in the Context of the COVID-19 Crisis'.
WHO 'Addressing Violence against Children, Women and Older People during the COVID-19 Pandemic: Key Actions' COVID-19: Risk Communication and Community Engagement (2020).
WHO Health Workforce www.who.int/health-topics/health-workforce#tabtab_1
World Health Organization 'WHO Director-General's Opening Remarks at the Mission Briefing on COVID-19'.
Zambia, Ministry of Health 'Standards and Guidelines for Reducing Unsafe Abortion, Morbidity and Mortality in Zambia' (2009).

14

ROLE OF REGIONAL HUMAN RIGHTS BODIES AND NATIONAL COURTS IN ADDRESSING HUMAN RIGHTS IN THE CONTEXT OF COVID-19 PANDEMIC

Ebenezer Durojaye

14.1 Introduction

The COVID-19 pandemic brought to the fore again the need for regional human rights bodies such as the African Commission on Human and Peoples' Rights to play a more active role in setting norms and standards to address such pandemics. The African Commission was established under the African Charter on Human and Peoples' Rights in 1987. Since then, it has remained one of the important human rights bodies in Africa charged with the promotion and protection of human rights. The Commission has been playing an important role in the promotion and protection of the right to health over the years. While the efforts of the African Commission in realizing the right to health is worthy of note, much more is still required to ensure that all Africans truly enjoy this right, in particularly regarding the different pandemics and epidemics that have confronted the region so far. Indeed, as will be discussed later, given that Africa has a rich experience dealing with pandemics and epidemics, the African Commission could have handled the COVID-19 pandemic much better. It should be noted that there are three major human rights bodies in Africa: the African Commission on Human and People's Rights, the African Committee of Experts on the Rights and Welfare of the Child, and the African Court on Human and Peoples' Rights. The focus of this chapter will be on the African Commission, however, where necessary reference will be made to the other human rights bodies to draw lessons and make comparisons.

Against this backdrop, this chapter examines the role of regional human rights bodies and national courts in addressing human rights violations in the context of the COVID-19 pandemic. It focuses on the promotional and

DOI: 10.4324/9781032671437-17

protective mandate of the African Commission on Human and Peoples' Rights, one of the most experienced human rights bodies in the region. In this regard, it assesses the role played by the Commission during the pandemic and argues that the Commission could have done better than it did in setting norms and standards to protect the human rights of vulnerable and marginalized groups in the region. Using South Africa, Kenya and Malawi as case studies, the chapter further discusses the role of national courts in protecting human rights in the wake of imposition of lockdowns by African countries. It examines whether national courts have held governments accountable to protecting human rights during public health emergencies such as the COVID-19 pandemic. It concludes by making recommendations on how regional human rights bodies and national courts can be more effective in ensuring the protection of human rights during future pandemics.

14.2 The mandate of the African Commission and its potential to address public health emergencies

The African Commission is the body charged with the responsibility of overseeing the implementation of the African Charter and for the time being the Maputo Protocol. The Commission was established in 1987 pursuant to Article 30 of the African Charter. It has both a promotional and a protective mandate. The Commission usually consists of 11 members who are expected to have distinguished themselves in their field of endeavour. The members are to serve in their individual capacity through secret ballot election conducted by the Assembly of Heads of State of the African Union. Article 45 of the African Charter empowers the Commission to provide interpretative guidance to the provision of the African Charter and by extension the Maputo Protocol. Relying on this provision, the African Commission has adopted important resolutions and general comments to provide further understanding of the provisions on the right to health in the Charter and the Maputo Protocol.

The Protective Mandate of the Commission includes receiving state reports and issuing concluding observations to states with a view to ensuring better protection of human rights at the national level. Also, the Commission's communication procedure provides a good opportunity to develop right jurisprudence on human rights in Africa and hold states accountable to violations of rights. Over the years, the Commission has handed down influential decisions in relation to socio-economic rights, including the right to health. Some of these important decisions include the *Purohit* case, where the Commission held that forced institutionalization and maltreatment of persons with mental disabilities by the Gambian government constituted a gross violation of Article 16 of the African Charter, the *SERAC* case, and the *Pen International* case. These decisions remain a beacon of hope for victims of human rights violations in the region.

14.3 The African human rights system and previous epidemics and pandemics

14.3.1 African Commission and HIV/AIDS

Africa is one of the regions that have long and rich experiences in dealing with pandemics and epidemics. In the 1990s, Africa was known as the epicentre of the HIV pandemic. This disease caused the death of millions of Africans and negatively impacted the labour force. The impact of the HIV pandemic was great such that it affected nearly every area of human endeavour. More importantly, the HIV pandemic raised some important human rights issues which further exacerbated stigma and discrimination in the context of the epidemic.

Examples of how HIV-positive persons or those affected by the epidemic were subjected to serious human rights abuses have been well documented.[1] This cut across almost every area of human endeavour, including housing, health, religion, family, and community sport. The fact that the origin of HIV was first detected among homosexuals in the US further aggravated the stigma and discrimination associated with it. Thus, many people living with HIV were made subjects of human rights abuses and denied their fundamental rights.[2] These include denial of employment, housing, healthcare services, and marriage and exclusion from social services and other benefits.[3] In some extreme situations, people living with HIV suffered violence, especially women living with HIV, and were made subjects of violence.[4] These range from physical, psychological, and emotional violence such as ejection from homes and denial of property rights upon the death of their husbands. While majority of people living with HIV are found in Africa, only few of them have access to life-saving medications.[5] This was due to the fact that pharmaceutical companies owned by developed countries insisted on patent rights to these life-saving medication under the Trade-Related Aspects of Intellectual Property Rights (TRIPS) Agreements[6] within the World Trade Organization (WTO) scheme. Many activists and civil society organizations protested this grave injustice and denial of life-saving medications as a gross violation of human rights of Africans.

In response to the human rights challenges posed by the HIV pandemic, the African Commission adopted a number of resolutions, calling on states to decisively and holistically address the human rights issues raised by the pandemic and curb its spread. Thus, as far back as 2002, the African Commission issued its first resolution calling on African states to adopt a rights-based approach to tackling the pandemic[7]. This was followed by the resolution on access to medicines in the context of HIV. As noted earlier, this resolution specifically addressed the high cost of life-saving medications for Africans, due to the patent rights enjoyed by pharmaceutical companies[8]. It called on African countries to ensure that trade agreements do not become barriers to access to life-saving medications.[9] It further enjoined African governments to explore the flexibility provisions in the TRIPS Agreement in order to ensure access to life-saving medications for their citizens as a human rights imperative.[10] In another resolution, the Commission addressed the disturbingly high cases of involuntary sterilization of HIV-positive women as a human rights violation.[11] According to the African Commission, involuntary sterilization of HIV-positive women undermines a number of rights guaranteed in the African Charter.[12] These include the rights to non-discrimination, dignity, health, found family, freedom from torture, and inhuman and degrading treatment.[13] The resolution urges African governments to put in place mechanisms that will ensure that HIV-positive women are not subjected to coercive forms of sterilization. More importantly, the Commission enjoined states to ensure the participation of women living with HIV in the development of laws, policies, and programmes relating to their sexual and reproductive health.[14]

Furthermore, the African Commission in 2010 adopted a resolution on the establishment of the Committee on the Protection of the Rights of People Living with HIV (PLHIV) and those at Risk, Vulnerable to and Affected by HIV (the HIV Committee) as one of its special mechanisms to deal specifically with human rights violations arising from HIV.[15] The Committee was charged, among other things, with addressing human rights abuses experienced by vulnerable and marginalized groups in the context of the pandemic. Since its establishment, the Committee has played an important role in developing norms and standards to combat the HIV pandemic. For instance, together with the Special Rapporteur on the rights of women in Africa, the Committee was involved in the drafting of the General Comments 1 on Article 14 (1) (d) and (e) of the Maputo Protocol.[16] This provision is the first to explicitly protect women from sexually transmitted infections, including HIV. Thus, it requires further clarifications on the nature and role of states in the effective implementation at the national level. This guidance is provided by GC 1, where the Commission elaborates on what is expected of states in ensuring that women are protected from sexually transmitted infections including HIV. It is also to be noted that the HIV Committee took the leading role in the drafting of resolution 260 on involuntary sterilization discussed earlier.

The Committee has equally embarked on mission visits to a number of countries to engage with states and other stakeholders to address critical issues in relation to human rights violations arising from HIV. More importantly, the Committee has carried out a compressive study on the human rights, laws, and challenges posed by the HIV pandemic in Africa.[17] This study detailed some of the human rights challenges in relation to HIV, suggesting a holistic approach by states, regional bodies, and other stakeholders in addressing these challenges. The study documented how sexual minorities and other vulnerable and marginalized groups should receive greater attention when developing policies, laws, and programmes to address HIV in the region.[18]

In addition, the African Commission has had opportunities to examine state report and provide useful concluding observations in relation to HIV. In some of its concluding observations to states, the Commission has requested governments for a more pragmatic approach to reducing the HIV epidemic,[19] to allocate more resources to address the epidemic,[20] for rights-based and gender-sensitive approaches to addressing the epidemic,[21] and to intensify preventive measures in order to curb the spread of the epidemic.[22]

14.3.2 African Commission and Ebola virus

With regard to addressing the Ebola virus disease epidemic, the African Commission issued a press release where it highlights some of the important challenges posed by the epidemic.[23] According to the Commission, states are to avoid any interventions that can potentially slow down the progress of effective curtailment of the virus. The Commission further called on African Union member states to explore regional and sub-regional cooperation with a view to addressing the epidemic. It further urged states to mobilize resources with a view to addressing the virus in a decisive manner. The Commission called on states and civil society groups to intensify efforts towards prevention and creating awareness, including sensitization campaigns to ensure protection of individuals from the virus.

In a resolution adopted to specifically address the impact of the virus in the Democratic Republic of Congo (DRC),[24] the Commission strongly condemned attacks on healthcare centres and health personnel charged with responding to the Ebola virus.[25] The Commission paid tribute to healthcare personnel who lost their lives in the course of treating people infected with Ebola. It then urged the government of DRC to 'take the necessary measures to protect the health of the populations and avoid any decision likely to impede an effective response to the Ebola virus'.[26] The Commission urged state parties to the African Charter to strengthen their health systems in order to prevent and curtail the spread of the epidemic and future epidemics.

14.4 The COVID-19 pandemic and the response from the African Commission

The COVID-19 pandemic affects various human rights; however, it directly impacts on the enjoyment of the right to health, guaranteed in the three major human rights instruments in the region. The right to health is guaranteed in Article 16 of the African Charter on Human and Peoples' Rights.[27] This article provides that every individual shall be entitled to the right to health. Although this provision is phrased in a slightly different manner from

Article 12 of the International Covenant on Economic, Social, and Cultural Rights (ICESCR),[28] it has been given the same interpretation as that for the Covenant. The African Commission has explained in the *Purohit* case that the right to health implies access not only to health care but also to goods and services related to health care.[29] As noted earlier, the Commission in the past has played an important role in setting standards and norms to address epidemics and pandemics such HIV/AIDS. Perhaps one of the criticisms of the Commission in this regard has been its rather 'slow' and 'reactionary' approach to such pandemics and epidemics. For instance, the Commission could have taken a more proactive and holistic approach to addressing the Ebola virus epidemic that raged the continent a few years back. The fact that the Commission failed to adopt norms and standards to address the deadly disease is an indication of its inconsistencies in dealing with public health emergencies in the region.

After the WHO declaration of COVID-19 as a pandemic, the Commission responded by issuing its first statement detailing the human rights concerns that the pandemic might raise.[30] In the statement, the Commission notes that the pandemic is a threat to the well-being and survival of many Africans and would require progressive and proactive measures to curb its spread.[31] The Commission further observes why urgent measures must be taken to curb the spread of the pandemic and that such measures must be consistent with respect for human rights as guaranteed in the Charter and other human rights instruments.[32] This would seem to be an attempt to strike the balance between individual rights and the need to curb the pandemic. It is always a contentious issue trying to ensure respect for human rights during public health emergencies. While some have argued that the need to protect the public should always take precedence over individual rights, others have contended that this should be based on balancing of the rights approach. In other words, one would need to adopt the proportionality test as provided in the Siracusa Principles. The essence of these principles is to recognize that states are obligated to protect the lives and property of the public during a public health emergency; however, this must be done with minimum infractions of fundamental rights of individuals. This set of principles adopted by the Human Rights Committee proposes that in order to restrict rights during public health emergencies, the following must be taken into consideration.

The statement identified the vulnerability of millions of Africans to diseases, including COVID-19, by decrying living conditions in many parts of the region such as the lack of access to basic sanitation and water, healthcare services, education, and decent housing.[33] The Commission therefore proposes holistic and proactive measures by African governments to tackle the pandemic.[34] This includes preventive measures such as the provision of access to water, sanitation, and information; community participation; and compliance with human rights.

A month after this statement, the Commission issued another statement on effective response to the pandemic.[35] In this statement, the Commission reiterated the importance of a rights-based approach to addressing the pandemic by noting the relevance of the various rights guaranteed under the Charter. These include Article 4, the right to life; Article 9, the right to access to information; and Article 16, the right to health. The Commission expressed concern about the weak state of the healthcare systems in the region, including lack of testing facilities and treatment to address the pandemic. It further bemoaned the slow and poor efforts by African governments to address the pandemic. The COVID-19 pandemic indeed exposed the poor state of the healthcare systems in many African countries. While the region was not as adversely affected as other regions, it still recorded a high mortality rate due to the poor state of the healthcare systems. Many of the deaths that occurred in the region could have been avoided but for the lack of infrastructure and healthcare providers in the region. For many years, the healthcare systems in African countries remained underfunded, lacking in basic facilities and suffering from a dearth of qualified healthcare personnel. This deplorable situation was more of a ticking time bomb waiting to explode, which eventually exploded as a result of the devastating effects of COVID-19 on the healthcare systems in the region. Commentators have decried the lack of political will on the part of African governments to commit adequate resources to the health sector. At the Abuja Declaration more than two decades ago, African governments agreed to commit 15% of their annual budgets to the health sector in order to address various diseases, including HIV, tuberculosis, and malaria.[36] However, many of these governments have fallen short of this commitment, an indication that they might be paying lip service to improving the healthcare systems.

More importantly, the Commission called on African governments to ensure that measures adopted to curb the spread of the pandemic are consistent with respect for the human rights of individuals. In this regard, states are urged to 'comply with the principles of legality, non-discrimination and equality, ensuring access to information, primacy of preventive and containment measures, to address non-implementation and non-compliance' in the context of the pandemic.[37] This is an important call given the manner many of African governments went about addressing the pandemic. Due to the lack of oversight from other arms of governments, the executive arm became very powerful and made executive decisions which could have serious implications for the fundamental rights of the people. Some of the measures adopted to curb the spread of the pandemic were excessive, stringent, and draconian, undermining the enjoyment of human rights.[38] Kilonzo has argued that the responses of the Kenyan government to addressing the pandemic fell short of respect for the human rights of the citizens.[39]

In another statement on the impact of the pandemic on general elections in Africa, the Commission expresses concerns about the impact of COVID-19 on elections in Africa.[40] It notes that the pandemic may affect the right of individuals to regular, free, fair, and transparent elections. The Commission notes that the right to regular, free, fair, and credible election is the most sacred democratic norm that serves as a primary means for the exercise of the right to self-government guaranteed in Article 20 of the African Charter and the right to participation in Article 13 of the same Charter as well as the provisions of the African Charter on Democracy, Elections, and Good Governance.[41] According to the Commission, public health measures, such as lockdowns and others, to safeguard the lives of the people in the context of COVID-19 may have negative effects on the right to vote and participation.[42] Indeed, these measures may limit the exercise of the right to vote and participation. The Commission enjoins states to take into consideration some salient points when contemplating whether to embark on elections in the context of public health emergencies such as COVID-19. These include observing laid down COVID-19 protocols such as maintaining public distance, use of sanitizers, considering the position of vulnerable and marginalized groups, and considering alternative means of voting that does not require physical presence at the polling booths, where possible.

The Commission through some of its special mechanisms has issued statements/press release to address the impact of COVID-19 on the specific mandate of these mechanisms. For instance, the Special Rapporteur on freedom of information in one of the press releases noted with concern the restrictions to access to Internet by some governments in a bid to curb the spread of the pandemic.[43] The Special Rapporteur enjoined states to ensure that 'members of the public receive accurate, regular, accessible and science-based information on the threat COVID-19 poses to their health'.[44] It is further noted that efforts by states to limit or obstruct access to Internet would impact negatively on access to health-related information that is crucial to protection from contracting COVID-19.[45] The Special Rapporteur concludes by noting that states should continue to respect the right to freedom of expression and access to information, including respect for rule of law, during the pandemic and refrain from exploiting the pandemic to undermine human rights.[46]

14.4.1 Resolution 449 on human and peoples' rights as the central pillar of successful response to COVID-19 and recovery from its socio-political impacts

Perhaps one of the important norms developed by the Commission during the pandemic was the adoption of Resolution 449 on human and peoples' rights as the central pillar of a successful response to COVID-19 and recovery from its socio-political impacts.[47] In noting the importance of a right-based approach to responding to the pandemic, the Commission calls calls on African states to adhere to recommended public health measures to address the pandemic such as wearing of masks, use of sanitizers, social distancing, opening of events in public spaces and disinfecting public places in or to ensure the right to health and life guaranteed in the Charter.[48] The Commission enjoins states to prioritize the protection of rights of groups most vulnerable to the pandemic, such as the elderly and persons with underlying medical conditions.[49] Recognizing the important role of healthcare workers in addressing the spread of the pandemic and saving lives, the Commission urges African governments to provide needed facilities, resources, and support to healthcare providers in order to discharge their duties effectively.[50] Irrespective of the measures adopted by African governments to address the pandemic, the Commission urges states to ensure that access to healthcare services, including sexual and reproductive healthcare services, non-COVID-19 services, and services for pregnant women and people living with HIV, are not hindered or interrupted.[51]

The resolution also affirms that states should ensure access to public services such as water, soap, and sanitations, especially for those in informal settlements. States are to respect individuals' right to consent to any medical treatment, and more importantly, states are to ensure that measures taken to curb the pandemic are consistent with the principles of legality, necessity, proportionality, and accountability and do not endanger human life. At the minimum, measures adopted by states must meet human rights standards and norms recognized in the Charter. Thus, states are to ensure that the implementation or enforcement of measures to address the pandemic does not undermine rights of individuals, particularly vulnerable groups such as persons with disabilities, women, girls, adolescents, refugees and asylum seekers, homeless people, and internally displaced persons.[52] It is commendable that the Commission adopts a holistic and broad approach to promoting and protecting human rights in the context of the pandemic by emphasizing the need to give attention to the rights of vulnerable groups.

There is no doubt that the resolution is comprehensive and seeks to address various aspects of human endeavour to mitigate the impact of the pandemic on Africans. Sadly, however, experience has shown that efforts by African governments to address the pandemic fell short of the norms and standards recommend by the African Commission. Studies have shown that healthcare services, including services for sexual and reproductive health and rights, were obstructed during the pandemic in many African countries.[53] Also, the imposition of lockdown and other restrictions were poorly implemented and gross human rights violations were reported, particularly due to the high-handedness of security agents.[54] More importantly, the rights of vulnerable and marginalized groups were seriously undermined during the pandemic as African government failed to adopt appropriate measures and programmes to secure the rights of these groups. In particular, the socio-economic rights of these groups were treated with levity.

14.4.2 Engagement with states during periodic reports

The states' report procedure is one of the important protective mandates of the African Commission in ensuring accountability from states regarding the promotion and protection of human rights. This process ensures that states submit periodic reports to the African Commission every two years. In response to the reports, the African Commission issues concluding observations detailing both positive aspects of the reports and shortcomings. Beyond the adoption of statements and the resolution to address the pandemic, the Commission did not effectively explore using its protective mandate through the state reporting process to engage with states on the efforts they have taken to address COVID-19. On few occasions, the Commission did require states to take measures regarding the pandemic, but this was not done consistently or forcefully. For instance, in response to the Namibia government's 7th combined report, the Commission merely requested the government to adopt measures to protect the rights of women prisoners during COVID-19. In another concluding observation on the report of Malawi, the Commission merely commended the efforts of the government to 'the Re-Admission Policy in 2016 which provides for the readmission of girls back into school after pregnancy during the COVID-19 lockdown'.[55] One would have expected a more rigorous engagement with the efforts made by the Malawian government to address COVID-19. It was indeed a missed opportunity for the Commission not to engage consistently with African governments on measures taken to address the pandemic. The Commission could have used the reporting process to evaluate the efforts of African governments to protect human rights in the context of the pandemic. Moreover, the Commission could have assessed measures taken by African governments to cushion the effects of the pandemic on the socio-economic rights of Africans, especially the vulnerable and marginalized groups. It may be argued that due to the unimpressive records of African governments on submitting periodic reports to the African Commission, the Commission could have been deprived the opportunity to engage with these governments regarding their efforts towards addressing the pandemic. It is a known fact that many African governments are behind in their reporting obligations to the Commission, and a few others have yet to submit any report.[56] This has serious implications for the oversight role of the Commission to ensure the effective implementation of the Charter and the Maputo Protocol.

14.4.3 Communication procedure

Regarding the communication procedure of the African Commission, no reported case was recorded dealing with COVID-19. It should be noted that communication can only be submitted to the Commission after the exhaustion of local remedies. Given the lengthy process to exhaust local remedies in many African countries, it is not unexpected that no case on COVID-19 made it to the Commission. This could have provided an opportunity for the Commission to clarify the nature of states' obligations in not only addressing the virus but also safeguarding the fundamental rights of the people. The Commission in the past has rich jurisprudence on securing the fundamental rights of individuals, including the right to health.[57] Most of its landmark jurisprudence has focused on socio-economic rights, including the right to health. The Commission has adopted the interrelatedness and indivisibility approach in its jurisprudence.[58] In comparison to other regional bodies, it can be argued that the response of the Commission leaves much to be desired.

14.5 National courts and the COVID-19 pandemic

Courts are often referred to as the last hope of the masses. They play an important role in ensuring that the rights of vulnerable and marginalized groups are protected and promoted. Sometimes referred to as the refuge of the weak and poor, courts play a crucial role in safeguarding human rights of all during a difficult time as the COVID-19 pandemic. As noted earlier, during the pandemic many African governments resorted to the use of lockdowns and other measures to address the spread of the pandemic. Some of the measures undermined the enjoyment of rights and further pushed vulnerable and marginalized groups below the margins of the society. In response to this, courts in some African countries were called upon to clarify the lawfulness or otherwise of some of the measures adopted by African governments to curb the spread of the pandemic. This discussion that follows examines how courts in three African countries responded to cases in relation to human rights issues raised by measures adopted by governments during the pandemic.

14.5.1 South Africa

South Africa is one of the African countries that was negatively affected by the COVID-19 pandemic. It recorded one of the highest number of people infected and deaths in the region. According to WHO, over four million cases of infections and over 100,000 deaths were recorded in the country.[59] In terms of dealing with the pandemic, the country has two options as provided by the Constitution. It could go the route of either declaring a state of emergency under section 37 of the Constitution or declaring a state of disaster under the Disaster Management Act (DMA) 57 of 2002. The country chose the latter and declared a state of disaster under the DMA, thereby limiting the enjoyment of fundamental rights to curb the spread of the pandemic. In addition to invoking the DMA, the president established the National Coronavirus Command Council (NCCC) to make decisions that affected the issuance and implementation of the regulations.[60] Some attempts were made to challenge the legality or otherwise of the measures adopted by the South African government.

In *Mohamed and Others v President of the Republic of South Africa and Others*, the applicants challenged the constitutionality of the regulations that restricted gatherings in religious places of worship as a violation of the rights to religion, freedom of movement, and dignity.[61] The issue was whether the restrictions on gatherings in places of worship were unconstitutional. The court held that in the spirit of making sacrifices for the greater good, and in view of the limitations clause, the restrictions were neither unreasonable nor unjustifiable. It is argued that the court maintained the status quo. The point of departure was the use of the limitations clause as the yardstick for maintaining the status quo.

Another interesting case that deals with the legality of the measures adopted by the government is the *De Beer and Others v Minister of Cooperative Governance and Traditional Affairs*.[62] In this case, the applicants sought a declaration that both the national state of disaster and the promulgated regulations are unconstitutional, unlawful, and invalid; in the alternative, the applicants sought an order that gatherings be declared lawful subject to conditions. The court held that several regulations fell short of the rationality test. It gave an example of irrationality in the restriction of movements – persons were prohibited from gathering in workplaces, but burials were allowed to be attended by 50 people. However, the court did not accord this expansive evaluation to other restrictions. It suffices to note that the court at least evaluated the enjoyment of rights – something that it did not do in the early stages of the restrictions.

In a similar case by the Supreme Court of Appeal on a case emanating from the Western Cape High Court, namely *Esau and Others v Minister of Co-operative Governance and Traditional Affairs and Others*,[63] the rationality of the lockdown regulations was questioned. The applicants had contested the lawfulness of the establishment and functioning of the NCCC, which the president set up to play a central role in the response to COVID-19. The issues for determination in this case were that, firstly, whether the Disaster Regulations of 29 April 2020 were consistent with sections 26 and 27 of the DMA; secondly, whether the Minister of Co-operative Governance and Traditional Affairs (the COGTA Minister) acted in a procedurally fair and rational manner when she made those regulations; and thirdly, whether some of the regulations were unreasonable and unjustifiable infringements of rights and, as such, invalid on that account. The fourth issue was whether the directions issued by the Minister of Trade, Industry, and Competition were invalid for want of legality and rationality.

The High Court found in favour of the respondents on all four issues, leading to the appeal. On appeal at the Supreme Court, the case was dismissed on the grounds that level 4 regulations were enacted legally, procedurally, and fairly and were rational, save for the provisions on exercise and the selling of hot food. Three facets of this decision may be examined: The government's views on the position of the NCCC, the role of the executive, and the question of rationality in comparison to the *De Beer* case. The court affirmed the constitutionality of the NCCC, noting that this could be established with the discretion of the executive. It further noted that the exercise of executive authority 'is a collaborative venture in terms of which the President acts together with the other members of the Cabinet'[64]; consequently, ministers are collectively and individually accountable to the parliament under section 92(2) of the Constitution.[65] With regard to the rationality principle, the court found that the rationality had to be found in the making of the regulations and not just their content. There was evidence to indicate that the minister had considered the participation and representation of the public through teams comprising officials from her department and the Department of Trade, Industry, and Competition.[66]

From the above cases, it is clear that the courts in South Africa played an important role in assessing the legality of the measures adopted by the government and considering its implications for enjoyment of the right. Where necessary, the courts have considered the balancing of rights to ensure that the measures adopted by the government are not excessive and within the limitation of rights provisions of the Constitution.[67]

14.5.2 Kenya

With the first reported case of COVID-19 occurring in Kenya in March 2020, the government took some measures with a view to controlling the spread of the pandemic. The government issued directives that, inter alia, discontinued learning in all educational institutions, suspended travel into Kenya, imposed a dusk-to-dawn curfew, curtailed movement in and out of selected regions, and closed places of worship and entertainment. Overall, the country recorded over 300,000 infections and over 5,000 deaths.[68] Just as in the case of South Africa, while the Kenyan government has the option of declaring a state of emergency as outlined in the Constitution or imposing curfews in line with the Public Order Act, the Kenyan government chose the latter and imposed curfews and other restrictions on movement and other activities in the country to curb the spread of the virus. The order initially applied between 7 p.m. and 5 a.m., but over time the hours have been altered depending on the spread and effect of COVID-19. There have been attempts by various individuals to challenge the measures adopted by the government to address the pandemic. One of the first cases in this regard is that of *National Super Alliance (NASA) Kenya v Cabinet Secretary for Interior and Co-ordination of National Government & 3 Others* [2017]. In that case, the High Court held that '[the] imposition of a curfew order is a stop-gap measure' which cannot be compared to a state of emergency contemplated under Article 58 of the Constitution.

Perhaps one of the most important challenges to the legality of the imposition of curfews to curb the spread of the virus was the case of *LSK v Hillary Mutyambai*, 2020. In that case, the Law Society of Kenya petitioned the high court to declare the curfew order illegal because, according to the Law Society, curfews can be declared only for the purposes of tackling crime, not disease. It was contended by the state that the imposition of the curfews became necessary in order to protect public safety and lives in light of the COVID-19 pandemic. The court held that the Public Order Act can be applied to public health emergencies such as the one posed by the COVID-19 pandemic and that the provisions of the Act complemented those of the Public Health Act.[69] However, the court noted that the curfew order 'does not only upset the people's way of life, but it also negatively impacts constitutional rights and freedoms such as freedom of movement, the freedom of association, and the freedom of assembly'.[70] For this reason, it said the curfew order could be constitutional only if it met the constitutional muster set under Article 24(1) of the Constitution. In applying the proportionality test, the court noted that although the main objective of the curfew was to reduce the transmission of COVID-19, there was no evidence by the petitioners or respondents that demonstrated how the curfew would attain the objective or whether the reduction of transmissions, if any, 'outweighs the hardship visited upon the populace by the curfew'.[71] Guided by the precautionary principle, the court came to the conclusion that the state cannot be faulted for taking precautionary and restrictive measures to slow down the spread of COVID-19.[72] It, however, was quick to point out that the implementation of the order must be consistent with respect for human rights.

In another case, *Joan Akoth Ajuang and another v Micheal Owuor Osodo and Others* (*Okoth*), the petitioners argued that the hushed burial of their loved one violated the deceased's right to human dignity and the surviving relatives' right to enjoy their culture through the exercise of cultural norms and beliefs regarding burial. While the court recognized the right to dignity to a deceased, through the respect of his wishes like testamentary dispositions, it also noted that the state did not follow the WHO Guidelines on the Management and Handling of Dead Bodies.[73] The measures included wearing of protective equipment like gloves to avoid physical contact with the deceased and social distancing of at least a metre from the body.[74] In comparison to Kenya's domesticated rules, it was clear that burial could only take place between 9 a.m. and 3 p.m. with about 15 people in attendance.[75] The state orchestrated burial after 8 p.m. was illegal, and it violated the enacted principles on the handling of burials during the COVID-19 period. The use of the precautionary approach was based on the uncertainty of the unknown concerning health risks associated with the exhumation of the deceased.[76]

Responding to the use of excessive force to implement the measures adopted by the government, the Court in *LSK v Hillary Mutyambai* (2020) noted that 'diseases are not contained by visiting violence on members of the public. . . . [T]he National Police Service must be held responsible and accountable for violating the rights to life and dignity among other rights'.[77] This a clear indication on the part of the court to monitor the implementation of the measures adopted by the executive arm to curb the spread of the pandemic. It shows the resilience of the courts in holding the government accountable by preventing abuse of powers.

14.5.3 Malawi

Like other African countries, Malawi also bore the brunt of the COVID-19 pandemic, albeit at a much lower rate compared to South Africa and Kenya. The total number of infections was estimated at 8,000, while 2,000 deaths were recorded.[78]

It used the Public Health Act to declare the pandemic a 'formidable disease' to enable the Minister of Health to issue directives to mitigate the spread of the disease.[79] Based on these rules, the minister passed the Public Health (Coronavirus Prevention, Containment, and Management) Rules, 2020, of infectious disease.[80] The requisite sections provide that

> the Minister may by notice declare . . . a formidable epidemic or endemic disease for the purpose of this Part.[81]
>
> purposes, namely-. . .[82]

Just like Kenya and Uganda, the rules provided for the declaration of a national lockdown, except for persons specified as providers of essential persons.[83] All persons were as a result confined to their residences unless they were essential persons, were seeking medical attention, or going to pharmacies, food supply stores, banks, or conducting physical exercises.[84]

The first major application was in the *State (on the application of Esther Kathumba & Others) v The President*.[85] The applicant sought a judicial review of the president's declaration to institute a lockdown. At the core of the application, four main issues were raised: Firstly, whether the decision to declare a lockdown without the attendant declaration of a state of emergency was a derogation of the fundamental rights under the Constitution, and secondly, whether the decision to declare a lockdown without providing for social security interventions to marginalized groups was a punishment to Malawians. More importantly, the implications of the measures for the enjoyment of the socio-economic rights of the people have become a source of concern for marginalized groups.[86] The third issue was whether the decision to promulgate the Public Health (Coronavirus Prevention, Containment and Management) Rules without parliamentary oversight was a derogation of the fundamental rights in the Constitution. The fourth issue was whether the decision to promulgate and implement the COVID-19 Rules under section 31 of the Public Health Act was wrong as far as they authorized measures that were beyond the scope of the parent statutory provisions.[87]

14.6 The African Commission/national courts and future pandemics

While it can be said that the African Commission has made efforts in responding to the COVID-19 pandemic, these efforts are less than satisfactory. The Commission could have used it powers in developing norms and standards in setting new norms in relation to protecting human rights during public health emergencies. This could become the benchmark to assess states' response to future pandemics. Failure on the part of the Commission to establish new norms and standards to address pandemics such as the COVID-19 has created gaps in the jurisprudence of the Commission to address future pandemics. It is hoped that the approach of the African Commission will be different when addressing future pandemics. The Commission would be expected to be more proactive and progressive in monitoring states' responses to future pandemics and in ensuring due respect for the fundamental rights of individuals.

From the analysis of courts in the three countries above, it is clear that the courts to a great extent have risen up to upholding the rights of individuals during the pandemic. The courts have been bold in holding states accountable to their obligations to not only address the pandemic but also safeguard individual human rights. One would expect that for future pandemic, the courts will remain stronger and a refuge to vulnerable and marginalized groups whenever tension exists between measures adopted to address public health emergencies and protect human rights. As seen from the cases discussed earlier, in the early part of the pandemic, it would seem that the courts were more willing to defer to the executive arm by not interfering with the measures taken to address the pandemic. However, the courts became decisive and scrutinized the measures adopted by governments. In future, one would expect the courts to remain steadfast to its duty of assessing the legality or otherwise of governments' measures to address public health emergencies. A progressive and active court is a beacon of hope to vulnerable and marginalized groups during the period of public health emergencies.

14.7 Conclusion

Regional human rights bodies such as the African Commission and national courts remain sources of hope for vulnerable and marginalized groups during a period of public health emergencies. This is because sometimes measures adopted by states may tend to undermine the human rights of individuals. While governments are expected to take appropriate measures to address public health emergencies, such measures must be consistent with international norms and standards such as the Siracusa Principles and conform to fundamental rights as enshrined in the Constitution. As seen from the discussion above, the African Commission missed the opportunity to develop norms and standards to guide states in addressing the COVID-19 pandemic from a rights-based perspective. One hopes that the Commission will do better in the future when called upon to address similar pandemics. It will be important that the Commission adopts proactive measures that include adopting important guidelines or general comments that will holistically address human rights issues in the context of public health emergencies.

The discussion on the role played by the courts in the three countries indicates that they have not fared badly. However, one would expect the courts in the future to be more vigilant and firmer in curtailing the excessive use of powers by the executive arm in a bid to address any future pandemic. The courts would need to be more consistent in their approach in providing checks on the excessive use of powers by the executive. This will not only ensure certainty in protecting the rights of vulnerable and marginalized groups but also ensure that measures adopted are in conformity with the principles of proportionality and legality.

Notes

1 Global Commission on HIV and the Law *Risk, rights and health* (2012) 7.
2 As above.
3 As above.
4 As above.
5 See, V Balogun & E Durojaye 'The African Commission on Human and Peoples' Rights and the promotion and protection of sexual and reproductive health' (2011) 11(2) *African Human Rights Law Journal* 368.
6 TRIPS: Agreement on Trade-Related Aspects of Intellectual Property Rights, 15 April 1994, Marrakesh Agreement Establishing the World Trade Organization, Annex 1C, 1869 U.N.T.S. 1197 (1994) [hereinafter TRIPS Agreement].01.
7 Resolution on the HIV/AIDS Pandemic – Threat against Human Rights and Humanity adopted at the 29th Ordinary Session of the African Commission held in Tripoli, Libya ACHPR Res.53/(XXIX) 01.
8 Resolution 141 on Access to Health and Needed Medicines in Africa ACHPR/Res.141(XXXXIV).
9 As above.
10 As above.
11 Resolution 260 on Involuntary Sterilisation and the Protection of Human Rights in Access to HIV Services – ACHPR/Res. 260 (LIV) 2013.
12 As above.
13 As above.
14 As above.
15 ACHPR/Res.163(XLVII) 10.
16 The Protocol to the African Charter on the Rights of Women in Africa adopted by the African Union (AU) in 2003 entered into force on 27 November 2005.
17 A Study on HIV, the Law and Human Rights in Africa.
18 As above.

19 Concluding Observations and Recommendations on the 4th and 5th Periodic Report of the Republic of Sudan adopted during the 12th Extra-Ordinary Session of the African Commission on Human and Peoples' Rights held from 30 July to 4 August 2012, Algiers, Algeria para 46.
20 Concluding Observations and Recommendations on the Initial, 1st, 2nd, 3rd, and 4th Periodic Report of the Federal Democratic Republic of Ethiopia adopted during the 47th Ordinary Session of the African Commission on Human and Peoples' Rights held from 12 to 26 May 2010, Banjul, The Gambia para 68.
21 Concluding Observations on the 3rd Periodic Report of the Republic of Cameroon adopted during the 15th Extraordinary Session held from 7 to 14 March 2014, Banjul, The Gambia para XIV.
22 As above.
23 Statement by the African Commission on Human and Peoples' Rights on the Spread of the Ebola Virus September 2014.
24 Resolution on the Threat of the Ebola Epidemic Virus in the Democratic Republic of Congo (DRC) ACHPR/Res.424(EXT.OS/XXVI) 2019.
25 As above.
26 As above.
27 African Charter on Human and Peoples' Rights, adopted by the O.A.U. Summit at Nairobi, Kenya, 2–7 June 1981; O.A.U. Doc. CAB/LEG/6713r.
28 International Covenant on Economic, Social and Cultural Rights, adopted Dec. 16, 1966, preamble, G.A. Res. 2200A (XXI), U.N. GAOR, Supp. No. 16, U.N. Doc A/6316 (1966) (entered into force 2 September 1990).
29 *Purohit and Anor v Gambia* (Communication No. 241/2001) [2003] ACHPR 49; (29 May 2003).
30 Press Statement of the African Commission on Human and People's Rights on the Corona COVID-19 virus 28 February 2020.
31 As above.
32 As above.
33 As above.
34 As above.
35 African Commission on Human and People's Rights Press Statement on human rights-based effective response to the Novel COVID-19 virus in Africa 24 March 2020.
36 Abuja Declaration on HIV/AIDS, Tuberculosis and other Related Infectious Diseases.
37 African Commission (n 35 above).
38 See for instance, O Oluduro 'Walking a Tightrope: Balancing human rights concerns and public health measures during the Coronavirus (COVID-19) pandemic in Nigeria' in E Durojaye & D Powell (eds) *Constitutional resilience and the COVID-19 pandemic: Perspective from sub-Saharan Africa* (2022).
39 J Kilonzo 'A test of Kenya's constitutional and democratic resilience' in E Durojaye & D Powell (eds) *Constitutional resilience and the COVID-19 pandemic: Perspective from sub-Saharan Africa* (2022).
40 Statement of the African Commission on Human and Peoples' Rights on Elections in Africa during the COVID-19 Pandemic July 2020.
41 As above.
42 As above.
43 Press Release, African Commission on Human and People's Rights Special Rapporteur on Freedom of Expression and Access to Information in Africa, Commissioner Lawrence Mute 8 April 2020.
44 As above.
45 As above.
46 As above.

47 ACHPR/Res. 449 (LXVI) 2020.
48 Para 2.
49 Para 3.
50 Para 4.
51 Para 5.
52 Para 7.
53 As above.
54 As above.
55 See Concluding Observations and Recommendations on the 2nd and 3rd Combined Periodic Report of the Republic of Malawi on the Implementation of the African Charter on Human and Peoples' Rights (2015–2019) Adopted by the African Commission on Human and Peoples' Rights at the 70th Ordinary Session held from 23 February to 9 March 2022.
56 See E Durojaye 'The contribution of the African human rights system to the understanding of the right to health' (2021) 21(2) *African Human Rights Law Journal* 441.
57 See, *Purohit and Anor v Gambia* (n 29 above). See also, *Social and Economic Rights Action Center (SERAC) and Another v Government of Nigeria* Communication 155/96 decided at the 30th Ordinary Session of the African Commission held from 13 to 27 October 2001, Banjul, The Gambia.
58 See for instance *Free Legal Assistance Group and Others v. Zaire,* Communication. No. 25/89, 47/90, 56/91, 100/93.
59 World Health Organization 'Global report – South Africa' available at www.covid-19.who.int.
60 R De Coning 'South Africa's national response to COVID-19, with specific reference to sub-level governance in provinces' (2020) 3(1) *Africa Journal of Public Sector Development and Governance* 74–89.
61 *Mohamed and Others v President of the Republic of South Africa and Others* [2020] ZAGPPHC 120.
62 *De Beer and Others v Minister of Cooperative Governance and Traditional Affairs* [2020] ZAGPPHC 676 (23 October 2020).
63 *Esau and Others v Minister of Co-operative Governance and Traditional Affairs and Others* (611/2020) [2021] ZASCA 9 (28 January 2021).
64 As above, para 55.
65 As above.
66 As above, para 105.
67 More analysis on the measures adopted by the South African government during COVID-19, see R Nanima et al 'Constitutional and human rights issues arising from COVID-19 in South Africa' in E Durojaye & D Powell (eds) *Constitutional resilience and the COVID-19 pandemic: Perspectives from Africa* (2022).
68 See Worldometer Kenya available at www.worldometers.info/coronavirus/country/kenya/
69 *LSK v Hillary Mutyambai*, 2020, para 113.
70 As above, para 115.
71 As above.
72 As above, para 132.
73 *Okoth*, para 193.
74 As above.
75 Public Health (Prevention, Control and Suppression of Covid-19) Rules, Legal Notice 49 of 2020, Rule 8. *Okoth*, para 194.
76 *Okoth*, para 201, 248, 259 and 278.
77 Para 137.
78 Worldometer Malawi www.worldometers.info/coronavirus/country/malawi/.

79 The Public Health Act Chapter 34-01 available at https://bit.ly/36uLytV (accessed 2 October 2020).
80 T Gonese, A Shivamba & A Meerkotter 'A legal overview of the impact of COVID-19 on justice and rights in Southern Africa' available at www.southernafricalitigationcentre.org/wp-content/uploads/2020/05/Policy-brief-1-of-2020-COVID-laws.pdf (accessed 4 October 2020).
81 The Public Health Act Chapter 34-01, section 30.
82 As above, section 31.
83 Public Health (Corona Virus Prevention, Containment and Management) Rules, 2020.
84 As above.
85 *The State (on the application of Kathumba & Ors) v The President & Others* (Judicial Review Cause No. 22 of 2020) [2020] MWHC 8.
86 For a detailed discussion on the implications of measures on the enjoyment of socio-economic rights of marginalized groups, see R Nanima & E Durojaye *The socio-economic rights impact of COVID-19 in selected informal settlements in Cape Town* (2020).
87 For a detailed analysis of the position the constitutionality of the measures adopted by the government to curb the spread of COVID-19 in Malawi, see R Nanima & E Durojaye 'Exploring the constitutionality of the measures adopted by selected African countries in response to the COVID-19 pandemic' (2020).

15

THE NEXUS BETWEEN COVID-19 AND GENDER-BASED VIOLENCE AGAINST WOMEN

A case of Botswana, Kenya, and Nigeria

Keikantse Phele

15.1 Introduction

The COVID-19 pandemic brought to the fore and highlighted an important aspect of health in developing countries, the unreadiness of responding to an unknown pandemic because of limited and almost non-existent healthcare systems. Apart from being unready, the lack of adequate and functional health systems in many countries proved to be a major challenge. One of the key limitations of the pandemic was that since scientists were not aware of the transmission and fatality of the virus, countries closed their borders, intra-travel was restricted, and businesses closed to reduce the disease burden.

COVID-19 is not only a health crisis but also a far-reaching intricate pandemic that affected all areas of livelihood, which has exposed inequalities in society and further evidenced the existing inequalities, particularly against minority and vulnerable groups.[1] The lockdowns and travel restrictions affected imported goods, travel, and access to healthcare in many countries. The most basic types of equipment, like beds, masks, and personal protective equipment (PPE), were in short supply in Africa.[2] In Africa, the lack of basic medical equipment like oxygen[3] and adequate hospital beds led to preventable deaths. It is estimated that 163 million people died in Africa from COVID-19 between 2020 and 2022.

According to the International Monetary Fund (IMF), 'low-income countries have been hard hit by the pandemic and their large financing needs are only likely to grow as they deal with the crisis and its economic aftermath.'[4] The economic progress that was made by countries in the Global South has been backtracked by COVID-19. In sub-Saharan Africa (SSA), such countries will experience a negative decline in their economies, which

DOI: 10.4324/9781032671437-18

will take them back 25 years on the progress that has been made.[5] The effect of that sharp decline will have a ripple impact and negatively affect the accessibility of services, including access to healthcare services and health commodities, apart from deepening inequalities and poverty. Apart from the loss of millions of lives and the health effects of long COVID-19, the number of cases of gender-based violence (GBV) has risen sharply across the globe.[6] GBV is one of the most globally prevalent human rights violations that affects mainly girls and women of any social and economic status.[7] An estimated one in three women will experience physical or sexual abuse in her lifetime,[8] with the number doubling in SSA.

Historically, epidemics have led to increased rates of intimate partner violence (IPV), unintended pregnancies, sexual exploitation, and other forms of GBV.[9] Other factors, such as poverty, lack of education, socioeconomic opportunities, and impunity for crime and abuse, also tend to contribute to and reinforce a culture of violence and discrimination based on gender. Such factors are frequently aggravated in times of conflict and displacement as the rule of law is eroded as families and societies are torn apart.[10]Africa remains unstable with coups and humanitarian crises each year, a factor that makes response to health emergencies poor.

Other factors that aggravate GBV include proximity to perpetrators, lack of safe spaces and homes for those who have been violated, restricted movements and confinement in homes, the vulnerability of survivors, the closure of courts, and patriarchy.[11]

Lesbian, Gay, Bi-Sexual, Transgender, and Intersex (LGBTI) persons, sex workers, and persons who inject drugs are adversely affected by the gendered nature of GBV. COVID-19, therefore, has dire consequences for the right to health, sexual and reproductive health rights (SRHR), freedom of movement, and access to services. In addressing the effects of COVID-19, Madziyire provides an intersectional approach that can be used to resolve such consequences, stating:

> A maternal, sexual, and reproductive health framework emphasizing human rights, acknowledging intersecting injustices, and recognising power structures is essential for addressing and monitoring the inequitable gender, health, and social effects of the pandemic.[12]

15.2 Feminism and access to health: COVID-19 and GBV

This chapter will explore the intersection of feminist approaches to dealing with GBV, mainly how the absence of women in the COVID-19 response teams in Africa affected an effective and inclusive response.

The lack of visibility of women in many African COVID-19 response teams[13] is problematic as women are positioned as 'caregivers, nurturers at homes and in communities in most African nations.'[14] There are 'powerful narratives of the women living with a debilitating health crisis in a socio-cultural environment where traditional gender identities for both men and women are still the preferred and practiced norm.'[15] Thus, it may seem correct that women with their advancement in society are still left behind in all areas of the socio, economic, and political environment.[16]

Globally, the health sector boosts 70% of women,[17] who were also and continue to be the larger responders to COVID-19 in hospitals, mostly as nurses.[18] It is adequate that they must be part of response teams and contribute to health strategies at a higher level in health emergencies.

The lack of visibility of women in the countries discussed provides an opportunity to assess feminist voices to find solutions that can be used to recalibrate the overwhelming burden of patriarchy on women, reduce GBV in women and girls, promote Sexual and Reproductive Health Rights (SRHR), bodily autonomy, and holistic inclusion of women in various health and pandemic responses. Feminism assists in responding to the dictates of patriarchal dominance to make progress for women's equal participation and inclusion in society at large.[19] Patriarchy is propelled by culture and religion across the world, as this is not only peculiar to African nations.[20] Patriarchy has silenced the voice of women in various contexts and leverages that continue to systematically oppress and exclude women from positions of power and authority.[21] While feminism is shunned as a collective of 'being anti-culture, anti-male and anti-religion and a Western ideology, it censures a system that unrepentantly places women's needs as secondary to men's'.[22] In many cultures, as this is not the norm, patriarchy is not called out for what it is because women and girls are socialized from a young age to remain silent and show respect towards men.[23] We must carefully analyze and understand the capitalist social structures that go hand in hand with the resurgence of all types of fundamentalisms and their totalizing discourses. They threaten to roll back our achievements and silence us into total patriarchal submission."[24]

Tamale provides a reflection and solutions on how women should fight the silence expected and imposed on them by patriarchy:[25]

> The first thing we must do is set aside our reluctance to engage with political structures, systems, and institutions. Often, we openly declare our organizations to be 'non-political.'
>
> We do not want to be tarred with the brush of politics and we distance ourselves from formal politics as much as possible.
>
> However, how can we avoid politics when women's subordination and oppression are a political issue? How can we engage the powerful patriarchs in our countries without confronting politics?[26]

Despite laws and the advancement of women into different positions in society, the engraved systematic patriarchal practices and demands have at many times found women socialized into silence – from home, communities, corporates, and politics. The majority of lawmakers and politicians are male, who then make decisions and interventions that put women in disadvantaged positions – positions that women can hardly negotiate from.

This fundamentalism, as Tamale refers to it, is an area that must be consistently challenged and contested by women so that they can create spaces that are inclusive and accommodative to everyone, that recognize and take women's rights as equal human rights as those of men – an aspect that patriarchy profusely rejects.

15.3 Regional and international commitments to GBV

This chapter will highlight and discuss select regional and international commitments that are against GBV, which the countries discussed in this chapter are parties to: The Protocol to the African Charter on Human and Peoples' Rights on the Rights of Women in Africa (Maputo Protocol)[27] The African Union's Agenda 2063, Sustainable Development Goals.[28] Internationally, some of the leading instruments against GBV are Convention on the Elimination of All forms of Discrimination Against Women (CEDAW), the UN Resolution 1325 on Women Peace and Security, the 1995 Beijing Platform for Action, the International Convention on Civil and Political Rights (ICCPR),[29] the Convention on the Rights of Children,[30] which have specific provisions on equal protection and the right to be protected from inhumane and degrading treatment. At a regional level, the African Union's Agenda 2063 'identifies GBV as a major obstacle to human security, peace, and development, often fueled by armed conflict, terrorism, extremism, and intolerance.'[31] Therefore, the mentioned texts are key in providing guidance with respect to interventions to reduce GBV.

The application of international law in national jurisdictions must be applied alongside local laws to provide holistic and effective action in ending GBV, which is an economic, social, health, and development concern.[32] Despite the efforts being made GBV is a scourge that needs to be attended to proactively. The intersection of an emergency health crisis did not deter the continuation of GBV but showed gaps in the response to GBV and the challenges that women, girls, key and vulnerable populations experience as a result of GBV.

15.4 Health commitments in the region

Countries in the region have undertaken some initiatives because of the commitments emanating from various regional agreements. It is against this backdrop that the various health commitments can assist in how countries respond to COVID-19 and future pandemics. One such commitment is the Abuja Declaration on HIV/AIDS, tuberculosis, and other related infectious diseases which were agreed on in 2001.[33] African countries committed to allocating 15% of their annual financial budgets to the health sector as a means of holistically improving the health systems in Africa. Botswana has met the agreements stipulated in this commitment, and Kenya and Nigeria are yet to satisfy the ethos of the commitments.[34] While Botswana has satisfied the budget allocation, the resource allocation as was evidenced by COVID-19 showed inadequacies of basic medical equipment, with the result being that those developing countries, including Botswana, had to rely on PPE donations from other countries[35]

The Africa Health Strategy 2016–2030 (Strategy)[36] with an overall vision of 'health is a human right that must be accessed by all' gives a view into how Africa should be implemented to achieve the goals set out in the Strategy. However, this has been backtracked by COVID-19. The lessons learnt from COVID-19 must be used to plan for future health emergencies.

Reproductive health[37] rights are a state of complete physical, mental, and social well-being, not merely the absence of disease or infirmity in all matters relating to the reproductive system and its functions and processes. It, therefore, implies that people can have a satisfying and safe sex life and that they can reproduce and have the freedom to decide when and how often to do so.[38] Sexual rights are defined as a state of physical, emotional, mental, and social well-being about sexuality; it is not merely the absence of disease, dysfunction, or infirmity. Sexual health requires a positive and respectful approach to sexuality and sexual relationships, as well as the possibility of having pleasurable and safe sexual experiences, free of coercion, discrimination, and violence. For sexual health to be attained and maintained, the sexual rights of all persons must be respected, protected, and fulfilled.[39]

15.5 Access to SRHR services during COVID-19

Recent evidence suggests that despite some concentrated declines in access to health services, in April and May 2020, many countries were able to maintain or restore access to essential health services, including the provision of contraceptives that enhance family planning. However, the impact of COVID-19 on access to health services has various effects and consequences across countries and is still ongoing.[40] As a result of these disruptions, as many as 1.4 million unintended pregnancies may have occurred globally before women were able to resume the use of family planning services, and this number could be as high as 2.7 million at the higher end of projections or as low as 500,000 at the lower end of projections.[41]

It is estimated that cases of teen pregnancies, unsafe abortions,[42] child marriages, and female genital mutilation (FGM)[43] will increase because of a lack of access to sexual and reproductive health rights (SRHR) services and commodities. Marginalized, underprivileged, and vulnerable communities have been adversely affected by access to SRHR services in SSA. Unmet needs will have far-reaching consequences in the future for all those affected.[44]

The intersection of COVID-19, the right to health, and GBV shows an intricate and continuing problematic anecdote of systematic multi-layered adverse effects women suffer on a day-to-day basis. The comparative analysis of the countries provides similarities in how countries approached the lack of access to essential services and commodities during the pandemic. It further shows an increase in mental health issues, GBV, and the absence of timely responses to GBV. Invariably, the response to COVID-19 also showed grave inequalities in accessing essential health services in SSA.

15.6 Legal framework on GBV in Botswana

This chapter discusses and analyzes Botswana's GBV issues and how it responded to COVID-19

On 2 April 2020, Botswana, a nation of an estimated 2.3 million people, followed suit with the global lockdowns with its first 28-day mandatory lockdown and shut down all business and restricted movements[45] to contain the virus and rate of infection. Only essential services were open for business, which comprised mainly health services and national security institutions. Only public hospitals were open and restricted to emergency health issues.[46] During the period of the 28-day restriction, the country was divided into zones that restricted intra-travel except with permits.

Invariably, access to SHRH services was affected across the country. Coupled with Constitution[47] of Botswana's lack of the right to health and the right to sexual and reproductive rights, many citizens, particularly women, suffered many consequences resulting from COVID-19 restrictions.

Like other countries in Africa and globally, Botswana experienced an overwhelming surge in GBV against women and girls. In Botswana, over 67% of women have experienced abuse, which is over double the global average.[48] GBV undermines the health, dignity, security, and autonomy of its victims, yet it remains shrouded in a culture of silence and normalization.[49] Victims of violence, the majority of which are women and girls, can suffer sexual and reproductive health consequences, including forced and unwanted pregnancies, sexually transmitted infections, including HIV, and even death.[50] The surge of GBV between March and April 2020 resulted in the Botswana police recording 22 cases of rape, 2 cases of murder and suicide, and 23 cases of defilement.[51]

15.7 Botswana laws on GBV

According to UNFPA, two-thirds of women experience GBV in Botswana and have experienced violence from people who are close to them.[52] While the Constitution is limited in terms of socioeconomic rights, the Domestic Violence Act provides for GBV remedies, except for marital rape which is not recognized in the Botswana laws.[53] The Constitution recognizes the right to life, dignity, equal protection of the law, and the right to be protected from inhuman and degrading treatment. The rights provided for in the Constitution are inclusive of the right and processes to be protected from GBV. The same rights are provided in the ICCPR and the Universal Declaration of Human Rights, in which Botswana is a signatory. Apart from the Domestic Violence Act, Botswana has also acceded to the CEDAW in 1996, which in its holistic approach is to eliminate all forms of discrimination against women.

15.8 Efforts by Botswana to tackle GBV

Section 2 of the Domestic Violence Act provides for four areas of violence that the lower courts, being the Magistrates Court, can deliberate on an urgent basis of application:

> '[D]omestic violence' means any controlling or abusive behavior that harms the health or safety of the applicant and includes- (a) physical abuse or threat thereof; (b) sexual abuse or threat thereof; (c) emotional, verbal, or psychological abuse; (d) economic abuse; (e) intimidation; (f) harassment; (g) damage to property;(h) where the applicant and the respondent do not stay in the same home, entry into the applicant's home without his or her consent; (i) unlawful detainment; or (j) stalking.

As a result of the high number of GBV cases, civil society organizations (CSOs), mainly Botswana Gender-Based Violence Prevention and Support Centre (BGBVPSC)[54] and other CSOs, advocated for a comprehensive response from the government. At the onset of the pandemic, ministers of different portfolios were invited to address the country on national television on how their departments will respond to COVID-19. The minister whose portfolio includes gender did not mention how they would tackle GBV. It is only when CSOs working on GBV were seeking relief from the public as a result of police reports that action was taken. As a result of the accountability demanded by the CSOs, the Botswana Police Services, for the first time in history, provided a toll-free number for reporting GBV during COVID-19.[55] While this was a welcome development, the police service had not provided the necessary needed environment for reporting GBV cases and their conclusion. CSOs provided further support, and through Men for Gender Justice, they provided an intersecting link of campaigns that focused on men as key agents of addressing GBV. Accordingly, a multi-sectoral approach to tackling GBV is needed and must be enhanced because it is mainly men who are perpetrators of GBV.[56]

To adequately respond to the increase in GBV cases, in November 2020 ad hoc GBV courts were set up across the country to expedite and provide relief at Magistrates Courts, which are lower courts that are found in all the major villages in Botswana. 'The Government moved to establish the courts after women's rights advocates warned that lockdown curbs were exacerbating high rates of GBV by confining many women at home with abusers.'[57] This was a welcome move by CSOs, as this was one of the focal points of advocacy initiatives.

15.9 Safe spaces for women and children

There are only three organizations that operate safe shelters for survivors of GBV in Botswana, and these organizations were overwhelmed, and continue to be, because of the escalation of GBV cases. BGBVPSC[58] provides a temporary shelter for GBV survivors and, during the 28-day lockdown in April 2020, called for relief as their center was full of survivors of GBV.[59]

According to a UNFPA report[60], BGBVPSC reported that during April 2020 they provided 155 people with shelter compared to 50–60 clients each month pre-COVID-19, 67 people sought counseling through online services, and 50 people sought assistance through short messages (SMS). Seven temporary shelters for GBV survivors were opened across Botswana, with one shelter reserved for men. The discrepancy and surge are evidenced by the statistics, showing that not only are shelters needed but also there must be direct investment by the government to adhere to some of its global commitments like the Sustainable Development Goals (SDGs) 3–5, which focus on ending harmful practices, and goal 10, which aims to reduce inequalities in various issues, including the right to health and GBV.[61]

SOS Children's Villages Botswana provides short-term and long-term accommodation and care for children who are at risk of losing parental care or have lost it.[62] Childline Botswana is another organization that provides a safe space for abused children. Women Against Rape (WAR)[63] provides services and safe spaces for women and girls who have experienced sexual abuse, particularly rape. Similarly, like BGBVPSC, it was overwhelmed by the need to provide more space during lockdowns in Botswana because of the higher number of rape cases.[64]

Despite the efforts of CSOs, the government does not have any structures that provide interventions and solutions against GBV. The response to GBV in Botswana is minimal and needs more structure and timely response. This will allow identified gaps and challenges to be addressed. The travel restrictions and the size of gatherings permitted affected the community engagement work of many CSOs, resulting in the suspension of community dialogue, training, sensitization, and information dissemination on human rights.[65] In some areas, because of the negative impact of COVID-19 restrictions, people living with Human Immunodeficiency Virus (PLWHIV) were provided with a three-month supply of medication, while some organizations were also able to obtain movement permits to offer house-to-house delivery of antiretroviral treatment. The limitations on outreach activities have meant the number of people reached by various interventions has plummeted.[66]

15.10 The intersection of COVID-19 and GBV in Kenya and Nigeria: A comparative analysis

Since the outbreak of the coronavirus disease COVID-19, emerging data and reports from those on the frontlines have shown that all types of violence against women and girls (VAWG) intensified in countries affected by the pandemic.[67]

The African Union Guidelines have prioritized increased budgetary allocation from the various special funds set up at national or continental levels and mobilized more resources from international development partners and other sources to be dedicated specifically to national rapid responses to protect women and girls from GBV.[68]

According to a Global Fund Report, the economic fallout of the COVID-19 pandemic has also resulted in a general decline in household incomes, negatively affecting access to food and shelter and contributing to deteriorating mental health, with a disproportionate impact on LGBTI communities and sex workers.[69] Key informants and organizations that provide services for women facing GBV also described a significant increase in cases of GBV, domestic violence, and intimate partner violence among women, young girls, and LGBTI people, who have borne the brunt of abuse from family members during the lockdown. The intersection of poverty, lax GBV laws, patriarchy, and the lack of social and legal protection for women and girls has also led to an increase in GBV.

15.11 Kenya

This section will assess the local and international efforts made by Kenya to reduce GBV and draw a conclusion on the successes, if any, and failures in curbing GBV.

Kenya acceded to CEDAW in 1984 for the recognition of the necessary laws to recognize the needs for women's rights and protection in all spheres and has also ratified the Maputo Protocol – the two leading instruments for the protection of women globally and in Africa. One of the key progresses and acknowledgment of the existence of the dire consequences of GBV in Kenya saw the amendment of the Constitution in 2010 through Section 27, which provides for equal protection and equality before the law.[70] Section 29 provides for the security of persons, which is limited by GBV. The formulation of the Female Genital Mutilation Act of 2010 was to reduce the effects of GBV because of harmful cultural practices metered out against women and girls through FGM, which is a common and harmful practice in Kenya.[71] One of the strides made by Kenya is the enactment of Chapter 63 of the Kenya Protection Against Domestic Violence Act of 2015.[72]

In April 2020, the National Council on Administration of Justice reported that it dealt with 35.8% of cases of GBV out of the other cases they had received.[73] FGM is common in Kenya, and it was noted as a form of GBV that was on the rise too.[74] There is a significant spike in sexual offenses in many parts of the country.[75] Sexual offenses such as rape and defilement have constituted more than 35% of all reported cases.

LVCT Health, a local Kenyan NGO, stated that in the 1.5 months following the COVID-19 lockdown, 'a total of 793 adolescent and young women presenting to their clinics reported experiencing violence, a stark increase from pre-COVID times.'[76] More adolescents fell pregnant, and because of multi-layered discrimination and COVID-19, they did not access health facilities, and that was observed after schools were closed to contain the spread of COVID-19.

Adolescent pregnancies and defilement SGBV numbers increased and were more visible during COVID-19 restrictions, which showed 'gender-based structural inequalities and challenging already weak health and social protection systems in many parts of the world.'[77] Survivors were kept away from health facilities due to the fear of contracting COVID-19 or of being forced to test for COVID-19,[78] even if they had no symptoms and had come in for another ailment, and they would then be made to go to a quarantine center if they tested positive. With one of the world's highest maternal mortality rates, which added to limited movements, hospital fees, and fear of contracting the virus, an estimated 18% of women gave birth to stillborn or preterm babies and presented at hospitals the last minute for birth, thus endangering their lives. There was also a decline and limitation in accessing SRHR commodities.[79]

As reports of GBV surging in the country became prominent, stakeholders lobbied to keep the national hotline open.[80] Additional resources were provided by foreign donors to hire counselors, advertise services provided by the hotline, and strengthen referrals for survivors. Other service providers resumed operations and set up toll-free hotlines, phone calls, and other virtual platforms to offer counseling services to survivors.

President Kenyatta ordered an investigation[81] 'of violence against women and girls, including rape, domestic violence, female genital mutilation, and child marriage' because of the escalating numbers of GBV during COVID-19 restrictions, which were at 92%.[82] The commitments of Generation Equality Forum Kenya[83] to end GBV by 2022 coincided with the escalation of SGBV during COVID-19. The Forum's key focus areas are gender equality and ending FGM and all forms of GBV by 2026. Essentially, the country intends to achieve that by using existing laws, policies, available data, effective service delivery, accountability, adequate financing, and collaborations with international partners.[84] It is argued that this is an ambitious target, and even with its consistency, many Kenyan women and girls continue to suffer from gender and socioeconomic inequalities. It will take more than aspirations to achieve that, and the direct involvement of beneficiaries must be considered as well as financial resources, experts, facilities, and effective implementation, to make significant progress.

While Kenya has adopted the Generation Equality Forum, it does not mention LGBTI persons. According to the National Gay and Lesbian Human Rights Commission (NGLHRC), an NGO that advocates for LGBT rights in Kenya, despite the response by Kenya, LGBTI persons were not included and suffered exclusion, discrimination, transphobia, and homophobia. Access to health, particularly for those living with HIV, was difficult.[85]

The Generation Equality Forum Kenya allows Kenya to be inclusive in ending all forms of GBV and equality in Kenya. The exclusion of key and vulnerable communities is a step back, as a holistic approach is needed for gender equality and an inclusive nation that recognizes and protects all human beings.

The rise in GBV in Kenya during COVID-19 has defeated and undermined the efforts that have been made at the international and national levels that seek to lessen the burden of GBV on women, girls, and vulnerable groups. Sections 27 and 29 of the Constitution and the Prohibition of the Female Genital Mutilation Act, which are critical in this discourse, have not been adhered to protect everyone equally. Rhetorically, the question is, if in promulgating the laws and acceding to and ratifying international commitments, were there any meaningful structures put in place to counteract the consequences of GBV in emergencies like COVID-19? Despite all the commitments, Kenya does not recognize marital rape as a crime, furthering the acceptable norms around GBV, particularly among spouses.[86] More efforts need to be done to show commitment against GBV and dismantle patriarchy to protect women.

15.12 Nigeria

Similar to Botswana and Kenya, Nigeria has national and local commitments to reduce the consequences of GBV, which have become endemic. According to Enemo, the basic rights of women are violated with little attention from the state.[87] Some of the international obligations that Nigeria has acceded to that promote dignity, equality, and protection of rights, are the CEDAW, which it ratified in 1985, the Universal Declaration of Human Rights Treaty, the ICCPR, and the International Convention Against Torture and Other

Inhuman or Degrading Treatment or Punishment (Torture Treaty).[88] While it is important to draw inferences from international commitments, local efforts have been made to lessen the burden of GBV. The Constitution provides for the right to life and dignity, while the Violence Against Persons (Prohibition) Act of 2015 (VAPP) prohibits all forms of violence against persons. The VAPP, with good intentions, is only limited to the Federal Capital Territory, which includes only the states in the Central region of Nigeria, including the capital Abuja, and excludes other states within Nigeria, a clear weakness of the law in protecting all against GBV.[89] In contrast to these efforts, Section 55 of the Penal Code provides for wives to be chastised by their husbands and for assaults on women as misdemeanors.[90] This has a negative effect on women reporting GBV, as the law itself perpetuates violence against women.[91]

In Nigeria, a sharp rise in GBV cases by 56% was reported across 24 states during the first two weeks of April 2020 compared with the same period in March, after lockdown measures were enacted on 31 March 2020.[92] According to a UN Women's Report,[93] a change in household environment because of the proximity of families and being confined for longer periods was realized. The UNFPA Global Site Report 2020 provides that 'apart from the COVID-19 pandemic, the resulting loss of income and huge household stress suffered by women and girls has, in addition, presented a prevalence of SGBV challenges in the contexts of increased risks of domestic violence, intimate partner violence, and sexual exploitation and abuse, as well as barriers to help-seeking options for survivors'.

The tension between couples and emotional, physical, and sexual abuse were some of the forms of violence experienced by women.[94] The UN Women, UNFPA, UNODC, UNICEF UN System in Nigeria (2020) Briefing Paper maintained that as Nigeria began to feel the effects of the COVID-19 outbreak's interactions with limited healthcare infrastructure and multiple pre-existing inequalities and fragilities, the emergence of the Shadow Pandemic of GBV also threatened the health and well-being of already vulnerable women and girls. It added that due to pre-existing inequalities and vulnerabilities, groups of women and girls face heightened risks of experiencing SGBV during the pandemic.[95]

Women with disabilities as a vulnerable group did not escape the devastating effects of COVID-19. Affected groups also included refugees and internally displaced persons, women and girls living with disabilities, and informal workers.[96]

Misuse of funds by family members, lack of food, and lack of access to hospitals were experienced by women with disabilities. Access to health was hindered by expensive hospital fees, transport limitations, and movement restrictions. Those with maternal healthcare needs, such as pregnancy, faced challenges in registering pregnancies for natal check-ups due to restricted movements.[97] Thus, the effects of COVID-19 cut across all home environments, and in some households 'men were suddenly violent, and conflicts arose easily.'[98]

There was a disruption in access to SRHR commodities, which already have limited access because of existing inequalities.[99] Limitations brought by COVID-19 resulted in lack of contraception, low uptake where it was available and a decreased in the number of people using it. According to a study conducted in six countries, including Nigeria, to assess access to SRHR commodities, it was found that there was an increase in forced child marriages and adolescent pregnancies in North Nigeria,[100] thus endangering children and adolescents' reproductive and sexual health and lifetime mental health problems.[101]

As a result of COVID-19 burnout, illness, and the health budget for PPE equipment, Nigeria experienced a shortage of healthcare workers, which impeded access to health.[102] The lack of data on the extent of SGBV experienced in Nigeria by different communities is not documented, which is a gap in how future responses to GBV can be enhanced. The distortion and inaccuracy of data make advocacy campaigns difficult, as well as holding leaders accountable for inaction.[103]

The sharp increase in femicide, SGBV, and limitations on accessing SRHR services in Nigeria formed a movement that spread across Africa to call on Nigerian leaders to act and show commitment against GBV. In November 2020, Nigeria declared rape and GBV a state of emergency, in an endeavor to make better laws and protect women and girls from GBV. Social media, particularly Twitter, was used by Nigerian activists to demand action from the Nigerian government. The hashtag #withher was used during the Twitter campaign and is popularized by the Spotlight Initiative[104] movement, which focuses on campaigning globally for the reduction of GBV in 2030 in line with the SDGs.

15.13 Recommendations

The IMF has approved a far-reaching package of support that would expand low-income countries' access to financial assistance at zero-interest rates while 'providing stronger safeguards against taking on debt they cannot handle'. For these efforts to succeed, economically stronger member countries will have to play their part.[105]

There is an urgent need for countries to adhere to the commitments of the African and global health and rights commitments, which will reduce the disease burden in sub-Saharan Africa. Implementing the obligations will not be effective if it does not include key populations, vulnerable, and marginalized communities. The decriminalization of LGBTI is needed as a right and for the protection of human rights, dignity, and equality.

COVID-19 exposed inequalities in society, which highlighted, among others, poverty and a lack of access to basic health services. Investments in health systems must be made to promote the best-attainable state of well-being. The lessons learned from the HIV response in Africa must be applied to COVID-19 so that health systems can improve in the future. While COVID-19 and HIV may be parallel in their spread, knowledge about preparedness and approaches are lessons that can improve how to respond effectively in a health emergency. Many sub-Saharan African countries did not have the basic equipment, for instance, protective wear, for healthcare practitioners, which exposed many to COVID-19.

GBV is a product of patriarchy that is worsened by a lack of political will to enact laws that will deal with perpetrators of GBV. Apart from political will, the judiciary, police, and social welfare are core to GBV's response. Collaborative and well-funded structures that are focused on challenging GBV will provide a better future for women and girls. Without commitment, the cycle of GBV will continue as observed during COVID-19.

Recognition of women as equals in society and feminist values of equality and inclusivity must always be included in responses to pandemics and health emergencies by incorporating the principle of leaving no one behind and for us by us.

Direct funding of civil society organizations by national governments with transparency must be taken as collaboration partnerships and not tokens to serve political aspirations. Funding will give opportunities for safe spaces and shelters that can accommodate survivors of GBV with a wide array of specialized services.

The demilitarization of responses to national emergencies must be replaced by inclusive security policies that recognize that it is mainly poor people who are affected, most people who do menial jobs, and women who work at markets for survival.

Provision of social, economic, political, and cultural rights; improving lives through social contracts by politicians; and free and quality healthcare committed to the betterment of people's lives are the need of the hour. SRHR rights must be recognized as fundamental human rights and be promoted as such.[106]

According to Tamale, 'feminist agenda of all forms of fundamentalism, whether it is cultural fundamentalism (such as the revival of virginity tests), religious fundamentalism (such as the crippling of women's sexual and reproductive rights), or economic fundamentalism (such as neo-liberal structural adjustment policies), all pose a serious threat to the feminist agenda.

Increased crime rates, increased SRHR violations, SGBV, all forms of sexual and reproductive health rights violations, and sexual and GBV were reported to have been directly experienced by women and girls. The interventions were focused on the need to increase public awareness and to train and retrain law enforcement personnel and those involved in enforcing COVID-19 protocols, as well as religious leaders, traditional rulers, market leaders, and community educators on SRHR and SGBV as they relate to COVID-19 and its protocols. The second identified intervention was to set up clusters in public places, such as community markets and churches, to enable victims of gender and family violence to alert the authorities.

'Effective protection can be established only by preventing SGBV, identifying risks, and responding to survivors, using a coordinated, multi-sectoral approach. The present protection environment in Kenya is fraught with challenges and filled with opportunities, which should be carefully considered when devising responses. Whereas the Kenyan legal framework provides a mechanism for addressing SGBV, the extent to which the frameworks respond to the plight of the survivors of SGBV is debatable. The legal and policy framework mostly focuses on bringing the accused person to 'justice' without a corresponding obligation to alleviate the conditions of the survivor of SGBV. The survivor of SGBV is more of an alien to the criminal justice system because the offense is perceived by the system to have been committed against the state, not against the survivor of the SGBV as an individual.[107]

The interdependency between the provision of public services, GBV, and women's economic rights, including unpaid care work, must be recognized and addressed. GBV is not only about physical or sexual abuse but is becoming wider than this because women bear the brunt of the inadequate service delivery.[108]

Botswana's response to COVID-19 in closing the borders and implementing the recommended WHO protocols was made within a reasonable time in line with other SADC countries in April 2020. Technically, the response has progressed well. On the socioeconomic front, it is a gloomy picture, particularly in the sense that GBV is almost not addressed generally because of the silence around it and the patriarchal nature of the Botswana culture, which highlights in many ways the countries' priorities.

With only one GBV shelter in Gaborone, the capital city, and one rape crisis center in Maun – which are all donor-funded – survivors of GBV had nowhere to go for safety. Limited movements and the lack of toll-free lines or drop-in centers in a crisis have left survivors with dire mental health consequences.

Overreliance on South Africa for SRHR commodities and the closing of borders in the last two years have led to unwanted pregnancies and the unavailability of condoms in public health institutions[109] that are accessed for free across the country. With such a gap, there is a likelihood of an increase in HIV infections, STIs, and unwanted pregnancies. Botswana laws prohibit abortion with exceptions for fatal pregnancies, rape, and incest, and thus the procurement of abortion is not an option because it is criminalized.[110]

A committed political position to change the landscape of violence in sub-Saharan Africa by enacting policies, laws, and instituting effective mechanisms and structures – for instance, GBV courts, government-funded safe spaces, and shelters, and the inclusion of women in making decisions that affect them.

Above all, a gendered, inclusive, human rights-based approach to women-led response[111] in day-to-day lives and a robust one during pandemics will contribute to enhanced access to health services, a reduced number of GBV cases, and a better quality of life for women and girls. A dedicated budget and capacitated personnel in GBV, health, SRHR provision, counseling, and a wide array of non-discriminative and accommodative services are additional factors.

Botswana, Kenya, Nigeria, and Zimbabwe have similar responses to COVID-19. Kenya, with its internet access, has managed to roll out online GBV responses to survivors in the country. Women and girls in rural and indigenous areas may find it difficult to reach and access the services. However, it is a lesson learned from Kenya that can be used in innovative ways to use offline apps to be able to reach as many people as possible.

The response to COVID-19 must reflect the aspirations of the CEDAW, African health commitments, the Maputo Protocol, and the values of non-discrimination, equality, and the highest attainable health, and diversity and inclusion. The diversion of many health budgets to focus on COVID-19 disregarded SRHR needs and did not anticipate a sharp rise in GBV cases.[112] These are the recommitments that countries must make to ensure the response to COVID-19 is better in the future. There is an urgent need to brand access to health as inclusive and dignified. The focus on COVID-19 on health systems in the countries discussed and in African countries must be a lesson learned in how not to respond to one area of health and neglect others.

15.14 Future pandemics and the way forward

COVID-19, the right to health, and GBV have intersections that can be used for effective response and successful implementation of future pandemic interventions. SSA has the highest disease burden globally. SAA has experience with Ebola, Malaria, HIV, MDR TB, and now COVID-19, and with such experience, governments must be able to use multifaceted approaches to respond to future pandemics.

Any response to any future pandemics will be determined by various factors, including a collective top-down approach, from government to stakeholders to communities. The positive approaches that have been used in the past must be the basis for interventions in future pandemics. Because of the health inequalities and inequities in SSA, there are critical factors that must inform effective interventions in the future. Some of the factors are poverty, rural and indigenous communities, key and vulnerable communities, lack of water, access, and location to health facilities, and a budget for emergency health situations.

Achieving the SDGs needs strategic planning that encompasses all key respondents, and this will not be done without putting people first and directing and 'early quality investment in high tier facilities in public health care to tackle inequalities.'[113] Without investment, there will be a loss of lives, as in the past pandemic.

A human rights-based approach should be developed, promoted, and implemented so that everyone is included. Such development and promotion will lead to health equity that will 'support improved health governance and leadership allowing health systems to reflect better in the population they serve while reducing health inequalities.[114]

Future pandemics will need preparedness, a stable and improved political and socioeconomic environment, transparency by leaders, available expertise, and trained responders across all sectors. One of the key factors in SSA is that countries must share and learn from each other and be able to share expertise and provide capacity to one another, rather than relying on the Global North, as was observed during COVID-19. Local philanthropies and African-grown corporates are also key players governments can approach as part of their Environmental Social Governance (ESG) and sustainability processes to support responses to future pandemics.

15.15 Conclusion

The COVID-19 pandemic has shown that GBV is an urgent matter that must be addressed by all stakeholders. It is also evident that it is women, children, and vulnerable populations who are significantly affected than men and boys in all their diversity. Despite GBV national laws and international commitments that the countries discussed in this chapter have enacted and are parties to, national budgets, policies, laws, and accessible services are lacking to protect those who are adversely affected. Without deliberate efforts and political will, women, girls, and vulnerable populations will continue to suffer because of GBV.

While laws may exist, there must be a shift in society against the social construction of women and girls that their agency is not through a patriarchal binary lens but by self-determination. Countries must adhere to commitments they have made locally and internationally to lessen the burden of GBV. The numbers of GBV violations in each country indicate that it is time that countries provide safety and security to those who are adversely affected. There need to be clear laws, policies, accessible safety measures, and an effective justice system that will enable those who experience GBV to be provided with protection of the law to ensure dignity, safety, and promotion of bodily integrity as envisioned in national and international commitments on GBV.

Without an inclusive gendered response, women and girls will be excluded and cannot be part of an adequate and dignified response to COVID-19. The feminist approach must be applied in interventions against GBV to decrease and eliminate GBV that is aggravated by patriarchy.

The Maputo Protocol, SDGs, national laws, and visions in the three countries not only denote an interest in protecting women but also show invariably the lack of commitment of political leadership to provide needed systems and implementation of laws to break the barriers of patriarchy to protect women, girls, and vulnerable populations from the deeply problematic and entrenched GBV.

The devastating effects of COVID-19 were not only health-related but also emphasized increased GBV, lack of access to basic health services, and the failure of states to provide adequate services and support for those experiencing GBV, which has deepened the inequalities experienced by women and girls in all their diversities. The national laws and international laws are meant to provide a transformative power for women, girls, and vulnerable groups to be free from GBV, which, as articulated in this chapter, needs effort, deliberate attention, and action.[115]

Notes

1 Socio-economic impact of COVID-19 in Botswana available at www.google.com/search?q=Socio-Economic+Impact+of+COVID-19 (accessed 29 January 2022).
2 Corona virus disease (COVID-19) scorecard in Africa hospital conditions beds and critical care available at https://accountability.international/coronavirus/ (accessed 29 January 2022).
3 As above.
4 C Mumssen & S Nolan‘ Report: Stepping up to meet low-income countries' pandemic recovery needs'(2021) available at https://blogs.imf.org/2021/07/26/stepping-up-to-meet-low-income-countries-pandemic-recovery-needs/ (accessed 26 January 2022).
5 International Monetary Fund paves way to new era austerity post-Covid-19 available at www.oxfam.org/en/press-releases/imf-paves-way-new-era-austerity-post-covid-19 (accessed 19 January 2022).
6 As above.
7 As above.
8 As above.
9 https://africa.unwomen.org/sites/default/files/Field%20Office%20Africa/Attachments/Publications/2021/Policy%20Paper-%20GBV%20in%20Africa%20during%20COVID-19%20pandemic_EN%2018%20Feb_compressed.pdf (accessed 20 January 2022).
10 As above.
11 As above.
12 G Murewanhema & MG Madziyire 'Covid-19 restrictive measures and maternal sexual and reproductive health issues: Risk of a double tragedy for women in sub-Saharan' (2021) 40 *Africa Pan African Medical Journal* 122.
13 https://reliefweb.int/report/world/where-are-women-conspicuous-absence-women-covid-19-response-teams-and-plans-and-why-we (accessed 30 January 2022).
14 As above.
15 Mumbi Silence as power: Women bargaining with patriarchy in Kenya (2016) 35(1) 14.

16 S Tamale 'African feminism: How should we change' (2006) 49(1) *Development* 40.
17 Corona virus (COVID-19) scorecard for Africa nurses and midwives and doctors available at https://accountability.international/coronavirus/ (accessed 30 January 2022).
18 African UN Women (n 53 above). https://africa.unwomen.org/sites/default/files/Field%20Office%20Africa/Attachments/Publications/2021/Policy%20Paper-%20GBV%20in%20Africa%20during%20COVID-19%20pandemic_EN%2018%20Feb_compressed.pdf (accessed 20 January 2022).
19 As above.
20 As above.
21 Mumbi Silence as power: Women bargaining with patriarchy in Kenya (n 16 above) 14.
22 As above.
23 As above.
24 Tamale (n 17 above) 40.
25 As above.
26 Tamale (n 17 above) 41.
27 OAU Do CAB/LEG/66.6 (2003) entered into force 25 November 2005.
28 Sustainable development goals available at https://sdgs.un.org/goals (accessed 1 May 2022).
29 GA Res 2200 (XXI), 21 UN GAOR Supp (No 16) 52, UN Doc A/ 6316 (1966), 999 UNTS Entered into force 23 March 1976.
30 Convention on the Rights of the Child, GA Res 44/25, annex,44UN GAOR Supp (No49) 167, UN Doc A/44/49 (1989), entered into force 2 September 1990.
31 SADC regional strategy and framework for addressing GBV 2018–2020, 9 available at www.unodc.org/documents/southernafrica/Stories/2019/SADC_Regional_Strategy_and_Framework_for_Action_on_GBV_-_FINAL_September_2018_-_ENGLISH_VERSION.pdf (accessed 1 May 2022).
32 Enemo (n 1 above) 13.
33 African Union 'Paper: African Summit on HIV/AIDS, Tuberculosis and other related infectious diseases' (2001) available at https://au.int/sites/default/files/pages/32894-file-2001-abuja-declaration.pdf (accessed 26 January 2022).
34 As above.
35 https://africacdc.org/news-item/africa-cdc-receives-third-donation-of-medical-supplies-from-jack-ma-foundation-co-hosts-global-medixchange-webinar-on-covid-19/ (accessed 28 January 2022).
36 African Union 'Report: Africa health strategy 2016–2030' (2016) available at https://au.int/sites/default/files/documents/24098-au_ahs_strategy_clean.pdf (accessed 26 January 2022).
37 See also http://apps.who.int/iris/bitstream/10665/258738/1/9789241512886-eng.pdf?ua=1 See also www.un.org/popin/unfpa/taskforce/guide/iatfreph.gdl.html (accessed 24 August 2018).
38 Reproductive rights are human rights A handbook for national human rights institutions available at www.ohchr.org/Documents/Publications/NHRIHandbook.pdf 7 (accessed 24 August 2018).
39 As above.
40 www.unfpa.org/sites/default/files/resource-pdf/COVID_Impact_FP_V5.pdf (accessed 19 January 2022).
41 Reproductive rights are human rights A handbook for national human rights institutions (n 39 above).
42 www.mariestopes.org/what-we-do/our-services/safe-abortion-and-post-abortion-care/ (accessed 21 January 2022).
43 https://reliefweb.int/report/burkina-faso/resilience-action-lessons-learned-joint-programme-during-covid-19-crisis-unfpa (accessed 13 January 2022).

44 As above.
45 www.who.int/docs/default-source/coronaviruse/country-case-studies/botswana-c19-case-study-20-july.pdf? (accessed 27 January 2022).
46 UNFPA Botswana report available at https://botswana.unfpa.org/en/topics/gender-based-violence-1 (accessed 25 January 2022).
47 Constitution of Botswana CAP 00:00.
48 UNFPA Botswana Report (n 47 above).
49 As above.
50 As above.
51 www.mmegi.bw/news/worrisome-drug-use-on-the-rise-in-covid-19-lockdown/news (accessed 25 January 2022).
52 UNFPA Botswana Report (n 47 above).
53 CAP 28:05.
54 Botswana gender based violence prevention and support centre available at www.bgbvc.org.bw/index.php/about/our-history (accessed 20 January 2022).
55 https://allafrica.com/stories/202010160050.html (accessed 15 January 2022).
56 As above.
57 TM Obagboye 'Addressing gender-based violence in Africa (Nigeria and Botswana)' (2021) *Saudi Humanities Social Sciences Journal* 409.
58 Botswana Gender-Based Violence Prevention and Support Centre (n 55 above).
59 https://botswana.unfpa.org/en/news/much-more-needs-be-done-ending-gender-based-violence-botswana (accessed 23 January 2022).
60 As above.
61 UN sustainable development goals available at https://sdgs.un.org/goals (accessed 22 January 2022).
62 SOS Botswana available at www.sos-botswana.org/index.php/our-strategy (accessed 27 January 2022).
63 Women against rape Botswana available at www.womenagainstrape.org.bw/index.html (accessed 23 January 2022).
64 As above.
65 Mid-term assessment Botswana global fund report available at www.theglobalfund.org/media/10862/crg_2021-midtermassessmentbotswana_report_en.pdf (accessed 24 January 2022).
66 As above.
67 United Nations women Africa policy papers gender-based violence during COVID-19 pandemic available at https://africa.unwomen.org/sites/default/files/Field%20Office%20Africa/Attachments/Publications/2021/Policy%20Paper-%20GBV%20in%20Africa%20during%20COVID-19%20pandemic_EN%2018%20Feb_compressed.pdf (accessed 26 January 2022).
68 Mid-term Assessment Botswana Global Fund Report (n 66 above).
69 As above.
70 Kenya Constitution of 2010.
71 Tanui-Too et al. 'Gender equality and empowerment of women and girls: The implementation of SGD 5 in Kenya' (2021) *Africa Habitat Review* 17.
72 No 2 of 2015.
73 Generation equality forum Kenya road map available at www.genderinkenya.org/wp-content/uploads/2021/06/Generation-Equality-Forum_Kenya-Roadmap_Policy-Brief.pdf 7 (accessed 29 January 2022).
74 As above.
75 McGovern et al. 'COVID-19 and gender-based violence (GBV): Hard-to-reach women and girls, services, and programmes in Kenya' (2021) (29) *Gender & Development* 1 60.
76 As above, 58. https://africa.unwomen.org/sites/default/files/Field%20Office%20Africa/Attachments/Publications/2021/Policy%20Paper-%20GBV%20

in%20Africa%20during%20COVID-19%20pandemic_EN%2018%20Feb_compressed.pdf.

77 McGovern et al. (n 76 above) 59.

78 As above, 65.

79 J Thorpe 'The reproductive health fall- out of a global pandemic' (28) *Sexual and Reproductive Health Matters* 1.

80 McGovern et al. (n 76 above) 66.

81 As above.

82 Generation equality forum Kenya's roadmap for gender equality available at www.genderinkenya.org/publication/generation-equality-forum-kenyas-roadmap-for-gender-equality/ (accessed 29 January 2022).

83 Generation Equality Forum Kenya Road Map (n 74 above).

84 As above, 3–4.

85 The impact of COVID-19 on human rights of LGBT persons available at www.ohchr.org/Documents/Issues/SexualOrientation/IESOGI-COVID-19/CSOs/NGLHRC.pdf (accessed 27 January 2022).

86 Tanui-Too et al. (n 72 above).

87 Enemo (n 1 above) 13.

88 Resolution 3452 (XXX) entered into force on 26 June 1987.

89 Enemo (n 1 above) 6.

90 Act of 1960 See also www.equalitynow.org/discriminatory_law/northern_nigeria_the_penal_code/ (accessed 1 May 2022).

91 Enemo (n 1 above) 4.

92 https://africa.unwomen.org/sites/default/files/Field%20Office%20Africa/Attachments/Publications/2021/Policy%20Paper-%20GBV%20in%20Africa%20during%20COVID-19%20pandemic_EN%2018%20Feb_compressed.pdf (accessed 26 January 2022).

93 Experiences of women with disabilities in Nigeria during COVID-19 available at https://reliefweb.int/sites/reliefweb.int/files/resources/Brief-Experiences-of-women-with-disabilities-in-Nigeria-during-COVID-19-en.pdf (accessed 28 January 2022).

94 As above.

95 UN Women Briefing Paper UN System 21 (2020).

96 Jenyo 'An assessment of the Covid-19 pandemic on sexual and gender based violence in Nigeria' (2020) 7(1) *International Journal of Peace and Conflict Studies* 12.

97 As above.

98 As above.

99 Effects of COVID-19 on sexual and reproductive health; Case study available at https://reliefweb.int/report/world/effects-covid-19-sexual-and-reproductive-health-case-study-six-countries (accessed 28 January 2022).

100 As above.

101 As above.

102 As above.

103 Gender and COVID-19 in Nigeria available at www.genderandcovid-19.org/wp-content/uploads/2020/10/Gender-and-COVID-19-in-Nigeria.pdf (accessed 29 January 2022).

104 With her www.spotlightinitiative.org/withher/withher (accessed 30 January 2022).

105 Nolan et al. 'Stepping up to meet low-income countries' pandemic recovery needs' available at https://blogs.imf.org/2021/07/26/stepping-up-to-meet-low-income-countries-pandemic-recovery-needs/ (accessed 27 January 2022).

106 A feminist response to COVID-19 available at https://equipop.org/for-a-feminist-response-to-covid-19/ (accessed 19 January 2022).

107 Aura, situational analysis and legal framework available at http://kenyalaw.org/kl/index.php?id=4512 (accessed 27 January 2022).
108 Stopping abuse and female exploitation (SAFE) Zimbabwe technical assistance facility violence against women and girls during the COVID-19 crisis in Zimbabwe: Analysis of practice-based data from women's coalition of Zimbabwe (analysis of data: March – May 2020) (July 2020) available at www.adultrapeclinic.org.zw/wp-content/uploads/2020/09/SAFE-Report-on-Gender-Based-Violence-Data-in-Zimbabwe-during-C19-for-publication-with-logo.pdf (accessed 27 January 2022).
109 Condom shortage BONELA calls for action available at www.mmegi.bw/news/condom-shortage-bonela-calls-for-action/news (accessed 29 January 2022).
110 Section 224 Penal Code.
111 New Zealand positioned itself as a model of how female leadership bring inclusivity and a feminist lens to acute health pandemics available at www.feministcovidresponse.com/wp-content/uploads/2020/12/Feminist-Response-to-COVID-19-Advocacy-Monitoring-Toolkit-English-2.pdf (accessed 30 January 2022).
112 Effects of COVID-19 on sexual and reproductive health; Case study (n 100 above).
113 Falchetta et al. 'Planning universal accessibility to public health care in Sub-Saharan Africa' (2020) *PNAS* 31764.
114 George et al. 'Addressing neglected tropical diseases in Africa: A health equity perspective' (2023) 8 *Global Health Research and Policy* 5, Article number: 30.
115 Enemo (n 1 above) 1.

BIBLIOGRAPHY

Journal articles

P Enemo 'Effectiveness of Nigeria's International Obligations in Curbing Domestic Violence' (2018) 9(1) *Nnamdi Azikiwe University of International Law and Jurisprudence* 1–13.

G Falchetta, A Hammond, & S Shayeh 'Planning Universal Accessibility to Public Health Care in Sub Saharan Africa' (2020) 117(50) *Proceedings of the National Academy of Sciences* 31760–31769.

NS George, SC David, M Nabiryo, BA Sunday, OF Olanrewaju, Y Yangaza, & DO Shomuyiwa 'Addressing Neglected Tropical Diseases in Africa: A Health Equity Perspective' (2023) 8(30) *Global Health Research and Policy* 1–7.

G Gwatiri & K Mumbi 'Silence as Power: Women Bargaining with Patriarchy in Kenya' (2016) 35(1) *Social Alternatives* 13–18.

O Jenyo 'An Assessment of the Covid-19 Pandemic on Sexual and Gender Based Violence in Nigeria' (2020) 7(1) *International Journal of Peace and Conflict Studies* 12–25.

G Murewanhema & MG Madziyire 'Covid-19 Restrictive Measures, and Maternal Sexual and Reproductive Health Issues: Risk of a Double Tragedy for Women in Sub-Saharan' (2021) *Africa Pan African Medical Journal* 122–126.

J Neetu, C Roy, M Mwangi, N Raval, & T McGovern 'COVID-19 and Gender-Based Violence (GBV): Hard-to-Reach Women and Girls, Services, and Programmes in Kenya' (2021) 29(1) *Gender & Development* 55–71.

TG Obagboye 'Addressing Gender Based Violence in Africa (Nigeria and Botswana)' (2021) 6(10) *Saudi Journal of Humanities for Social Sciences* 405–413.

S Tamale 'African Feminism: How Should We Change?' (2006) 49(1) *Development* 38–41.

P Tanui-Too & J Chelang'a 'Gender Equality and Empowerment of Women and Girls: The Implementation of SGD 5 in Kenya' (2021) *Africa Habitat Review* 13–21.

International instruments and documents

Africa Agenda 2063.

African Charter on Human and Peoples' Rights, adopted 27 June 1981 OAU Doc CAB/ LEG/67/3 Rev 5, 21 ILM 58 (1982) entered into force 21 October 1986.

Convention on the Elimination of All Forms of Discrimination Against Women, Adopted 18 December 1979, GA Res 34/180, UN GAOR,34th session, UN Doc A/34/46(1980), entered into force 3 September 1981.
Convention on the Rights of the Child, GA Res 44/25, annex, 44UN GAOR Supp (No49) 167, UN Doc A/44/49 (1989), entered into force 2 September 1990.
International Covenant on Civil and Political Rights, GA Res 2200A(XXI), 21 un GAOR Supp. (No 16) 52, UN Doc A/ 6316(1966)993 UNTS 3 (entered into force 3 January 1976).
Programme of Action of the International Conference on Population and Development, Report of the International Conference on Population and Development, 5–13 September 1994, UN Doc A/CONF. 171 13.
Protocol to the African Charter on Human and Peoples' Rights on the Rights of Women in Africa OAU Doc CAB/LEG/66.6 (2003) entered into force 25 November 2005.
UN Sustainable Development Goals.
Universal Declaration of Human Rights, adopted and proclaimed by the United Nations Assembly in Resolution 217 A (III) 1948.

Legislation

Botswana Domestic Violence Act of 2009.
Constitution of the Federal Republic of Nigeria of 1999(As amended).
Constitution of the Republic of Botswana of 1966 (As amended).
Constitution of the Republic of Kenya of 2010.
Matrimonial Causes Act of 2004 of Nigeria.
Penal Code of Botswana Chapter 08:01.
Penal Code of Kenya of 2012.
Prohibition of Female Genital Mutilation Act of 2015.
Violence Against Persons (Prohibition) Act of 2015.

Reports

African Union 'Paper: African Summit on HIV/AIDS, Tuberculosis and Other Related Infectious Diseases' (2001) https://au.int/sites/default/files/pages/32894-file-2001-abuja-declaration.pdf (accessed 26 January 2022).
African Union 'Report: Africa Health Strategy 2016–2030' (2016) https://au.int/sites/default/files/documents/24098-au_ahs_strategy_clean.pdf (accessed 26 January 2022).
Bothoko P Mmegi Online 'Worrisome Drug Use on the Rise in Covid 19 Lockdown' www.mmegi.bw/news/worrisome-drug-use-on-the-rise-in-covid-19-lockdown/news (accessed 25 January 2022).
Gays and Lesbians of Zimbabwe 'Report: COVID-19 SOCIO-ECONOMIC IMPACT LGBTIQ+ on Lockdown in Zimbabwe A GALZ Report on the Socio-Economic Challenges Experienced by the LGBTIQ+ Community in Zimbabwe during the Covid-19 Lockdown Isolation Period' (2020) https://galz.org/wp-content/uploads/2020/06/COVID-REPORT-01.pdf (accessed 29 January 2022).
A Mersie 'Teenage Pregnancies Rise in Parts of Kenya as Lockdown Shut Schools' www.reuters.com/article/us-health-coronavirus-teenage-pregnancie/teenage-pregnancies-rise-in-parts-of-kenya-as-lockdown-shuts-schools-idINKBN27W11H.
Mid-Term Assessment Botswana Global Fund's Report Mid-Term Assessment Botswana (2021) www.theglobalfund.org/media/10862/crg_2021-midtermassessment botswana_report_en.pdf (accessed 24 January 2022).
MSI Reproductive Choices www.mariestopes.org/what-we-do/our-services/safe-abortion-and-post-abortion-care/ (accessed 21 January 2022).

C Mumssen & S Nolan 'Report: Stepping up to Meet Low-Income Countries' Pandemic Recovery Needs'(2021) https://blogs.imf.org/2021/07/26/stepping-up-to-meet-low-income-countries-pandemic-recovery-needs/ (accessed 26 January 2022).

'New Zealand Positioned Itself as a Model of How Female Leadership Brings Inclusivity and a Feminist Lens to Acute Health Pandemics' www.feministcovidresponse.com/wp-content/uploads/2020/12/Feminist-Response-to-COVID-19-Advocacy-Monitoring-Toolkit-English-2.pdf (accessed 30 January 2022).

K Odada 'Impact of COVID-19 on Young People's Access to Contraceptives and Contraceptive Services' www.srhm.org/news/the-impact-of-covid-19-on-young-peoples-access-to-contraceptives-and-contraceptive-services/ (accessed 24 January 2022).

'Report: The Impact of COVID-19 on Human Rights of LGBT Persons' www.ohchr.org/Documents/Issues/SexualOrientation/IESOGI-COVID-19/CSOs/NGLHRC.pdf (accessed 27 January 2022).

United Nations Population Fund 'Report: Botswana' https://botswana.unfpa.org/en/topics/gender-based-violence-1 (accessed 22 January 2022).

United Nations Population Fund 'Report: Resilience in Action: Lessons Learned from the Joint Programme during the COVID-19 Crisis (UNFPA-UNICEF Joint Programme on the Elimination of Female Genital Mutilation: Accelerating Change' (2020) https://reliefweb.int/report/burkina-faso/resilience-action-lessons-learned-joint-programme-during-covid-19-crisis-unfpa (accessed 13 January 2022).

United Nations Population Fund's 'Technical Note: Impact of COVID-19 on Family Planning: What We Know One Year into the Pandemic' (2021) www.unfpa.org/sites/default/files/resource-pdf/COVID_Impact_FP_V5.pdf (accessed 26 January 2022).

World AIDS Day and the Intersectionality of Gender Based Violence 'COVID-19 and HIV/AIDS' https://galz.org/worlds-aids day-and-the-intersectionality-of-gender-based-violence-covid-19-and-hiv-aids/ (accessed 27 January 2022).

World Health Organisation 'Report: Sexual Health and Its Linkages to Reproductive Rights: An Operational Approach' (2017) http://apps.who.int/iris/bitstream/10665/258738/1/9789241512886-eng.pdf?ua=1 (accessed 29 January 2022).

World Health Organisation 'Report: BOTSWANA Bordering Africa's Epicenter: How Early Action and Careful Border Control Policies have So Far Contained COVID-19 to Clusters' (2020) www.who.int/docs/default-source/coronaviruse/country-case-studies/botswana-c19-case-study-20-july.pdf? (accessed 27 January 2022).

Websites and internet sources

https://africa.unwomen.org/sites/default/files/Field%20Office%20Africa/Attachments/Publications/2021/Policy%20Paper-%20GBV%20in%20Africa%20during%20COVID-19%20pandemic_EN%2018%20Feb_compressed.pdf Page 8 (accessed 26 January 2022).

https://africacdc.org/news-item/africa-cdc-receives-third-donation-of-medical-supplies-from-jack-ma-foundation-co-hosts-global-medixchange-webinar-on-covid-19/ (accessed 28 January 2022).

African Union 'Policy Paper: Gender Based Violence in Africa during the Covid 19 Pandemic' (2020) https://africa.unwomen.org/sites/default/files/Field%20Office%20Africa/Attachments/Publications/2021/Policy%20Paper-%20GBV%20in%20Africa%20during%20COVID-19%20pandemic_EN%2018%20Feb_compressed.pdf (accessed 26 January 2022).

https://allafrica.com/stories/202010160050.html

www.bgbvc.org.bw/index.php/about/our-history (accessed 20 January 2022).

https://botswana.unfpa.org/en/news/much-more-needs-be-done-ending-gender-based-violence-botswana (accessed 23 January 2022).

Corona Virus (COVID-19) Scorecard for Africa Nurses and Midwives and Doctors https://accountability.international/coronavirus/ (accessed 30 January 2022).
https://equipop.org/for-a-feminist-response-to-covid-19/ (accessed 19 January 2022).
https://galz.org/galz-provides-relief-packages-for-members-during-covid-19-lockdown/
www.genderandcovid-19.org/wp-content/uploads/2020/10/Gender-and-COVID-19-in-Nigeria.pdf (accessed 29 January 2022).
www.genderinkenya.org/publication/generation-equality-forum-kenyas-roadmap-for-gender-equality/ (accessed 29 January 2022).
Nolan et al 'Stepping up to Meet Low-Income Countries' Pandemic Recovery Needs' https://blogs.imf.org/2021/07/26/stepping-up-to-meet-low-income-countries-pandemic-recovery-needs/
www.oxfam.org/en/press-releases/imf-paves-way-new-era-austerity-post-covid-19 (accessed 19 January 2022).
https://reliefweb.int/report/world/effects-covid-19-sexual-and-reproductive-health-case-study-six-countries (accessed 28 January 2022).
https://reliefweb.int/report/world/where-are-women-conspicuous-absence-women-covid-19-response-teams-and-plans-and-why-we (accessed 30 January 2022).
https://reliefweb.int/sites/reliefweb.int/files/resources/Brief-Experiences-of-women-with-disabilities-in-Nigeria-during-COVID-19-en.pdf (accessed 28 January 2022).
https://sdgs.un.org/goals
www.sos-botswana.org/index.php/our-strategy (accessed 27 January 2022).
www.spotlightinitiative.org/withher/withher (accessed 30 January 2022).
www.womenagainstrape.org.bw/index.html (accessed 23 January 2022).

INDEX